Techniques of Abdominal Wall Hernia Repair

Pradeep Chowbey · Davide Lomanto
Editors

Techniques of Abdominal Wall Hernia Repair

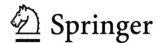 Springer

Editors
Pradeep Chowbey
Metabolic and Bariatric Surgery
Max Super Specialty Hospital
New Delhi
India

Davide Lomanto
Minimally Invasive Surgical Centre
KTP Advanced Surgical Training Centre
Yong Loo Lin School of Medicine
National University Health System
National University of Singapore
Singapore

ISBN 978-81-322-3942-0   ISBN 978-81-322-3944-4   (eBook)
https://doi.org/10.1007/978-81-322-3944-4

This Springer imprint is published by the registered company Springer Nature India Private Limited
The registered company address is: 7th Floor, Vijaya Building, 17 Barakhamba Road, New Delhi 110 001, India

Contents

About the Editors

Pradeep Chowbey is currently Chairman of the Max Institute of Minimal Access, and Chief of Surgery and Allied Surgical Specialties at Max Hospital, New Delhi, India. He is the Honorary Surgeon to **the President of India and Surgeon to His Holiness the Dalai Lama**. He is the Founder President of the Asia Pacific Hernia Society (2004) and Former President of the Asia-Pacific Metabolic and Bariatric Surgery Society (2010–2012), of the Pacific Chapter of the International Federation for the Surgery of Obesity and Metabolic Disorders (2011–2013), and of the International Federation for the Surgery of Obesity and Metabolic Disorders (2012–2013).

He established the Minimal Access, Metabolic & Bariatric Surgery Centre, Sir Ganga Ram Hospital, New Delhi, in 1996, the first of its kind on the Asian subcontinent. His current institute, the Max Institute of Minimal Access, is accredited as an International Centre of Excellence for Endohernia Surgery and Bariatric Surgery. He was on the steering committee for formulating the **Worldwide Guidelines and Recommendations** for inguinal hernia and ventral and incisional abdominal wall hernias published in the *Surgical Endoscopy* journal (Springer).

He is the Editor in Chief of the *Journal of Minimal Access Surgery*, the official publication of IAGES, a Section Editor (Ventral/Incisional Hernia Surgery) for *Hernia: The World Journal of Hernia and Abdominal Wall Surgery*, and an Associate Editor for the *International Journal of Abdominal Wall and Hernia Surgery*.

Davide Lomanto is currently a Professor of Surgery at the National University of Singapore and Director of the Minimally Invasive Surgical Centre (MISC) and of the KTP Advanced Surgery Training Centre (ASTC), National University Hospital (NUS). He is a Secretary-General and a Past President of the Endoscopic and Laparoscopic Surgeons of ASIA (ELSA); a Founding Member and Advisory President of the Asia Pacific Hernia Society (APHS); and a Founding Member and Past-President of the Asia-Pacific Metabolic and Bariatric Surgery Society (APMBSS). He has been awarded Honorary Memberships in several endolaparoscopic societies: Japan (JSES), India (IAGES), Indonesia (PBEI, PERHERI), the Philippines (PCS, PALES), and Thailand (RCST). He recently been awarded the prestigious Honorary Fellowship Ad Hominem from the Royal College of Surgeons of Edinburg (FRCS) and from the European Association for Endoscopic Surgery (EAES).

He serves as Experts in several Guidelines Committee for Inguinal and Abdominal Wall Hernia.

He currently serves as Managing Editor of the Asian Journal of Endoscopic Surgery; Associate Editor of Hernia: The World Journal of Hernia and Abdominal Wall Surgery; and International Editorial Member for Surgical Endoscopy and Asian Journal of Surgery. He was knighted by the Italian Government on 26 December 2009.

Part I

General

The Economics of Hernia Surgery

1

Jose Macario Faylona

1.1 Introduction

Hernia surgery is one of the most common operations being done worldwide. Statistics from the different countries varies but in the US, China, and India, inguinal hernia surgery can go as high as one million cases per year [1]. Throughout the lifetime of an individual, the chance of having a hernia operation is 27% for males and 3% for females [2]. Hernia surgery involves not only inguinal hernia but also ventral or incisional hernias. Through the years, the management of hernias has evolved from tissue repairs to prosthetic repairs and laparoscopic repairs. With the advent of all of these technological breakthroughs and new techniques in hernia surgery, it is necessary to assess the economic impact of these things in terms of health care cost, as well as costs that the patients will incur.

1.2 Health Economics

In terms of health economics, different countries will have different systems of funding health care, but they have one thing in common; health care resources are limited and needs to be spent rationally for the benefit of more people. In line with this, health economists need to make crucial decisions as to which will be funded and which will be rejected. In the case of hernia surgery, there are so many variables that need to be considered in deciding the most economical choice for a hernia patient. Things that need to be considered are the following:

1. Tissue repair vs. prosthetic repair
2. Open vs. laparoscopic repair
3. Type of mesh to use
4. Type of fixation
5. Day case or in-hospital procedure
6. Type of anesthesia
7. Antibiotic use
8. Impact on patients' quality of life and return to work

With all these things to consider, it is essential for the decision-makers of health care to understand the concepts of health economics. Decision should be based on several concepts:

1. Cost-minimization analysis
2. Cost-effectiveness analysis
3. Cost-utility Analysis
4. Cost-benefit analysis

J. M. Faylona (✉)
Department of Surgery, UP College of Medicine,
University of the Philippines-Manila,
Manila, Philippines

© Springer Nature India Private Limited 2020
P. Chowbey, D. Lomanto (eds.), *Techniques of Abdominal Wall Hernia Repair*,
https://doi.org/10.1007/978-81-322-3944-4_1

1.3 Cost-Minimization Analysis

Cost-minimization is defined by achieving a defined objective at the least cost. This type of analysis is used only in situations where the benefits of alternative treatments have been proven to be identical. It is required that rigorous evaluation of the health benefits is needed so that the measures being compared are proven to be clinically equivalent [3].

1.4 Cost-Effectiveness Analysis

The NICE defines cost-effective analysis as an economic study design in which consequences of different intervention are measured using a single outcome. This type of analysis compares the costs and health effects of an intervention in order to assess the extent to which it is providing value for money. This involves getting the direct costs, indirect costs as well as intangibles that affect the outcome. This type of analysis involves computing for the cost-effectiveness ratio (CER) and the incremental cost-effectiveness ratio (ICER). This is best used for the analysis of different treatment regimens for treating the same condition (Fig. 1.1) [4].

1.5 Cost-Utility Analysis

This type of analysis combines multiple outcomes into a single measure. It needs to use several parameters such as the quality-adjusted life years (QALY), which measures health as a combination of the duration of life and the health-related quality of life. It also utilizes ICER. Once the analysis is complete, this is compared to a threshold ICER wherein anything that falls below the threshold is funded and anything above is not. This type of analysis was developed so that decision-makers will have a basis for comparing the value of different alternative interventions that have very different health benefits [5].

1.6 Cost-Benefit Analysis

This type of analysis links cost and outcomes by expressing both in monetary units. Any intervention that has a result of the benefit exceeding the cost is said to be advantageous to the patient and is worthwhile to consider [6].

Hernia surgery involves so many variables as well as many outcome measures such as recurrences, chronic inguinal pain, and numbness. It is therefore the role of the researcher to use the different models of economic analysis to get the necessary information and make the necessary recommendations to health care providers and financers of health.

1.7 Guidelines and Economics in Hernia Surgery

With the rapid development in hernia surgery, the European Hernia Society (EHS) and the Asia Pacific Hernia Society (APHS) have created several guidelines [1, 7, 8]. These guidelines intend to provide surgeons on how to decide and proceed with the different aspects in the management of this problem. With regards to economics in hernia surgery, the following are several issues that need to be addressed.

1.8 Watchful Waiting or Surgery

There were two publications that tackled the issue on watchful waiting for inguinal hernia. The Fitzgibbon trial in 2006 recommended that watchful waiting is acceptable in the management of asymptomatic or minimally symptomatic inguinal

Cost Effectiveness Ratio (CER) = Cost of intervention/Health effects produced

Incremental cost-effectiveness ratio (ICER) = Difference in costs between programs P1 and P2/Difference in health effects between programs P1 and P2

Fig. 1.1 Cost effective analysis formula

hernia patients. In this study, 23% of the observed patients crossovered to surgery [9]. In the O'Dwyer trial 29% crossovered to surgery, of which three had serious hernia-related adverse events. O'Dwyer thus recommended that if there is a significant comorbidity, there might be a benefit for early elective hernia surgery [10]. The European Hernia Society 2009 guidelines states that watchful waiting is recommended for minimally symptomatic or asymptomatic inguinal hernia. This was revised in 2014 wherein the recommendation is that surgical repair should be done to medically fit patients with painless hernia [8]. The revision in the guideline is due to the publication of Chung et al., who did a long-term follow-up of patients with painless hernia. In this chapter, the rate of conversion from observation to surgery is 16% at 1 year, 54% at 5 years, and 72% at 7.5 years [11]. The APHS recommendation, however, states that surgical treatment be recommended as most will develop symptoms over time.

In the economic perspective, latest guidelines would state that inguinal hernia patients even if asymptomatic should be offered surgical repair. It will be costly for the patients if the patient comes in as an emergency due to incarceration or strangulation. The surgery that will be performed will be more difficult and will entail hospitalization, general or regional anesthesia, antibiotic use, longer hospital stay, and convalescence. Elective hernia surgery can be performed as a day case surgery under local anesthesia without antibiotics. These will be discussed further.

1.9 Diagnostics in Hernia Surgery

Diagnosing inguinal hernias is not costly. Evident hernias are easily detected by physical examination [12, 13]. There is no role for CT Scan in diagnosing hernias, but magnetic resonance imaging has a high sensitivity and specificity (>94%) for detecting hernias as well as other musculoskeletal and tendon pathologies [13–15]. EHS guideline recommends that investigation is preferred only in patients with obscure pain or swelling [7]. A surgeon only needs to do the

proper physical examination to detect an inguinal hernia and do additional tests like the MRI if the surgeon is entertaining the possibility of other musculoskeletal problems causing inguinal pain. This approach is more cost-effective in terms of health care cost and financing.

1.10 Day Surgery for Inguinal Hernia

In terms of economics in hernia surgery, it is more cost-effective to the day case than an in-hospital case. There are several studies that prove that day surgery is more cost-effective than in-hospital surgery [16]. In a large cohort study done in the United States (US), it was found that there is a 56% higher cost with in-hospital hernia surgery procedures than day case surgery. Another study done in Germany confirms these findings in the US [17, 18]. There are also indirect cost benefits such as freeing the hospital bed for the use of other patients that will need hospitalization, which will be advantageous to the rational use of limited health resources. EHS and APHS guidelines both state that doing inguinal hernia surgery is safe in an ambulatory setting [1, 7]. This was also proven by several studies not only for performing day case surgery under local anesthesia but different anesthetic techniques (general anesthesia and regional) for different types of hernia surgery including endoscopic techniques [18, 19]. Formerly, day case surgery is reserved only for ASA I and ASA II patients, but current evidence states that it can also be done for higher ASA patients provided there is satisfactory care at home [20–22]. What is important is that candidates for day case surgery should be evaluated properly preoperatively by the anesthesiologist and prepared adequately for the surgery.

1.11 Tissue Versus Mesh in Hernia Surgery

Mesh repair for inguinal hernia has already been proven by several studies as well as guidelines to be superior over tissue repair [1, 7]. The only tissue repair that is acceptable and gives satisfactory results based on evidence is the shouldice repair. Shouldice repair, however, requires expertise since recurrences were noted to be higher in centers that are not experts in the shouldice repair [23, 24]. In the case of mesh repair, recurrences will be decreased and there is a decreased incidence of chronic inguinal pain [25]. This will translate to early return to work of patients. With reduced recurrences health resources can be channeled to other health problems and the patient will also be productive with no loss of man-hours due to recurrences. In the Philippines, the government will spend around $400 per case of hernia surgery and another $400 for every case of recurrent hernia [26]. Extrapolating data from population studies, the Philippine government health insurance will spend a total of 60 million dollars per year if there are 150,000 cases of hernia per year [1]. A big number of hernia cases in the Philippines are still done using non-mesh repairs, especially the modified bassini technique. If we extrapolate that 70% of cases are done using non-mesh technique and with a conservative estimate of 20% recurrence, then the government will spend an additional eight million dollars to cover for the recurrences, and this does not include the man-hours lost in productivity if the patient is part of the working group.

1.12 Economics of Prosthetic Material

Since the introduction of polypropylene in the 1950s, the design and composition of prosthetic materials have evolved to provide better biocompatibility for hernia patients. Guidelines would state that material reduced meshes have some advantage with respect to chronic pain and foreign body sensation in the first year after open surgery, which is not applicable for endoscopic repair. Use of lightweight mesh is also cautioned for large hernias especially for open inguinal hernia repair [8]. In terms of health resource funding, the cheapest flat mesh maybe

justifiable for funding since the end result will be the same.

Modified meshes such as the self-adhering mesh, mesh plug, and bilayer mesh systems have the same comparable result as the Lichtenstein technique and thus may not be amenable for funding in limited health resources due to the additional cost it will entail [8].

1.13 Type of Anesthesia

In any economic model, it is definitely more cost-effective to the hernia case under local anesthesia. Local anesthesia has already been proven to be safe and effective in primary unilateral inguinal hernias [27–29]. Local anesthesia has the advantage of less anesthesia-related complaints, less urinary retention problems, shorter recovery and faster discharge from the hospital [30–34]. The cost-effectivity of local anesthesia has been proven by several studies when compared to regional or general anesthesia [32, 35]. The only problem with local anesthesia is that it is not suitable for the stoppa technique and the endoscopic technique.

1.14 Open Versus Laparoscopic Technique

Guidelines would state that both open mesh technique and endoscopic technique have similar results in terms of recurrences and chronic inguinal pain. There are additional advantages for endoscopic technique such as lower incidence of wound infection, hematoma formation, and faster return to normal activities. The open mesh technique has the advantage of shorter operative time and can be done under local anesthesia [1, 7, 8].

Using the economic models, open mesh technique will always be less costly than the laparoscopic technique. The National Institutes of Health and Case Excellence (NICE) conducted cost-effectiveness analysis of laparoscopic surgery versus open hernia techniques [36]. Theater costs and in-hospital costs are similar for both open and endoscopic technique. Additional cost for laparoscopic procedures is 167 lb per procedure if using reusable equipment and 788 lb per procedure if using disposable equipment. This was also reflected in the study done by the Medical Research Council Groin Hernia Trial Group, which showed that laparoscopic hernia procedure would cost 1112.64 lb compared with 788.79 lb for open hernia operations [37].

Comparing Transabdominal Preperitoneal Approach (TAPP) and Totally Extraperitoneal Approach (TEP) in terms of costs showed that TEP is the more cost-effective option due to limited use or non-use of fixation device as well as less complications in the long run in terms of visceral injuries, vascular injuries, port site hernias, and adhesions [7, 36, 38].

Fixation techniques vary for both TEP and TAPP. TEP may have no fixation with equivalent results as shown in different studies [39–41]. This actually makes TEP cheaper than TAPP. Fibrin Glue fixation may have and initial benefit with regards to inguinal pain when compared with traumatic fixation devices but in the long term, the results are the same [42]. Kukleta et al., published data on the use of *n*-butyl cyanoacrylate for mesh fixation, which showed that it is safe and effective [43]. Cyanoacrylate is cheaper than fibrin glue and thus may be a good alternative for fixation.

One possible advantage of laparoscopy over the open technique is the possibility of detecting an occult hernia on the other side, which can be repaired simultaneously in the laparoscopic technique and thus prevent another operation in the future, which is not a possibility in the open technique. This concept, however, does not consider the possibility that the occult hernia may not develop symptoms during the patient's lifetime. Laparoscopy may also have the advantage of detecting a femoral hernia in women, which may be missed in the anterior repair. Guidelines recommend that the preperitoneal approach is better for women. With this approach, recurrences and missed hernias will be avoided and additional expense for reoperation can be prevented when using the anterior approach [7].

1.15   Antibiotic Prophylaxis

Wound infection risk for hernia surgery is between 2.4 and 4.3% based on randomized controlled studies [44–52]. 2009 EHS guidelines recommend that antibiotic prophylaxis is needed only for patients with risk factors for wound infection [8]. This, however, was revised in 2014, which states that in institutions with high rates of wound infection (>5%), the use of antibiotic prophylaxis is necessary. This is very important in terms of hernia economics, since antibiotics are expensive and surgeons should be able to discern if patients need prophylactic antibiotics or not.

1.16   Conclusion

There are different economic models that can be used in analyzing the cost-effectivity of the different operations for inguinal hernia surgery. These models can be utilized by government health financing institutions to decide on the procedures that need to be funded. Laparoscopic surgery is a more expensive option than open mesh surgery, and more studies are needed to study the indirect benefits in cost of laparoscopy in terms of early return to work as well as the benefits of less incidence of chronic inguinal pain and numbness in relation to work-related financial outcomes.

References

1. Lomanto D, Wei-Keat C, Faylona JM, Huang CS, Lohsiriwat D, Maleachi A, Yang GPC, Li MKW, Tumtativitikul S, Sharma A, HArtung RU, Choi BY, Sutedja B. Inguinal hernia repair: towards Asian guidelines. Asian J Endosc Surg. 2015;8:16–23.
2. Primatesta P, Goldcare MJ. Inguinal hernia repair: incidence of elective and emergency surgery, readmission and mortality. Int J Epidemiol. 1996;25:835–9.
3. Haycox A. What is cost minimization analysis. 2009. www.medicine.ox.ac.uk/bandolier/painres/download/whatis/what_is_cost-min.pdf.
4. Phillips C. What is cost effectiveness. 2009. www.medicine.ox.ac.uk/bandolier/painres/download/whatis/Cost-effect.pdf.

5. McCabe C. What is cost utility analysis. 2009. www.medicine.ox.ac.uk/bandolier/painres/download/whatis/What_is_util.pdf.

6. Campbell HE. Health economics and surgical care. Surgery. 2003;21(6):133–6.

7. Simons MP, Aufenacker T, Bay-Nielsen M, Bouillot JL, Campanelli G, Conze J, de Lange D, Fortelny R, Heikkinen T, Kingsnorth A, Kukleta J, Morales-Conde S, Nordin P, Schumpelick V, Smedberg A, Smietanski M, Weber G, Miserez M. European Hernia Society Guidelines on the treatment of inguinal hernia in adult patients. Hernia. 2009;13:343–403.

8. Miserez M, Peeters E, Aufenacker T, Bouillot JL, Campanelli G, Conze J, Fortelny R, Heikkinen T, Jorgensen LN, Kukleta J, Morales-Conde S, Nordin P, Schumpelick V, Smedberg S, Smietanski M, Weber G, Simons MP. Update with level 1 studies of the European Hernia Society Guidelines on the treatment of inguinal hernia in adult patients. Hernia. 2014;18:151–63.

9. Fitzgibbon RJ Jr, Giobbie-Hurder A, Gibbs JO, Dunlop DD, Reda DJ, McCarthy M Jr, Neumyer LA, Barkun JS, Hoehn JL, Murphy JT, Sarosi GA Jr, Syme WC, Thompson JS, Wang J, Jonasson O. Watchful waiting versus repair of inguinal hernia in minimally symptomatic men: a randomized clinical trial. JAMA. 2006;295:285–92.

10. O'Dwyer PJ, Ching L. Watchful waiting was as safe as surgical repair for minimally symptomatic inguinal hernias. Evid Based Med. 2006;11:73.

11. Chung L, Norrie J, O'Dwyer PJ. Long-term follow-up of patients with a painless inguinal hernia from a randomized clinical trial. Br J Surg. 2011;98(4):596–9.

12. Kraft BM, Kolb H, Kuckuk B, Haaga S, Leibl BJ, Kraft K, Bittner R. Diagnosis and classification of inguinal hernias. Surg Endosc. 2003;17:2021–4.

13. Van Den Berg JC, de Valois JC, Go PM, Rosenburch G. Detection of groin hernia with physical examination, ultrasound and MRI compared with laparoscopic findings. Invest Radiol. 1999;34:739–43.

14. Leander P, Ekberg O, Sjorberg S, Kesek P. MR imaging following herniography in patients with unclear groin pain. Eur Radiol. 2000;10:1691–6.

15. Barile A, Erriquez D, Cacchio A, De Paulis F, Di Cesare E, Masciocchi C. Groin pain in athletes: role of magnetic resonance. Radiol Med (Torino). 2000;100:216–22.

16. Ramyil VM, Ognonna BC, Iya D. Patient acceptance of outpatient treatment for inguinal hernia in Jos, Nigeria. Cent Afr J Med. 1999;45:244–6.

17. Mitchell JB, Harrow B. Costs and outcomes of inpatient versus outpatient hernia repair. Health Policy. 1994;28:143–52.

18. Weyhe D, Winnemöller C, Hellwig A, Meurer K, Plugge H, Kasoly K, Laubenthal H, Bauer KH, Uhl W. (section sign) 115 b SGB V threatens outpatient treatment for inguinal hernia. Analysis of outcome and economics. Chirurg. 2006;77:844–55.

19. Engbaek J, Bartholdy J, Hjortsø NC. Return hospital visits and morbidity within 60 days after day surgery: a retrospective study of 18,736 day surgical procedures. Acta Anaesthesiol Scand. 2006;50:911–9.

20. Davies KE, Houghton K, Montgomery JE. Obesity and day-case surgery. Anaesthesia. 2001;56:1112–5.

21. Jarrett PE. Day care surgery. Eur J Anaesthesiol Suppl. 2001;23:32–5.

22. Prabhu A, Chung F. Anaesthetic strategies towards developments in day care surgery. Eur J Anaesthesiol Suppl. 2001;23:36–42.

23. Beets GL, Oosterhuis KJ, Go PM, Baeten CG, Kootstra G. Longterm followup (12–15 years) of a randomized controlled trial comparing Bassini-Stetten, Shouldice, and high ligation with narrowing of the internal ring for primary inguinal hernia repair. J Am Coll Surg. 1997;185:352–7.

24. Simons MP, Kleijnen J, van Geldere D, Hoitsma HF, Obertop H. Role of the Shouldice technique in inguinal hernia repair: a systematic review of controlled trials and a meta-analysis. Br J Surg. 1996;83:734–8.

25. Grant A. Mesh versus non mesh repair of groin hernia meta-analysis of randomized trials leased on individual patient data. Hernia. 2002;6:130–6.

26. PHIC list of procedure case rates 2013. www.philhealth.gov.ph/circulars/2013/annexes/circ35_2013/Annex2_ListOfProceduresCaseRates.pdf.

27. Callesen T, Bech K, Kehlet H. One-thousand consecutive inguinal hernia repairs under unmonitored local anesthesia. Anesth Analg. 2001;93:1373–6.

28. Kark AE, Kurzer MN, Belsham PA. Three thousand one hundred seventy-five primary inguinal hernia repairs: advantages of ambulatory open mesh repair using local anesthesia. J Am Coll Surg. 1998;186:447–55.

29. Kehlet H, Bay Nielsen M. Anaesthetic practice for groin hernia repair—a nation-wide study in Denmark 1998–2003. Acta Anaesthesiol Scand. 2005;49:143–6.

30. Ozgün H, Kurt MN, Kurt I, Cevikel MH. Comparison of local, spinal, and general anaesthesia for inguinal herniorrhaphy. Eur J Surg. 2002;168:455–9.

31. Schmitz R, Shah S, Treckmann J, Schneider K. Extraperitoneal, "tension free" inguinal hernia repair with local anesthesia—a contribution to effectiveness and economy. Langenbecks Arch Chir Suppl Kongressbd. 1997;114:1135–8.

32. Song D, Greilich NB, White PF, Watcha MF, Tongier WK. Recovery profiles and costs of anesthesia for outpatient unilateral inguinal herniorrhaphy. Anesth Analg. 2000;91:876–81.

33. Teasdale C, McCrum AM, Williams NB, Horton RE. A randomised controlled trial to compare local with general anaesthesia for short-stay inguinal hernia repair. Ann R Coll Surg Engl. 1982;64:238–42.

34. van Veen RN, Mahabier C, Dawson I, Hop WC, Kok NF, Lange JF, Jeekel J. Spinal or local anesthesia in Lichtenstein hernia repair: a randomized controlled trial. Ann Surg. 2008;247:428–33.

35. Nordin P, Zetterström H, Carlsson P, Nilsson E. Cost-effectiveness analysis of local, regional and general

anaesthesia for inguinal hernia repair using data from a randomized clinical trial. Br J Surg. 2007;94:500–5.

36. National Institute for Clinical Excellence. Laparoscopic surgery for inguinal hernia repair. Technology Appraisal 83.2004. National Institute for Clinical Excellence http://www.nice.or.uk/pdf/TA083guidance.pdf.

37. MRC Laparoscopic Groin Hernia Trial Group. Cost utility analysis of open versus laparoscopic groin hernia repair: results from a multicenter randomized clinical trial. Br J Surg. 2001;88:653–61.

38. Schmedt CG, Sauerland S, Bittner R. Comparison of endoscopic procedures vs Lichtenstein and other open mesh techniques for inguinal hernia repair: a meta-analysis of randomized controlled trials. Surg Endosc. 2005;19:188–99.

39. Tam KW, Liang HH, Chai CY. Outcomes of staple fixation of mesh vs. nonfixation in laparoscopic total extraperitoneal inguinal repair: a meta-analysis of randomized controlled trials. World J Surg. 2010;34(12):3065–74.

40. Teng YJ, Pan SM, Liu YL, Yang KH, Zhang YC, Tian JH, Han JX. A meta-analysis of randomized controlled trials of fixation vs. nonfixation of mesh in laparoscopic total extraperitoneal inguinal hernia repair. Surg Endosc. 2011;25(9):2849–58.

41. Lovisetto F, Zonta S, Rota E, Mazzilli M, Bardone M, Bottero L, Faillace G, Longoni M. Use of human fibrin glue (Tissucol) vs. staples for mesh fixation in laparoscopic transabdominal preperitoneal hernioplasty: a prospective, randomized study. Ann Surg. 2007;245(2):222–31.

42. Kukleta JF, Freytag C, Weber M. Efficiency and safety of mesh fixation in laparoscopic inguinal hernia repair using n-butyl cyanoacrylate: long term biocompatibility in over 1,300 mesh fixations. Hernia. 2012;16:153–62.

43. Aufenacker TJ, van Geldere D, van Mesdag T, Bossers AN, Dekker B, Scheijde E, van Nieuwenhuizen R, Hiemstra E, Maduro JH, Juttmann JW, Hofstede D, van Der Linden CT, Gouma DJ, Simons MP. The role of antibiotic prophylaxis in prevention of wound infection after Lichtenstein open mesh repair of primary inguinal hernia: a multicenter double-blind randomized controlled trial. Ann Surg. 2004;240:955–60.

44. Celdrán A, Frieyro O, de la Pinta JC, Souto JL, Esteban J, Rubio JM, Señarís JF. The role of antibiotic prophylaxis on wound infection after mesh hernia repair under local anesthesia on an ambulatory basis. Hernia. 2004;8:20–2.

45. Morales R, Carmona A, Pagán A. Utility of antibiotic prophylaxis in reducing wound infection in inguinal or femoral hernia repair using polypropylene mesh. Cir Esp. 2000;67:51–9.

46. Oteiza F, Ciga MA, Ortiz H. Antibiotic prophylaxis in inguinal hernioplasty. Cir Esp. 2004;75:69–71.

47. Perez AR, Roxas MF, Hilvano SS. A randomized, double-blind, placebo-controlled trial to determine effectiveness of antibiotic prophylaxis for tension-free mesh herniorrhaphy. J Am Coll Surg. 2005;200:393–7.

48. Platt R, Zaleznik DF, Hopkins CC, Dellinger EP, Karchmer AW, Bryan CS, Burke JF, Wikler MA, Marino SK, Holbrook KF, Tosteson TD, Segal MR. Perioperative antibiotic prophylaxis for herniorrhaphy and breast surgery. N Engl J Med. 1990;322:153–60.

49. Sanchez-Manuel FJ, Seco-Gil JL. Antibiotic prophylaxis for hernia repair. Cochrane Database Syst Rev. 2004;(4):CD003769.

50. Schwetling R, Bärlehner E. Is there an indication for general perioperative antibiotic prophylaxis in laparoscopic plastic hernia repair with implantation of alloplastic tissue? Zentralbl Chir. 1998;123:193–5.

51. Tzovaras G, Delikoukos S, Christodoulides G, Spyridakis M, Mantzos F, Tepetes K, Athanassiou E, Hatzitheofilou C. The role of antibiotic prophylaxis in elective tension-free mesh inguinal hernia repair: results of a single-centre prospective randomised trial. Int J Clin Pract. 2007;61:236–9.

52. Yerdel MA, Akin EB, Dolalan S, Turkcapar AG, Pehlivan M, Gecim IE, Kuterdem E. Effect of single-dose prophylactic ampicillin and sulbactam on wound infection after tension-free inguinal hernia repair with polypropylene mesh: the randomized, double-blind, prospective trial. Ann Surg. 2001;233:26–33.

Surgical Anatomy of Groin and Groin Hernia

2

Shintaro Sakurai

2.1   Introduction

J. Hureau [1] stated the following in 2001: "Too often has it been said that all aspects of anatomy have been described. As soon as a new surgical technique appears or a new tool of morphological investigation is designed, our level of understanding appears suddenly deficient." The same can be said of the anatomy of the inguinal region, as the development of laparoscopic techniques and preperitoneal approaches to surgical hernia repair has necessitated a renewed understanding of inguinal anatomy.

The three-dimensional anatomy of the inguinal region may initially seem confusing and overwhelming. For instance, some structures, while continuous, have different names depending on their anatomical location. Additionally, in fetal life, the testes develop near the kidney before descending to the scrotum, bringing along the processus vaginalis and several fasciae. Yet, if one realizes that the structures enveloping the peritoneal cavity, e.g., the peritoneum and various fasciae, exhibit localized protrusion but the structural components maintain their relationships vis-à-vis one another, the anatomy of the inguinal region will not appear as challenging to understand.

2.2   Surface Anatomy and Landmarks of Clinical and Operative Significance (Fig. 2.1)

The pubic tubercle is a triangular process lateral to the superior margin of the pubic bone where the inguinal ligament is attached. The anterior

S. Sakurai (✉)
Hernia Center, St. Luke's International Hospital, Tokyo, Japan

Department of Rehabilitation, Kotoh Rehabilitation Hospital, Kotoh-ku, Tokyo, Japan
e-mail: 21sakurai21@jcom.home.ne.jp; ss3169427@docomo.ne.jp

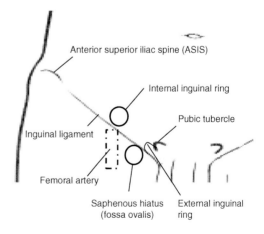

Fig. 2.1 Surface anatomy and landmarks of clinical and operative significance. Anatomical landmarks palpable from the body surface are shown. The internal inguinal ring and the saphenous hiatus are also shown, even though they are not palpable. Sakurai S. Anatomy of groin. Operation. 69, 4: 491–523, 2015. Fig. 1, p. 491

© Springer Nature India Private Limited 2020
P. Chowbey, D. Lomanto (eds.), *Techniques of Abdominal Wall Hernia Repair*,
https://doi.org/10.1007/978-81-322-3944-4_2

superior iliac spine (ASIS) is a bony projection from the anterior extremity of the ileum.

The inguinal ligament is located on the caudal edge of the external oblique aponeurosis. The ligament is slightly cranial to the skin fold that results upon bending the thigh, on an imaginary line between the pubic tubercle and the ASIS. Although the internal inguinal ring is not palpable externally, it is located approximately at the midpoint of the inguinal ligament. The external inguinal ring is lateral to the pubic tubercle. In male patients with external inguinal hernias, it is possible to palpate the margins of the dilated external inguinal ring using one's fingertips, by pushing and inverting the scrotal skin in a superior and lateral direction. Asking the patient to apply abdominal pressure is a useful tool in diagnosing small hernias, as the added pressure causes the hernia sac to protrude and facilitates palpation.

The femoral artery can be palpated caudal to the inguinal ligament.

The location between the femoral artery and the pubic tubercle is the saphenous hiatus (or oval fossa) where femoral hernias protrude, although it is not palpable without hernia.

2.3 Difference Between a Fascia and an Aponeurosis (Tendon)

Fascia is most commonly confused with aponeurosis, but the understanding of the difference between them is very important. According to Condon [2], fascia is a condensation of connective tissue into a definable, homogenous layer. Fascia may vary from a diaphanous layer of no intrinsic strength to a more easily discerned and thicker lamina. They invest or cover the muscle and aponeurosis, but they lack the organization and intrinsic tensile strength. An aponeurosis is the flat, dense, white tendon of insertion of muscle. It is composed of strong collagenous tissue.

2.4 The Subcutaneous Adipose Tissue and Superficial Abdominal Fascia

The subcutaneous adipose tissue consists of two layers of superficial abdominal fasciae: Camper's fascia (superficial layer) and Scarpa's fascia (deep layer). The former is a thick layer of adipose tissue located between the epidermis and Scarpa's fascia, and it is difficult to identify a well-demarcated membranous structure. The latter is a milky-white, homogenous membrane with no defined structure, and it can be distinguished from the external oblique aponeurosis as the fibers are not angled diagonally. Scarpa's fascia can easily be grasped using forceps, and it can be moved from side to side with the overlying skin. In between the two layers of superficial abdominal fascia, there are one or two superficial epigastric vessels that run perpendicular to the site of incision.

The medial aspect of the superficial fascia is fixed to the linea alba. The inferior aspect of Scarpa's fascia traverses the inguinal ligament to become the cribriform fascia, or it traverses the external inguinal ring to become the Dartos fascia, which is found in the subcutaneous layer of the scrotum.

2.5 The Innominate Fascia, the Intercrural Fiber, the External Spermatic Fascia, and the Fascia Lata (Figs. 2.2, 2.3, and 2.4)

The external oblique, internal oblique, and transversus abdominis muscles are all surrounded by two layers of investing fasciae (Figs. 2.2 and 2.3) [2, 3]. The external investing fascia of the external oblique muscle is called the innominate fascia (Figs. 2.3 and 2.4), a translucent membranous tissue that adheres to the external oblique muscle and aponeurosis. Superior and lateral to the external inguinal ring, this fascia intersects the fibers of

Fig. 2.2 Investing fasciae of each of the three layers of anterolateral abdominal musculature. McVay CB. Abdominal wall. In Anson and McVay Surgical Anatomy, 6th ed. Philadelphia, WB Saunders Co. 1984, pp 484–584

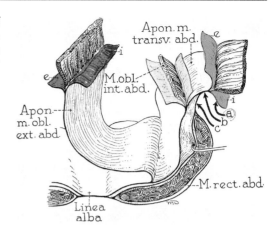

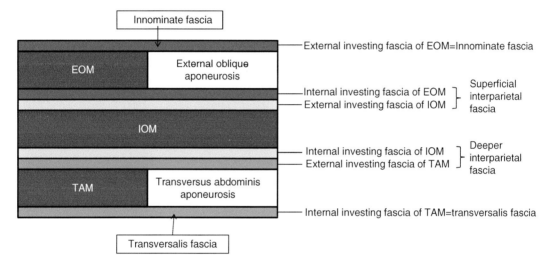

Fig. 2.3 Each three layers of abdominal wall muscle are enveloped by two layers of investing fasciae. The Internal investing fascia of EOM and the external investing fascia of IOM fuse and form the superficial interparietal fascia. The internal investing fascia of IOM and the external investing fascia of TAM fuse and form the deeper interpa-rietal fascia. The internal investing fascia of TAM is the transversalis fascia. *EOM* external oblique muscle, *IOM* internal oblique muscle, *TAM* transversus abdominis muscle. Sakurai S. Anatomy of groin. Operation. 69, 4: 491–523, 2015. Fig. 5, p 493

the external oblique aponeurosis perpendicularly to form the intercrural fiber (Figs. 2.4 and 2.5). The innermost layer of this fiber forms a semicircular "external inguinal ring" above the spermatic cord (Figs. 2.4 and 2.5). Inferior and medial to the external inguinal ring, the innominate fiber forms the external spermatic fascia, which envelops the spermatic cord and the cre-

master muscle that have protruded from the inguinal canal (Fig. 2.5).

Caudally, the innominate fascia extends to the thigh and becomes the fascia lata.

The fascia lata has the circular apertures, directly above the femoral vein, called the saphenous hiatus (or fossa ovalis) (Fig. 2.5). The great saphenous vein, superficial epigastric blood vesa

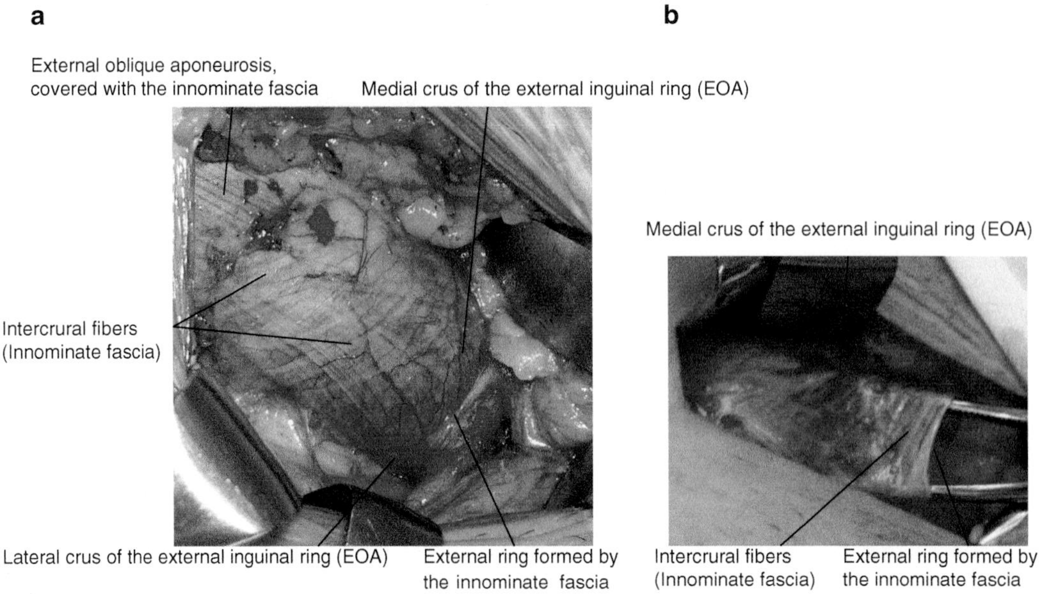

External oblique aponeurosis,
covered with the innominate fascia   Medial crus of the external inguinal ring (EOA)

Intercrural fibers
(Innominate fascia)

Lateral crus of the external inguinal ring (EOA)   External ring formed by
                                                     the innominate fascia

b

Medial crus of the external inguinal ring (EOA)

Intercrural fibers   External ring formed by
(Innominate fascia)   the innominate fascia

Fig. 2.4 (**a**) Innominate fascia, intercrural fiber, external oblique aponeurosis (EOA), medial and lateral crus of EOA. Sakurai S. Anatomy of groin. Operation. 69, 4: 491–523, 2015. Fig. 7, p 494. (**b**) External ring formed by the innominate fascia. Sakurai S. Anatomy of groin. Operation. 69, 4: 491–523, 2015. Fig. 7, p 494

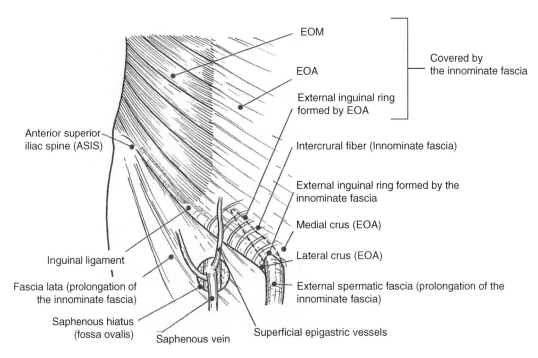

EOM

EOA

External inguinal ring
formed by EOA

Covered by
the innominate fascia

Anterior superior
iliac spine (ASIS)

Intercrural fiber (Innominate fascia)

External inguinal ring formed by the
innominate fascia

Medial crus (EOA)

Inguinal ligament

Lateral crus (EOA)

Fascia lata (prolongation of
the innominate fascia)

External spermatic fascia (prolongation of the
innominate fascia)

Saphenous hiatus
(fossa ovalis)   Saphenous vein   Superficial epigastric vessels

Fig. 2.5 Anatomy of the external oblique muscle (EOM) and aponeurosis (EOA), covered by the translucent innominate fascia. Sakurai S. Anatomy of groin. Operation. 69, 4: 491–523, 2015. Fig. 6, p 494

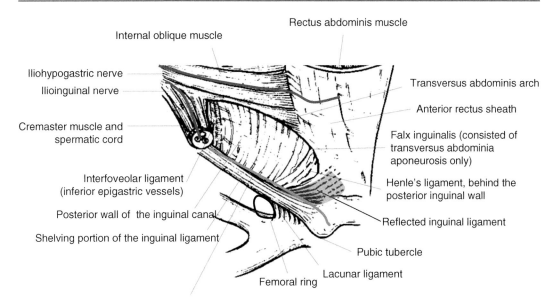

Fig. 2.6 Anatomy of the area around the posterior wall of the inguinal canal. "Blue line": genital branch of the genito-femoral nerve and inferior epigastric vessels

sels, and superficial circumflex iliac blood vessels branch off the femoral blood vessels, and this is the protrusion site for femoral hernias.

2.6   The External Oblique and Its Aponeurosis, the External Inguinal Ring, and the Inguinal Ligament
(Figs. 2.1, 2.4, 2.5, 2.6, and 2.7)

The area of the external oblique muscle that surrounds the inguinal region originates from the anterior two-thirds of the iliac crest, the iliopsoas fascia, and the iliopectineal arch. Medial to the line connecting the costal arch and the ASIS, the external oblique muscle transitions into the external oblique aponeurosis.

The medial aspect of the external oblique aponeurosis fuses with the internal oblique aponeurosis to form the anterior rectus sheath, before fusing with the contralateral fascia to form the linea alba.

Superior and lateral to the pubic tubercle, the external oblique aponeurosis splits into the medial and lateral crus, thereby forming a trian-

gular space (Figs. 2.1, 2.4, and 2.5). This opening is also referred to as the "external inguinal ring," but the anatomical entity responsible for the formation of a semicircular structure is the aforementioned external inguinal ring, which is formed by the intercrural fibers [2].

The medial crus is attached to the pubic crest, and the lateral crus to the pubic tubercle. Part of the lateral crus inverts superiorly and medially, then surrounds the lateral region of the pubic tubercle before adhering to the linea alba, forming the reflected inguinal ligament, also known as Colles' ligament (Fig. 2.6).

Before adhering to the pubic tubercle, the most inferior regions of the lateral crus split in a fan-like manner and attach to the superior pubic ramus. This area is called the lacunar ligament, or Gimbernat's ligament (Fig. 2.6).

The most inferior aspect of the external oblique aponeurosis thickens in the area between the ASIS and the pubic tubercle, and this anatomical structure is called the inguinal ligament (Figs. 2.1, 2.5, 2.6, and 2.7). It is rolled posteriorly and superiorly on itself and forms a groove to hold the spermatic cord and is called the "shelving portion" and its posterior

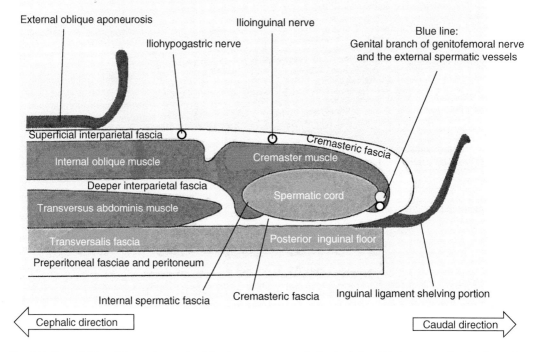

External oblique aponeurosis

Iliohypogastric nerve

Ilioinguinal nerve

Blue line:
Genital branch of genitofemoral nerve
and the external spermatic vessels

Superficial interparietal fascia

Cremasteric fascia

Internal oblique muscle

Cremaster muscle

Deeper interparietal fascia

Spermatic cord

Transversus abdominis muscle

Transversalis fascia

Posterior inguinal floor

Preperitoneal fasciae and peritoneum

Internal spermatic fascia

Cremasteric fascia

Inguinal ligament shelving portion

Cephalic direction

Caudal direction

Fig. 2.7 Superficial and deeper interparietal fasciae and cremasteric fascia. Sakurai S. Anatomy of groin. Operation. 69, 4: 491–523, 2015. Fig. 12, p 496

margin is called "shelving edge" (Figs. 2.7 and 2.8). The shelving edge is not fixed to any anatomical structures and has free edges, but it is attached dorsally to the innominate fascia, which is located between the shelving edge and the iliopubic tract [2, 3].

2.7 The Internal Oblique Muscle and the Interparietal Fasciae
(Figs. 2.3, 2.6, 2.7, and 2.8)

The internal oblique muscle in the inguinal area originates from the anterior two-thirds of the pubic crest, from the lumbodorsal fascia, and from the iliopsoas fascia or iliopectineal arch beneath the lateral half of the inguinal ligament, although there are no origins or insertions involving the inguinal ligament [3].

In most individuals, the internal oblique in the inguinal region consists of muscle fibers. After forming the superior margin of the inguinal canal, the muscle fibers transition into aponeurotic fibers that fuse with the deep layers of the transversus abdominis aponeurosis to form the anterior rectus sheath. The internal oblique aponeurosis also fuses medially with the external oblique aponeurosis. If the internal oblique had already transitioned from muscle fibers to aponeurotic fibers at the posterior wall of the inguinal canal, fusing with the transversus abdominis aponeurosis to attach to the pubic tubercle, it was called a conjoined tendon. However, such conjoined tendons occur in only 3% cases in Condon's dissection [2]. According to McVay [3], there is no fusion of these aponeurotic layers along the inguinal canal, so the use of the term "conjoined tendon" is a misnomer.

The internal investing fascia of the external oblique muscle and the external investing fascia of the internal oblique muscle fuse to form the superficial interparietal fascia, which surrounds the internal oblique muscle and the iliohypogastric nerve. The internal investing fascia of the internal oblique muscle and the external investing fascia of the transversalis abdominis muscle fuse to form the deeper interparietal fascia (Figs. 2.3, 2.7, and 2.8) [2].

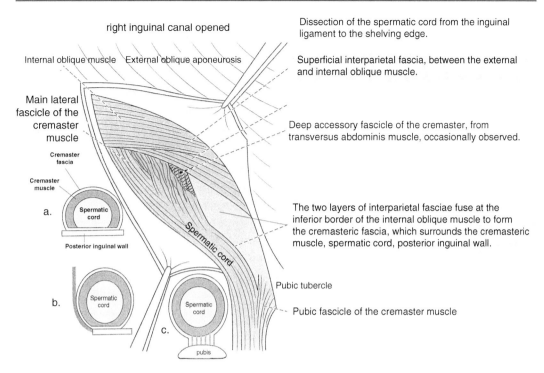

right inguinal canal opened

Dissection of the spermatic cord from the inguinal ligament to the shelving edge.

Internal oblique muscle   External oblique aponeurosis

Superficial interparietal fascia, between the external and internal oblique muscle.

Main lateral fascicle of the cremaster muscle

Deep accessory fascicle of the cremaster, from transversus abdominis muscle, occasionally observed.

Cremaster fascia

Cremaster muscle

a.   Spermatic cord

Spermatic cord

The two layers of interparietal fasciae fuse at the inferior border of the internal oblique muscle to form the cremasteric fascia, which surrounds the cremasteric muscle, spermatic cord, posterior inguinal wall.

Posterior inguinal wall

Pubic tubercle

b.   Spermatic cord   Spermatic cord

Pubic fascicle of the cremaster muscle

c.

pubis

Fig. 2.8 Cremaster muscle and cremasteric fascia. Sakurai S. Anatomy of groin. Operation. 69, 4: 491–523, 2015. Fig. 13, p 496

2.8 The Cremaster Muscle and the Cremasteric Fascia (Figs. 2.6, 2.7, 2.8, and 2.9)

The lowest portion of the internal oblique muscle is the cremaster muscle, which originates from the psoas fascia beneath the inguinal ligament.

The cremaster muscle fibers, initially applied only the anterior surface of the spermatic cord (Figs. 2.7 and 2.8a), forming the main lateral fascicle of the cremaster muscle [4], spread out around the cord in its course through the inguinal canal (Fig. 2.8b). In rare instances, a contribution of muscle fibers from the transversus abdominis muscle located cranial to the spermatic cord is also included in the cremaster muscle [2, 4]. In such cases, the fibers are called the deep accessory fascicle of the cremaster muscle (Fig. 2.8) [4]. As the cremaster muscle approaches the external inguinal ring, the muscle fibers spread out thinly towards the posterior side of the spermatic cord. At the external inguinal ring, the muscle surrounds two-thirds of the spermatic cord, but the muscle is not fixed to the inguinal ligament or the posterior wall of the inguinal canal

(Figs. 2.7 and 2.8b) [2]. It is at the pubic tubercle that the cremaster muscle finally surrounds the spermatic cord entirely and forms an area of strong fixation (Fig. 2.8c). Fruchaud [4] calls this area the pubic fascicle of the cremaster muscle (Fig. 2.8). When attempting to sufficiently cover the pubic tubercle with an onlay patch, it is important to deliberately dissect the pubic fascicle of the cremaster muscle and to separate the spermatic cord from the pubic tubercle. In some cases, there may be a relatively thick blood vessel that penetrates through the posterior wall of the inguinal canal located within the fibers on the dorsal side of the spermatic cord, lateral to the reflected ligament. In such instances, it may be necessary to ligate and dissect the blood vessel.

The cremasteric fascia, formed by the fusion of two layers of interparietal fasciae, not only surrounds the spermatic cord, cremaster muscle, ilioinguinal nerve, genital branch of the genitofemoral nerve, and external spermatic vessels (the last two structures are referred to as the "blue line"; more on this issue will be mentioned later) but also attaches the spermatic cord to the posterior wall of the inguinal canal (Figs. 2.7, 2.8, and 2.9).

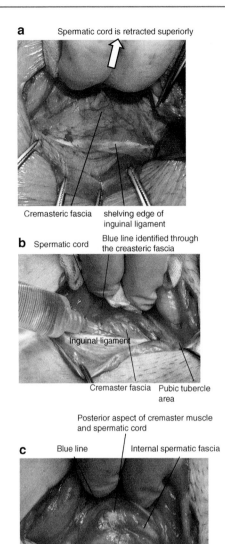

a Spermatic cord is retracted superiorly

Cremasteric fascia   shelving edge of
                      inguinal ligament

b Spermatic cord   Blue line identified through
                        the creasteric fascia

Inguinal ligament

Cremaster fascia   Pubic tubercle
                    area

Posterior aspect of cremaster muscle
and spermatic cord

c   Blue line   Internal spermatic fascia

Posterior wall of inguinal canal

Fig. 2.9 (**a**) Shelving portion and edge of the inguinal liga-ment and the cremasteric fascia. Spermatic cord is retracted superiorly by fingers and the cremasteric fascia connecting the spermatic cord and the shelving edge of the inguinal liga-ment is shown. The cremasteric fascia attaches the spermatic cord to the posterior wall of the inguinal canal. Sakurai S. Anatomy of groin. Operation. 69, 4: 491–523, 2015. Fig. 10, p 495. (**b**) The spermatic cord and the blue line are dissected from the posterior inguinal wall by injection of the local anesthetic agent beneath the cremasteric fascia. Sakurai S. Anatomy of groin. Operation. 69, 4: 491–523, 2015. Fig. 15, p 498. (**c**) After division of the cremasteric fascia, the demarcation line between the posterior inguinal wall and the internal spermatic fascia within the spermatic cord is easily identified. Note the blue line attached on inferior aspect of the spermatic cord. Sakurai S. Anatomy of groin. Operation. 69, 4: 491–523, 2015. Fig. 15, p 498

2.9   The Transversus Abdominis Muscle, Aponeurosis, and Fascia (Figs. 2.3, 2.6, 2.7, 2.9c, 2.10, and 2.11)

The transversus abdominis muscle and aponeuro-sis are the layer located deepest in the abdominal wall (Figs. 2.3, 2.6, 2.7, 2.9c, and 2.10). It originates from the lower six costal cartilages, the iliac crest, the lumbodorsal fascia, the ilio-psoas fascia and the iliopectineal arch, but is attached only to the upper-lateral one-third of the inguinal ligament. Thus, the middle-third of the inguinal ligament, lateral to the inferior epigas-tric vessels, is protected solely by the internal oblique muscle. This area, which includes the internal inguinal ring, is called the lateral triangle of the groin [5] (Fig. 2.11). It is the location where indirect inguinal hernias and interstitial hernias (hernias that protrude from between mus-cle fiber layers in the abdominal wall) may occur.

In the inguinal region cranial to the internal inguinal ring, the transversus abdominis muscle transitions into its aponeurosis. The inferior extremity of the aponeurosis curves cranially and forms the transversus abdominis arch (Fig. 2.10). According to a report by Condon [2], the insertion of the medial aspect of the arch is the rectus sheath, with 75% of cases attached more than 0.5 cm cra-nial to the superior margin of the pubic bone, and 14% of cases attached within 0.5 cm. Only 11% of cases displayed insertions to the superior margin of the pubic bone or Cooper's ligament and, in such cases, the area lateral to the insertion is called the falx inguinalis (Figs. 2.6 and 2.10).

2.10   The Transversalis Fascia (Figs. 2.3, 2.6, 2.7, 2.9c, 2.10, 2.12, and 2.14)

As with other muscle layers, the transversus abdominis muscle and its aponeurosis are sur-rounded by two layers (external and internal) of investing fasciae. In particular, the internal layer is called the transversalis fascia, which was believed to form the posterior wall (or floor) of the inguinal canal or the posterior inguinal wall

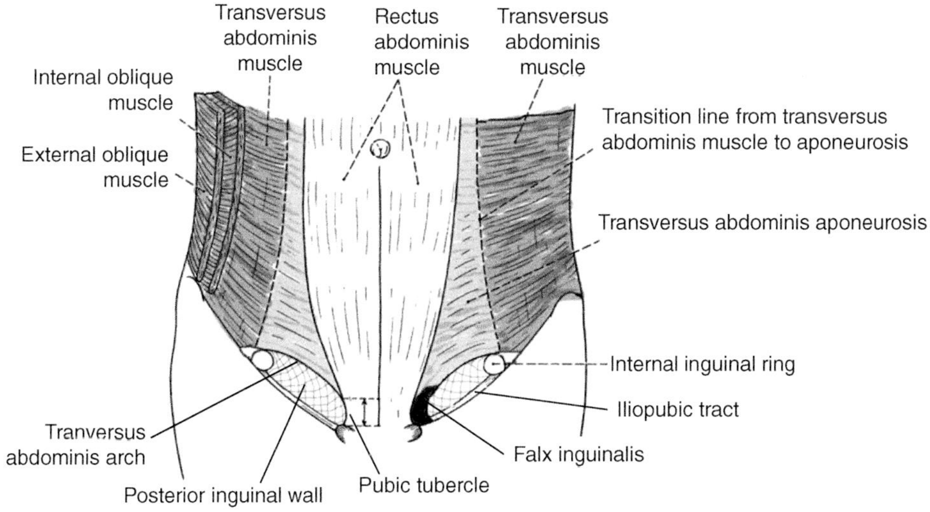

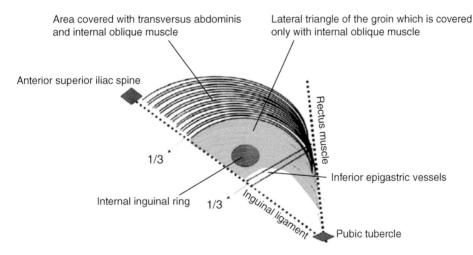

Fig. 2.10 Transversus abdominis arch, falx inguinalis, posterior inguinal wall. Right side of the body: the insertion of the medial aspect of the arch is the rectus sheath, with 75% of Condon's dissection attached more than 0.5 cm cranial to the superior margin of the pubic bone. Left side of the body: only 11% of Condon's dissection displayed insertions to the superior margin of the pubic bone or Cooper's ligament and, in such cases, the area lateral to the insertion is called the falx inguinalis. In the transversalis fascia of the posterior inguinal wall, the transversalis aponeurotic fibers form a mesh-like structure, thereby providing tensile strength. Sakurai S. Anatomy of groin. Operation. 69, 4: 491–523, 2015. Fig. 17, p 498

Fig. 2.11 Lateral triangle of the groin [5]. The transversus abdominis and internal oblique muscles originate from the upper one-third of the inguinal ligament. Only the internal oblique muscle originates from the middle-third of the inguinal ligament and this area is called the lateral triangle of the groin where indirect inguinal hernias and interstitial hernias may occur. From the lower third of the inguinal ligament, there is no muscle that protects the inguinal canal. Gilbert AI, Graham MF, Voigt WJ. The lateral triangle of the groin, Hernia, 4: 234–237, 2000

(Figs. 2.3, 2.6, 2.7, 2.9c, 2.10, 2.12, 2.13, and 2.14) [3]. Later studies, however, have suggested that the transversalis fascia envelops the entire abdominal cavity like a bag, and the structure has also been called the endoabdominal fascia, but this issue remains under debate [2, 3].

The transversalis fascia is a thin membrane and has no ability to resist increases in abdominal pressure. The transversalis fascia in the posterior inguinal wall is slightly thickened by apposition of its external surface of the deeper interparietal fascia. Reinforcement is also provided by the

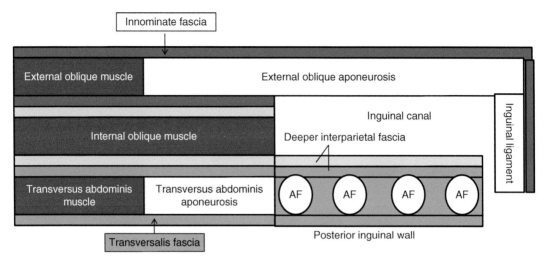

Fig. 2.12 In the transversalis fascia of the posterior inguinal wall, the transversalis aponeurotic fibers form a mesh-like structure, thereby providing tensile strength. AF represents the aponeurotic fibers from the transversus abdominis aponeurosis and from the iliopubic tract. Sakurai S. Fig. 12. Anatomy of groin. In Hernia Surgery, pp 7–35. Edited by Sakurai S, Nankodo, Tokyo, Japan, 2017

Fig. 2.13 The plane of the transversalis fascia and its downward extensions. Nyhus LM. An anatomical reappraisal of the posterior inguinal wall. Surg Clin North Am 5:1305, 1964

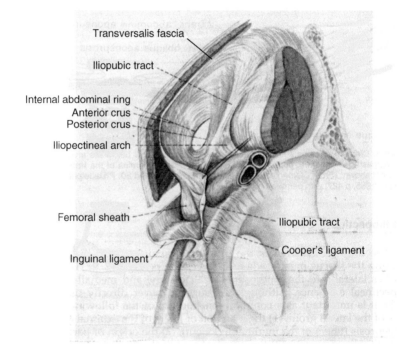

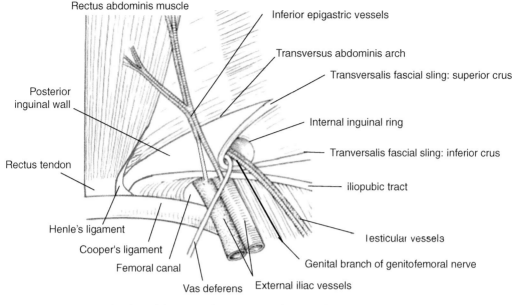

Rectus abdominis muscle

Inferior epigastric vessels

Transversus abdominis arch

Transversalis fascial sling: superior crus

Posterior inguinal wall

Internal inguinal ring

Tranversalis fascial sling: inferior crus

Rectus tendon

iliopubic tract

Henle's ligament

Testicular vessels

Cooper's ligament

Genital branch of genitofemoral nerve

Femoral canal

Vas deferens External iliac vessels

posterior view of the inguinofemoral region (right side)

Fig. 2.14 The transversalis fascia on the medial side of the internal inguinal ring forms a thick U-shaped cord-like structure laterally and superiorly, the transversalis fascial sling, holding the spermatic cord. Henle's ligament is a lateral expansion of the rectus abdominis tendon of insertion out onto Cooper's ligament. Sakurai S. Anatomy of groin. Operation. 69, 4: 491–523, 2015. Fig. 21, p 501

various number of aponeurotic fibers that bridge the gap between the transversus abdominis arch above and Cooper's ligament and the iliopubic tract below. These reinforcing fibers are usually directed obliquely from above downward and medially. Additional reinforcement is provided by aponeurotic fibers directed from below obliquely upward and medially. As a result, the transversalis aponeurotic fibers form a mesh-like structure, thereby providing tensile strength (Figs. 2.10 and 2.12) [2]. At the lateral aspect of the posterior inguinal floor, the adventitial fibers of the inferior epigastric vessels and the transversalis fascia fuse to form a ligament-like structure called the interfoveolar ligament, or the ligament of Hesselbach (Fig. 2.6) [2].

2.11 The Rectus Abdominis Muscle, the Posterior Rectus Sheath, the Arcuate Line, and the Rectus Fascia
(Figs. 2.6, 2.10, 2.14, and 2.15)

The rectus abdominis muscle arises from the fifth to seventh costal cartilages and from the xiphoid processus and inserts in the pubic crest and symphysis (Figs. 2.6, 2.10, and 2.14).

Above the midpoint between the umbilicus and the symphysis pubis, the rectus muscle is contained in the anterior and posterior rectus sheath, which are formed by the aponeurosis of the external oblique and the anterior lamina of the internal oblique and by the aponeurosis of the

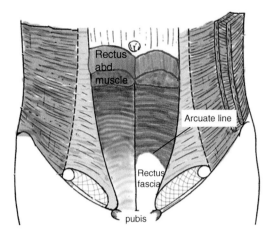

Rectus
abd.
muscle

Arcuate line

Rectus
fascia

pubis

Fig. 2.15 Variation in the position of the arcuate line, as well as the manner in which this line is formed. The left side of the body represents common case where the arcuate line is formed at the midway between the umbilicus and the pubis. The right side of the body represents the case where the density of aponeurotic fibers of the posterior rectus sheath decreases as the fibers approach the pubic bone and the fibers may reach the superior margin of the pubic bone or Cooper's ligament without forming an arcuate line. Right side of the body: no arcuate line formed. Left side of the body: arcuate line formed. Sakurai S. Anatomy of groin. Operation. 69, 4: 491–523, 2015. Fig. 17, p 498

posterior lamina of the internal oblique and the transversus abdominis, respectively. Below at about the midpoint between the umbilicus and the symphysis pubis, all three aponeuroses pass anterior to the rectus abdminis muscle, so that the inferior extent of the rectus abdominis muscle is devoid of a posterior rectus sheath. The lower margin of the posterior rectus sheath is called the arcuate line (the semicircular line of Douglas), usually located about midway between the umbilicus and the pubic crest (Fig. 2.15). Just like other muscle layers of the abdominal wall, the rectus abdominis muscle is enveloped by two layers of investing fasciae (transversalis fascia), even on the caudal end of the arcuate line which lacks the posterior rectus sheath. McVay [3] referred to the transversalis fascia in this region as the rectus fascia (Fig. 2.15). However, there is considerable variation in the position of the arcuate line, as well as the manner in which this line is formed. In 80% cases in McVay's dissection [3], there is a clear arcuate line located two-thirds

of the way up an imaginary line connecting the umbilicus and the pubic bone. There may be two arcuate lines, owing to failure of aponeurotic fibers of internal oblique to pass totally in front of the rectus muscle at a single point. Moreover, there may be cases where the density of aponeurotic fibers of the posterior rectus sheath decreases as the fibers approach the pubic bone (the apertures within the network of aponeurotic fibers are surrounded by the rectus fascia). In such instances, the fibers may reach the superior margin of the pubic bone or Cooper's ligament without forming an arcuate line (Fig. 2.15).

The insertion of the rectus abdominis muscle at the pubic bone becomes tendon-like and is called the rectus tendon. In cases where the investing fascia of the lateral margin of the tendon is thickened, this structure is called Henle's ligament (Fig. 2.14), and it has been observed in 46% of cases in Condon's dissection [2].

2.12 Particular Areas Formed from the Transversalis Fascia

2.12.1 The Internal Inguinal Ring and the Internal Spermatic Fascia (Figs. 2.1, 2.10, 2.11, 2.13, 2.14, 2.16, and 2.17)

The internal inguinal ring is an aperture found in the transversalis fasica on the lateral side of the inguinal canal. The vas deferens, the testicular artery and vein, the genital branch of genitofemoral nerve and the lymph channels pass through the preperitoneal space, and the internal inguinal ring becomes the hernial orifice for indirect inguinal hernias (Figs. 2.1, 2.10, 2.11, 2.13, 2.14, and 2.16).

The superior border of the internal inguinal ring consists of the transversus abdominis arch, and the inferior border consists of the iliopubic tract [2]. These two structures confer structural strength to the ring. The transversalis fascial sling (refer to section K-b below) forms the medial border. The lateral border is difficult to identify through observation from the peritoneal cavity, as

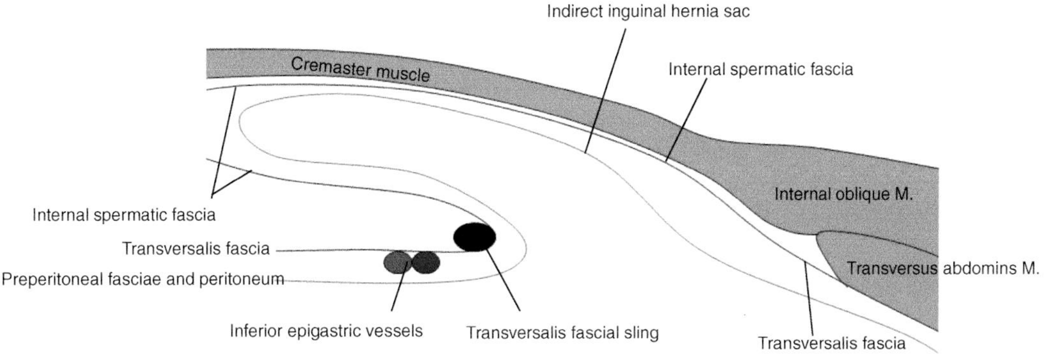

Indirect inguinal hernia sac

Cremaster muscle

Internal spermatic fascia

Internal oblique M.

Internal spermatic fascia

Transversalis fascia

Preperitoneal fasciae and peritoneum

Transversus abdomins M.

Inferior epigastric vessels   Transversalis fascial sling

Transversalis fascia

Fig. 2.16 A schematic representation of the horizontal cross-section at the level of the internal inguinal ring. Note the spermatic cord pierces through the abdominal cavity obliquely in a lateral-to-medial orientation. The

transversalis fascia on the medial side of the internal inguinal ring sags and becomes double-layered. Sakurai S. Anatomy of groin. Operation. 69, 4: 491–523, 2015. Fig. 22, p 501

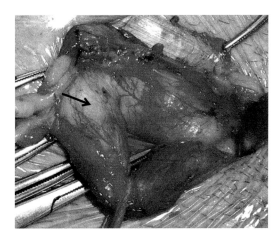

Fig. 2.17 After division of the main lateral fascicle of the cremaster muscle, the internal spermatic fascia (black arrow), containing the indirect inguinal hernia, vas deferens, testicular vessels, etc., is exposed. Sakurai S. Anatomy of groin. Operation. 69, 4: 491–523, 2015. Fig. 23, p 501

the spermatic cord pierces through the abdominal wall obliquely in a lateral-to-medial orientation (Figs. 2.13, 2.14, and 2.16).

The transversalis fascia passes through the internal inguinal ring and enters the inguinal canal while enveloping the spermatic cord, thereby forming a cylindrical protrusion medially at a slanted angle. Condon [2] called this cylindrical fascia the internal spermatic fascia, which measures less than 1 cm in healthy individuals

and fuses with the testicular blood vessels and adipose tissue. The indirect inguinal hernia is contained in the internal spermatic fascia (Figs. 2.9c, 2.16, and 2.17). There are also claims that the internal spermatic fascia is formed by the preperitoneal fascia (to be described later).

2.12.2 The Transversalis Fascial Sling
(Figs. 2.13 and 2.14)

Upon observing the internal inguinal ring from the preperitoneal space, one sees that the spermatic cord pierces through the abdominal cavity obliquely in a lateral-to-medial orientation. The transversalis fascia on the medial side of the deep inguinal ring sags and becomes double-layered, thereby forming a thick U-shaped cord-like structure laterally and superiorly, the transversalis fascial sling. The superior and inferior extensions of this sling are called the superior or anterior crus, and the inferior or posterior crus, respectively (Figs. 2.13 and 2.14). They provide the basis for the shutter mechanism that the approximation of the crura of the sling would partially close the internal ring, while the lateral sliding motion of the transversalis fascial sling would flatten the cord structures against the abdominal wall, increasing the obliquity of their course of exit [2].

2.12.3 The Iliopubic Tract and Cooper's Ligament

At the junction with the inguinal ligament, the transversalis fascia forms a aponeurotic band-like structure called the iliopubic tract (Figs. 2.10, 2.13, and 2.14). It joins the ASIS and the iliac crest laterally, runs above the iliopsoas muscle in a medial and inferior orientation. Part of the tract stretches dorsally to form the medial aspect of the iliopsoas fascia and the lateral wall of the femoral sheath. This structure is called the iliopectineal arch (Fig. 2.13). Another portion of the iliopubic tract runs over the anterior aspect of the femoral artery and vein to form the anterior margin of the femoral sheath. Then it curves posteriorly and inferiorly around the femoral canal; forming the medial margin of the femoral sheath. The tract then fans outs dorsally and ultimately forms Cooper's ligament at the superior pubic ramus (Figs. 2.16 and 2.17) [2].

2.13 The Inguinal Canal

The average length of the inguinal canal is said to be 4 cm in Caucasians [2].

It is commonly considered that the anterior wall of the inguinal canal was composed of the external oblique aponeurosis, the superior wall of the internal oblique muscle and traversus abdominis aponeurosis, the inferior wall of the inguinal ligament, the lacunar ligament and femoral sheath, and the posterior inguinal wall by the transversalis fascia and the aponeurotic fibers of the transversus abdominis muscle.

Yet, the presence of the two layers of preperitoneal fasciae between the posterior inguinal wall and the peritoneum (more on this topic will be discussed later) have been reported and recognized.

The posterior inguinal wall consists of the inferior border of the internal oblique muscle superiorly, the lateral border of the of the rectus sheath medially, the inferior epigastric blood vessels or the interfoveolar ligament laterally (Fig. 2.6).

In males, the inguinal canal contains the cremaster muscle, the cremasteric fascia, as well the vas deferens, the testicular artery, the pampiniform venous plexus, lymphatic channels, and adipose tissue that is continuous with the preperitoneal adipose tissue, surrounded by the internal spermatic fascia. Indirect inguinal hernias and the remnant of the processus vaginalis may also be included, and these structures are collectively referred to as the spermatic cord.

2.14 Myopectineal Orifice

Fruchaud [4] collectively referred to potential sites for groin hernia (indirect inguinal, direct inguinal, and femoral) as the myopectineal orifice (MPO). The myopectineal orifice presents irregular quadrilateral shape with four borders and an open central area. Its upper border is the inferior edge of the internal oblique muscle between the iliac fascia and the rectus sheath, and the lower border is Cooper's ligament. Its outer border is the iliac fascia, and the inner border is the lowermost part of the lateral edge of the rectus sheath.

2.15 Hesselbach Triangle

Hesselbach triangle is the location for direct inguinal hernia, and its well-known classic boundaries are the rectus abdominis muscle, inferior epigastric vessels, and the inguinal ligament. However, Hesselbach's 1814 definition of this triangle included the femoral region, much like the MPO [6]. Condon [2] noted that this anatomic boundaries of Hesselbach triangle should be redefined to be (1) the rectus sheath and falx inguinalis, (2) the inferior epigastric vessels, and (3) Cooper's ligament.

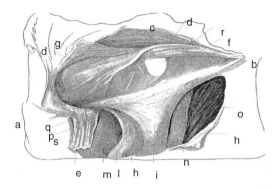

Fig. 2.18 Astley Cooper's engraving that shows two laminae of the transversalis fascia. An external view of a dissection of the left groin by Cooper. The inguinal ligament had been transected. (a) Pubes, (b) ilium, (c) abdominal muscles, (d) transversalis muscle and tendon, (e) external oblique muscle cut through and turned down, (f) external, (g) internal, (h) fascia lata turned back, (i) crural sheath covering the femoral artery, (l) saphena major vein, (m) some part of the semilunar edge of the fascia lata, (n) anterior crural nerve, (o) iliacus internus muscle, (p) seat of the crural arch to which the sheath adheres, (q) portion of the cural sheath passing behind the third insertion of the external oblique muscle, (r) opening of the fascia transversalis for the passage of the spermatic cord, (s) two lines that include the spot at which the crural hernia descends, and this is situated at the inner and upper part of the crural sheath. Cooper AP. Fig. 5 of PlateXII. In The anatomy and surgical treatment of abdominal wall hernia. 2nd ed. London, Longman & Co., 1827

2.16 Western Perspectives on the Fascial Structures and Cleavable Anatomical Spaces Located Between the Transverse Fascia and Peritoneum

The transversalis fascia was described (1804) [7] and named (1827) [8] by Cooper, and is said to be comprised of an external (outer) portion and an internal (inner) portion (Fig. 2.18). The existence of the internal portion was subsequently refuted and, until recently, the transverse fascia was thought to consist only of a single external portion [9, 10]. In the interim, several layers of fascia were thought to exist between the peritoneum and transverse fascia (Table 2.1), but many unknowns remain. For instance, it is unclear whether these fasciae are identical or distinct.

According to Tobin [11] (1944), the anterior and posterior leaves of the perirenal fascia (Gerota's fascia) enclose the kidneys, with the left and right fasciae merging at the midline (Fig. 2.19). Inferiorly, the two fasciae remain an open potential space, containing the ureter and testicular vessels to the iliac fossa.

They extend with the testicular vessels and vas deferens through the internal ring and the inguinal canal, all the way into the scrotum.

In 1945, Lytle [12] claimed the posterior inguinal floor l consists of two layers—the superficial "transversalis muscle layer" composed of the conjoined tendon and the transversalis muscle fascia, and the deep "transversalis fascia," each having a middle inguinal ring and internal inguinal ring (Fig. 2.20). The inferior epigastric vessels were said to be located between these two layers. However, current understanding of anatomy indicates that the superficial layer actually consists of the transverse fascia and the internal ring proper or transversalis ring, while the deep layer consists of the extraperitoneal fascia or preperitoneal fascia and secondary internal ring or preperitoneal fascial ring [9, 13, 14].

In 1975, Fowler [14] claimed that there were two preperitoneal fasciae behind the inguinal transverse fascia—a superficial membranous layer and a deep areolar layer—forming the preperitoneal space where the vas deferens course thorough (Fig. 2.21). The former comprises a "secondary" internal (inguinal) ring, in a deep layer located superior and lateral to the traditional inguinal ring. The inferior epigastric vessels were said to run between the transverse fascia and the membranous layer.

Table 2.1 Fasciae between the transversalis fascia and peritoneum, described in Western articles

Author	Superficial layer		Deep layer
Tobin (1944)	Perirenal fascia-posterior leaf		Perirenal fascia-anterior leaf
Fowler (1975)	Preperitoneal fascia-membranous layer		Preperitoneal fascia-areolar layer
Read (1992)	Cooper's Transversalis fascia-Posterior lamina		
Stoppa (1997)	A thin fibro-cellular layer, could be considered as Cooper's second lamina	Urogenital fascia Spermatic sheath Umbilico-prevesical fascia	Urogenital fascia Spermatic sheath Umbilico-prevesical fascia
Arregui (1997)	Transversalis fascia-posterior lamina (attenuated posterior rectus sheath)		Umbilical Prevesicular fascia
Mirilas, Slandalakis (2010)	Transversalis fascia-posterior lamina?	Umbilical prevesical fascia	Umbilicovesical fascia (contiguous with the Vesical fascia)

Sakurai S. Table 1. p 593. Anatomy of groin. Operation. 69, 4: 491–523, 2015

Perirenal fascia – anterior leaf   ----envelop kidney----   Perirenal fascia-posterior leaf

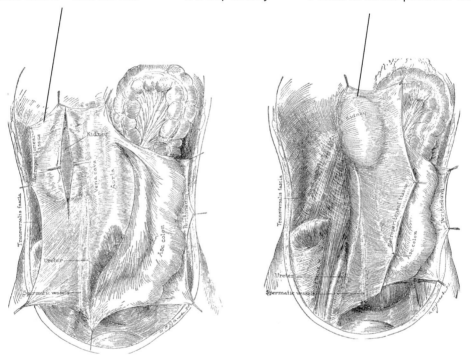

Fig. 2.19 Perirenal fascia (Gerota's fascia) reported by Tobin. Inferiorly, perirenal fascia remains an open potential space, containing the ureter and spermatic vessels. It extends with the spermatic vessels and vas deferens into the scrotum. Tobin CE. The renal fascia andits relation to th transversalis fascia. Anat Rec 89: 295–311, 1944

During hernia repair using a preperitoneal approach, Read [9, 10] noted in 1992 the presence of a novel fascia behind transversalis fascia of the posterior inguinal wall, inferior epigastric vessels, and rectus fascia. As this novel fascia ter-minates at the arcuate line, linea alba, Cooper's ligament, and secondary internal ring, he claimed this was Cooper's long-refuted internal portion of the transversalis fascia. Read called this the posterior lamina of the transversalis fascia, empha-

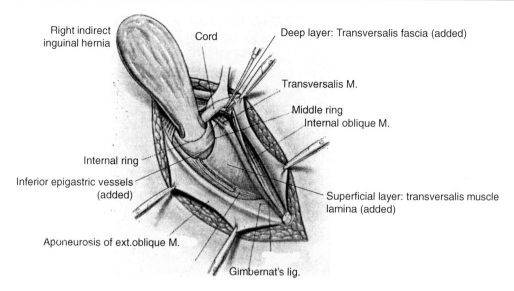

Fig. 2.20 Two layers of fasciae to the posterior wall of the inguinal canal by Lytle, some names have been added. Lytle describes two layers of fasciae to the posterior wall of the inguinal canal. Superficial layer, called as transversalis muscle lamina, and the deep layer, called as transversalis fascia. Current understanding of anatomy indicates that the superficial layer is the transverse fascia and the internal ring proper or transversalis ring, while the deep layer is preperitoneal fascia and secondary internal ring or preperitoneal fascial ring. Lytle WJ. Internal inguinal ring. Br J Surg. 32: 441–446, 1945

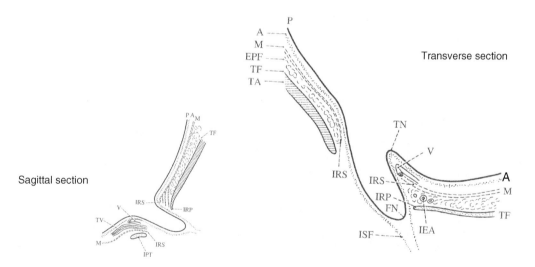

Fig. 2.21 Two layers of preperitoneal fascia behind the transveralis fascia of posterior inguinal wall. Folwer described two preperitoneal fasciae, a superficial membranous layer and a deep areolar layer—forming the preperitoneal space where the vas deferens courses through. The former comprises a "secondary" internal (inguinal) ring, in a deep layer located superior and lateral to the traditional inguinal ring. The inferior epigastric vessels run between the transverse fascia and the membranous layer. *P* peritoneum, *A* preperiotneal fascia-areolar layer, *M* preperitoneal fascia-membranous layer, *EPF* extraperitoneal fat, *TF* transversalis fascia, *TA* transversus abdominis muscle, *TN* true neck of sac, *IRS* secondary internal ring, *IRP* internal ring proper, *FN* false neck of sac, *IEA* inferior epigastric artery, *ISF* internal spermatic fascia, *V* vas deferens, *TV* testicular vessels, *IPT* iliopubic tract. Fowler R. The applied surgical anatomy of the peritoneal fascia of the groin and the "secondary" internal ring. Aust NZ J Surg. 45: 8–14, 1975

sizing that the transversalis fascia consists of two layers. The inferior epigastric vessels penetrate the posterior lamina of the transversalis fascia immediately after branching from the external iliac vessels, and run between the anterior and posterior laminae of the transversalis fascia at the posterior wall of the inguinal canal.

Stoppa, Diarra [15, 16] described in 1997 the perirenal fascia as the urogenital fascia (thus named because it envelops mesodermal urologic organs such as the kidney and ureter, as well as genital organs such as the testicle and vas deferens), based on their intraoperative observations during the giant prostheses for the reinforcement of the visceral sac, as well as their observations of cadaveric dissections (Figs. 2.22, 2.23, and 2.24). The urogenital fascia extends from the two layers of the perirenal fascia. The portion of the fascia extending from the retroperitoneal side of the internal inguinal ring to the inguinal canal is referred to as the spermatic sheath (Call this sheath as Stoppa's spermatic sheath, hereafter) as it envelops the vas deferens and testicular vessels (Fig. 2.25). The inner border is at the vas deferens, with the external border extending beyond the testicular vessels to the

midaxillary line. Anteriorly, the triangular area that surrounds both sides of the medial umbilical fold (remnants of the umbilical artery), with the umbilicus as the apex, was named the umbilico-prevesical fascia, which is comprised of two layers of fascia. The median umbilical fold includes the bladder and remnants of the urachus, which stem from the endodermal cloaca [17]. They are therefore not contained within the mesodermal umbilico-prevesical fascia, and is found between the peritoneum and the umbilico-prevesical fascia (Figs. 2.23 and 2.24).

The space between the transversalis and umbilico-prevesical fascia has an abundance of adipose tissue and is easily dissectable, and it contains the inferior epigastric vessels proximal to where they penetrate the transversalis fascia. However, the inferior epigastric vessels are not covered by the umbilico-prevesical fascia between the medial umbilical fold and the internal inguinal ring (Fig. 2.24). In some cases, there is a thin fibro-cullular layer between the umbilico-prevesical fascia and the transveraslis fascia. This layer may be the posterior lamina of the transversalis fascia, but this possibility has not been explored [16].

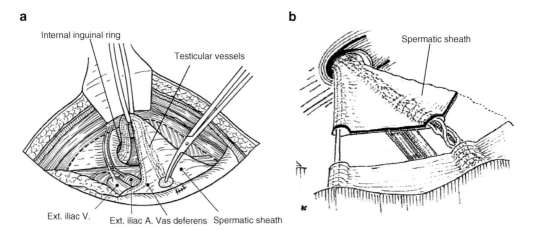

Fig. 2.22 Spermatic sheath, pointed out by Stoppa. Preperitoneal view of the right inguinal region during the parietalization of the cord components in the Giant prosthetic reinforcement of the visceral sac. (**a**) The spermatic sheath, the prolongation of two layers of the urogenital fasciae, ensheath the vas deferens and the testicular ves-

sels. (**b**) The inner border of the spermatic sheath is at the vas deferens, with the external border extending beyond the testicular vessels to the midaxillary line. Stoppa R, Diarra B, Mertl P. The retroparietal spermatic sheath—An anatomical structure of surgical interest. Hernia 1:55–59, 1977

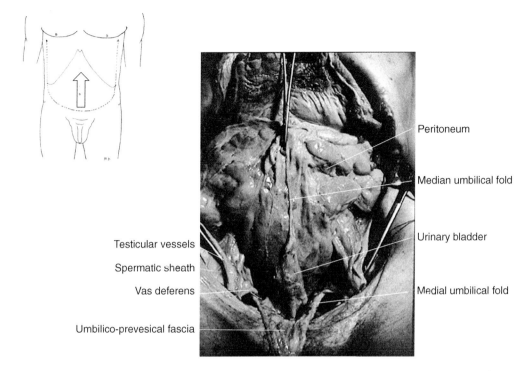

Fig. 2.23 Urogenital fascia, described by Stoppa. A large "U" incision on the abdominal wall is made and the flap includes the skin, muscles, and transversalis fascia is reflected upward, showing the preperitoneal space. Stoppa. The retroperitoneal spermatic sheath-An anatomical structure of surgical interest. Hernia, 1:55–59, 1977

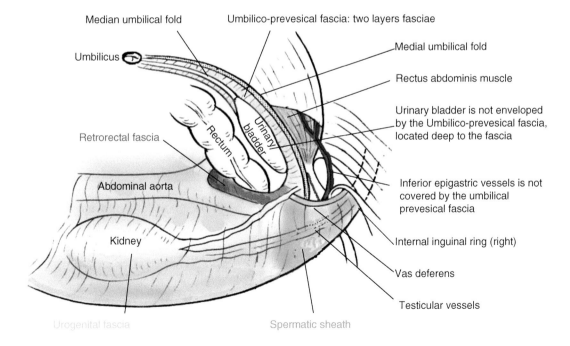

Fig. 2.24 Schema of the Urogenital fascia (two layer fascia) described by Stoppa, illustrated by Sakurai. The peritoneum had been removed. Sakurai S. Anatomy of groin. Operation. 69, 4: 491–523, 2015. Fig. 34, p 508

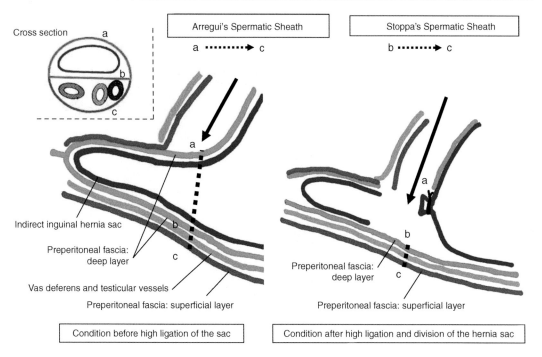

Fig. 2.25 Difference between Stoppa's spermatic sheath and Arregui's spermatic sheath. Sakurai S. Anatomy of groin. Operation. 69, 4: 491–523, 2015. Fig. 41, p 511

Like McVay et al. [3], Arregui [18] noted in 1997 that there are cases where a clear arcuate line is not observed. Rather, there may be a gradual reduction in fiber density, merging with several layers of fascia to reach the pubis. These fasciae were referred to as the "attenuated posterior rectus sheath" (Figs. 2.26 and 2.27) comprised of the posterior aponeurosis of the rectus sheath which is fused with the anterior lamina of the transversalis fascia (description as the rectus fascia is appropriate here) and the posterior lamina of the transversalis fascia. The posterior rectus space is between the attenuated rectus sheath and the rectus muscle, and it contains the inferior epigastric vessels which supply the rectus muscles (Figs. 2.26 and 2.27). What is often referred to as the preperitoneal space, described by Bendavid [19] as the inguinal space of Bogros containing the epigastric vessels and its branches, is actually a continuation of the posterior rectus space [18]. Dorsal to the attenuated posterior rectus sheath is a pre-peritoneal fascia called the umbilical prevesicular fascia. According to Arregui [18], the preperitoneal space is in between the attenuated posterior rectus sheath (including the posterior lamina of the transversalis fascia) and the umbilical prevesicular fascia, and is continuous with the retropubic space of Retzius (Figs. 2.26 and 2.27). The umbilical prevesicular fascia forms a conical sheath (Call this sheath as Arregui's spermatic sheath, hereafter) dorsal to the internal inguinal ring, which contains the spermatic cord, testicular vessels, and indirect hernia sac (if present) (Fig. 2.25). It extends into the inguinal canal and forms the internal spermatic fascia.

Stoppa's spermatic sheath ensheaths the vas deferens and testicular vessels, and is observed following high ligation of an external inguinal hernia and parietalization of the cord components. It does not include the hernia sac, and thus differs from Arregui's spermatic sheath (Figs. 2.22 and 2.25).

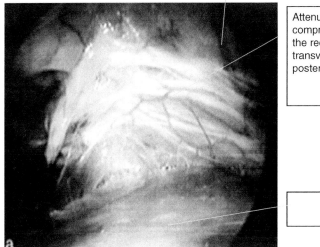
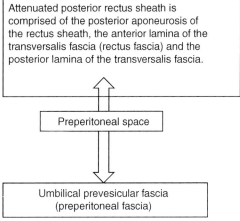

Attenuated posterior rectus sheath is comprised of the posterior aponeurosis of the rectus sheath, the anterior lamina of the transversalis fascia (rectus fascia) and the posterior lamina of the transversalis fascia.

Preperitoneal space

Umbilical prevesicular fascia (preperitoneal fascia)

Fig. 2.26 Extraperitoneal dissection in the midline lower abdominal wall, showing attenuated posterior rectus sheath, posterior lamina of the transversalis fascia and umbilical prevesicular fascia, by Arregui. Note the inferior epigastric vessels course in a space anterior to the attenuated posterior rectus sheath, which is the posterior rectus space. Arregui ME. Surgical anatomy of the pre peritoneal fasciae and posterior transversalis fasciae in the inguinal region. Hernia, 1: 101–110, 1997

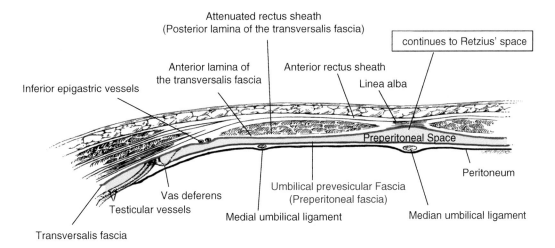

Fig. 2.27 Horizontal section of the lower anterior abdominal wall, by Arregui. Arregui ME. Surgical anatomy of the preperitoneal fasciae and posterior transversalis fasciae in the inguinal region. Hernia, 1: 101–110, 1997

Colborn and Skandalakis [20] (1998) concur with Read [9, 10] regarding the existence of the posterior lamina of the transversalis fascia, but question whether this is a distinct fascia or is simply a regional condensation of extraperitoneal tissue.

Mirilas and Skandalakis [13] (2010) theorize that the retroperitoneal organs (renal, adrenal, and gonadal) and extraperitoneal pelvic organs (bladder, lower colon) originate from the mesoderm during the embryonic stage. As these organs mature, extraperitoneal connective tissue is compressed against the muscles of the abdominal wall to form condensation fascia, such as the perirenal fascia. In the retropubic and perirectal spaces, condensation fascia provide flexible support to organs such as the bladder, ureter, and colon. Dorsal to the umbilicus, two fascia layers are formed between the bilateral medial umbilical ligaments. The deep umbilicovesical fascia or vesical umbilical fascia surrounds the median and medial umbilical ligaments, and these fasciae are continuous with the vesical fascia. The superficial umbilical prevesical fascia is a condensation fascia located in between the transversalis fascia and the bladder, and extends from the umbilicus to the lower wall of the bladder.

There is another condensation fascia in the inguinal region continuous with the perirenal fascia that forms the secondary internal inguinal ring, but this is not the posterior lamina of the transversalis fascia [21].

2.16.1 The Space of Bogros

Bogros, a French surgeon, published a report in 1823 on the surgical anatomy of the iliac region, describing a novel procedure for the ligation of the epigastric and external iliac arteries (Fig. 2.28) [10, 22]. He opened the inguinal canal by making a 5 cm transverse incision cephalic to the inguinal ligament, then widened the internal inguinal ring. Immediately behind the transversalis fascia, near the bladder, there is a more or less thicker layer of cellular tissue than in the rest of this

region. The first portion of the epigastric artery which is situated within this cellular layer, is more closely related to the transversalis fascia than to the peritoneum. The peritoneum, as it reflects from the iliac region of the anterior abdominal wall to the iliac fossa leaves in front a space 12–14 mm wide, where the external iliac artery ends and where the epigastric artery begins. He claimed that the inferior epigastric vessels could be ligated as near its origin as possible without opening the peritoneum.

The term "Space of Bogros (Espace de Bogros)" was first used by French anatomist, Rouviere in 1912 [1]. He described that "…….. the deep aspect of the inguinal wall…. The outer layer of the peritoneum is contact with soft tissues of the iliac fossa from 1 to 1.5 cm above the inguinal ligament. The peritoneum thus demarcates, with a dihedral angle formed by the fascia transversalis and the fascia iliaca inferiorly, a triangular, prismatic interval, filled with preperitoneal adipose tissue, called the space of Bogros" (Fig. 2.29). But this designation did not spread beyond France (Fig. 2.30).

Bendavid [19] (1992) reported that the space of Bogros is a lateral extension of the space of Retzius posterior to the inguinal canal, and contains a venous circle formed by the deep inferior gastric vein, iliopibic vein, rectusial vein, suprapubic vein, and retropubic vein.

However, Read [9, 10], as well as Arregui [18] (Figs. 2.26 and 2.27), Colborn and Skandalakis [20] claimed that the correct location of the Bogros space is between the posterior lamina of transversalis fascia and the peritoneum, and that the inferior epigastcic vessels (after penetrating the posterior lamina of the transversalis fascia) and Bendavid's venous circle are located outside (superficially to) the Bogros space, continuation of the posterior rectus space.

Stoppa [23] claim that the Bogros' space is further divided into a superficial and deep space by the spermatic sheath, the former containing the external iliac artery and nerve, while the latter is avascular where is the recommended placement of a large retroparietal (preperitoneal) mesh prosthesis (Fig. 2.31).

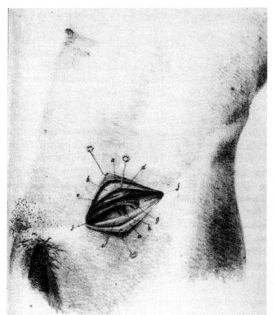 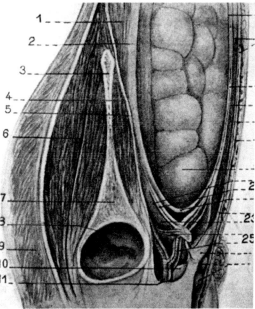

Fig. 2.28 "Essay on the surgical anatomy of the iliac region and description of a new procedure for the ligation of the epigastric and external iliac arteries" written by Bogros in 1823 (translated by Bendavid R). A 5 cm transverse incision cephalad to the inguinal ligament was made to open the inguinal canal, then the internal inguinal ring was widened. The peritoneum, as it reflects from the iliac region of the anterior abdominal wall to the iliac fossa leaves in front a space 12–14 mm wide, where the external iliac artery ends and where the epigastric artery begins. The epigastric artery was ligated as near its origin as possible without opening the peritoneum. Bogros JA, translation by Bendavid RA. Essay of surgical anatomy of the iliac region and description of a new procedure for the ligation of the epigstric and external iliac arteries. Special issue: The space of Bogros. In Postgraduate General Surgery. Bendavid RA (ed) 6: 4–14, 1995

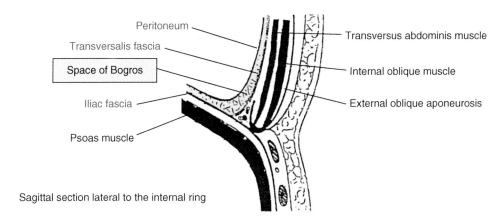

Peritoneum

Transversalis fascia

Space of Bogros

Iliac fascia

Psoas muscle

Transversus abdominis muscle

Internal oblique muscle

External oblique aponeurosis

Sagittal section lateral to the internal ring

Fig. 2.29 The space of Bogros, named by Rouviere in 1912. "……..the deep aspect of the inguinal wall…. The outer layer of the peritoneum is in contact with soft tissues of the iliac fossa from 1 to 1.5 cm above the inguinal ligament. The peritoneum thus demarcates, with a dihedral angle formed by the fascia transversalis and the fascia ili-aca inferiorly, a triangular, prismatic interval, filled with preperitoneal adipose tissue, called the space of Bogros". Hureau J: The space of Bogros and interparietoperitoneal spaces. In Bendavid R (ed), Abdominal Wall Hernias, Springer, 2001. pp 101–106

Fig. 2.30 "The Space of Bogros" in French Anatomy Textbook, by Paturet G., published in 1951: No description about boundaries of the space of Bogros is written. Hureau J: The space of Bogros and interparietoperitoneal spaces. In Bendavid R (ed), Abdominal Wall Hernias, Springer, 2001. pp 101–106

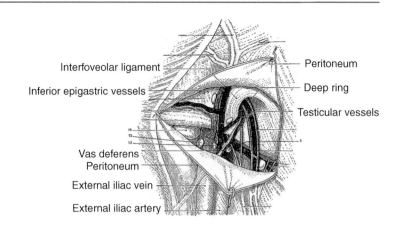

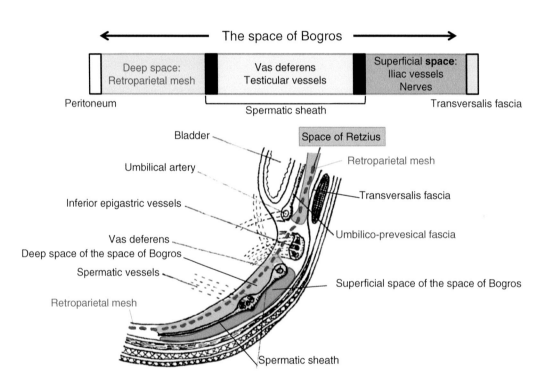

Fig. 2.31 Superficial and deep space of the space of Bogros by Stoppa [23]: Imaginary figure of the space of Bogros added. Stoppa R, Diarra B, Verhaeghe P, et al. Some problems encountered at re-operation following repair of groin hernia with pre-peritoneal prostheses. Hernia, 1998, 2:35–38

2.16.2 The Space of Retzius

Swedish anatomist and surgeon Retzius [24] published "some remarks on the proper design of the semilunar line of Douglas" in 1858 (the "semilunar line" is referred to as the "semicircular line of Douglas or the arcuate line" by contemporary anatomists) (Fig. 2.32). Caudad to the semicircular line, he noted that the fibers of the posterior rectus sheath are spread thin along the

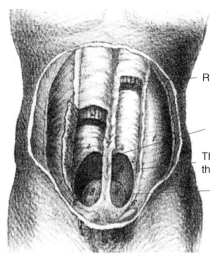

Rectus muscle cut through

The lineae of Douglas,
upper arcus

The preperitoneal cavity of
the bladder

Bladder only half
distended

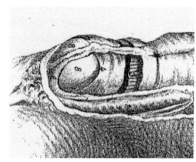

Fig. 2.32 "Some remarks on the proper design of the semilunar line of Douglas." (The name semilunar line of Douglas is changed to semicircular line of Douglas, at the present time) by Retzius A in 1858. The bladder is so distended that the whole of the cavity is quite filled, so that the linea alba makes a longitudinal impression on its anterior wall. (1) There must exist a preperitoneal cavity, in which the bladder could move by change of its volume. (2) The fascia of the transversus continues, investing the side wall of the said cavity for the bladder, and entering down very deep in the pelvic cavity. (3) The preperitoneal cavity of the bladder opens anteriorly into the sheath of the rectus muscles, which are filled with the same scarcely appreciated areolar tissue. Retzius AA. Some remarks on the proper design of the semilunar lines of Douglas. Edinburgh Med J, 3: 865–867, 1858

transversalis fascia, making it possible to manually palpate deep into the pelvis with light pressure, as far as the neck of the bladder. He observed the following:

1. Caudal to the semicircular line, there must exist a preperitoneal cavity, in which the bladder could move by change of its volume.
2. The fascia of the transversus continues, investing the side wall of the said cavity for the bladder, and entering down very deep in the pelvic cavity.
3. The preperitoneal cavity of the bladder opens anteriorly into the sheath of the rectus muscles, which are filled with the same scarcely appreciated areolar tissue.

Contemporary anatomy refutes claims 2 and 3, since the transversalis fasica does not surround the bladder, nor is it continuous with the rectus sheath. This inconsistency may be the reason why there remains much controversy regarding the definition and boundary of the so-called "Retzius space."

Read [10] (1997) claimed the transversalis and pre-umbilicovesical fasciae (noting that the umbilicovesical fascia consists of the pre-umbilicovesical and "true" lamina) form the Retzius space.

Diarra and Stoppa [16] (1997) claimed the Retzius space to be between the transversalis fascia and the bladder, and that it could be dissected into two distinct spaces along the umbilico-prevesical fascia. The superficial space is fatty and easily dissected, but the deep space contains dense connective tissue along with a venous plexus, making it difficult and dangerous to dissect.

Arregui [18] (1997) defined the space between the attenuated posterior rectus sheath and umbilical prevesicular fascia (preperitoneal fascia) as the preperitoneal space, and that this is continuous with the retropubic Retzius space (Fig. 2.27).

2.17 Japanese perspective on the dissection of fascial structures and cleavable planes located between the transversalis fascia and peritoneum (Fig. 2.33)

Japanese anatomist, Sato [25–30] noted that there are two layers of fascia between the peritoneum and transversalis fascia—the deep layer of subperitoneal fascia (anterior renal fascia or Gerota's fascia) and the superficial layer of subperitoneal fascia (posterior renal fascia or Gerota's fascia). He suggests that when the muscle layer is considered to be the central structure of the abdominal wall, the inner linings of the peritoneal cavity are comparable with the outer coverings of the abdominal wall, but reversed in orientation, in other word, layered symmetrically fashion (Fig. 2.34). So the peritoneum corresponds to the skin and the transversalis fascia corresponds to the innominate fascia. There are two layers of subperitoneal fasciae (called as preperitoneal fascia in Western countries) between the peritoneum and the transversalis fascia, corresponding to Camper's fascia and Scarpa's fascia.

The subperitoneal fasciae form the renal fascia, separating caudally to the gonadal vessel fascia, ureteric fascia, and aortic and vena caval fascia. In males, the gonadal vessel fascia form the triangular testiculodeferential fascia (likely identical to Stoppa's spermatic sheath [15, 16]) bounded by the testicular vessels and vas deferens with the internal ring as the apex. The deep layer of subperitoneal fascia covering the internal iliac artery (formerly called as the hypogastric artery) extends medially including the medial umbilical ligament and it passes anteriorly to the bladder to reach the umbilicus, while forming the two layer triangular shape vesicohypogastrica or the umbilical prevesical fascia, resembling to a washed sheet hanged on the line [31] (Figs. 2.35 and 2.36). The two subperitoneal fasciae contain the urachus at the midline, extending caudally to the levator ani, continuing as the vesical fascia posteromedially. The deep subperitoneal fascia medial to the ureteric fascia forms a thin vesical fascia that surrounds the lower part of the bladder, though it does not extend to the dome of the bladder, which is covered only by the peritoneum. References to "the fascia of the bladder" commonly involve the vesicohypogastric fascia [29].

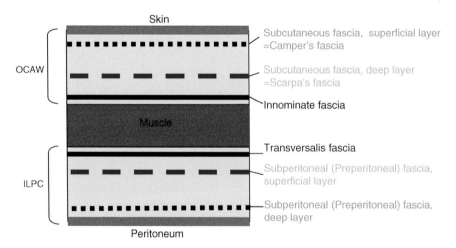

Fig. 2.33 Concept of structure of the abdominal wall by Sato, illustrated by Sakurai. *OCAW* outer coverings of the abdominal wall, *ILPC* inner linings of the peritoneal cavity. Sakurai S. Anatomy of groin. Operation. 69, 4: 491–523, 2015. Fig. 50, p 515

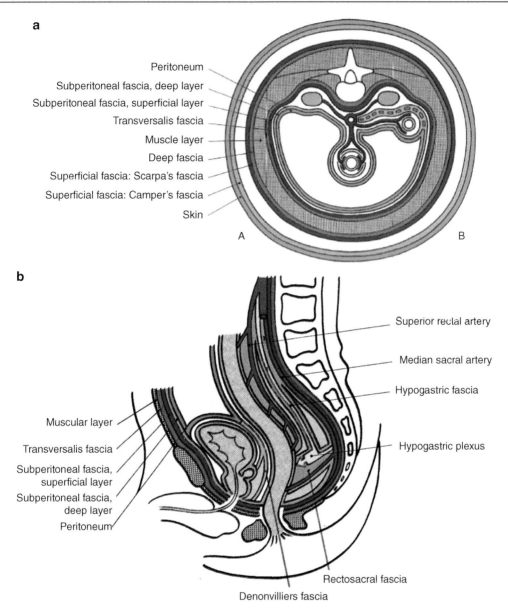

a

- Peritoneum
- Subperitoneal fascia, deep layer
- Subperitoneal fascia, superficial layer
- Transversalis fascia
- Muscle layer
- Deep fascia
- Superficial fascia: Scarpa's fascia
- Superficial fascia: Camper's fascia
- Skin

A   B

b

- Superior rectal artery
- Median sacral artery
- Hypogastric fascia
- Hypogastric plexus

- Muscular layer
- Transversalis fascia
- Subperitoneal fascia, superficial layer
- Subperitoneal fascia, deep layer
- Peritoneum

Rectosacral fascia
Denonvilliers fascia

Fig. 2.34 (**a**) Cross-section of the abdomen at the kidney level, by Sato. (**b**) Sagittal section of lower abdomen at midline, showing fascial structures by Sato. Sato T, Sato K. Regional anatomy for operative surgery of genitor-urinary organs.13. Fascial structures in the pelvis. Japanese Journal of Clinical Urology. 43: 576–584, 1989

Stoppa and Diarra [15, 16] did not refer to the vesical fascia per se, but noted that the umbilico-vesical fascia, which is continuous with the uro-genital fascia, does not envelop the bladder. This interpretation is largely consistent with Sato's description (Figs. 2.35 and 2.36). At the very least, it is clear that dissection posteriorly beyond the umbilical prevesical fascia runs the risk of bladder injury and should never be attempted during inguinal hernia surgery.

Sato did not specifically reference the posterior lamina of the transversalis fascia, which covers the inferior epigastric vessels dorsally at the posterior wall of the inguinal canal.

Fig. 2.35
Vesicohypogastric
fascia. Sato T. Regional
anatomy for operative
surgery of genitor-
urinary organs.14.
Urinary bladder and
prostate. Japanese
Journal of Clinical
Urology. 43:669–676,
1989

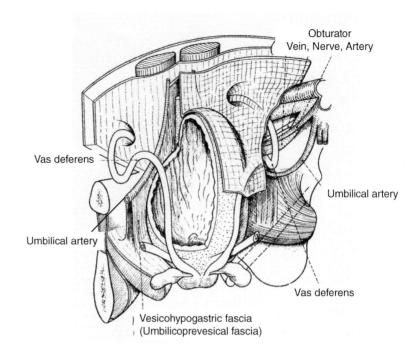

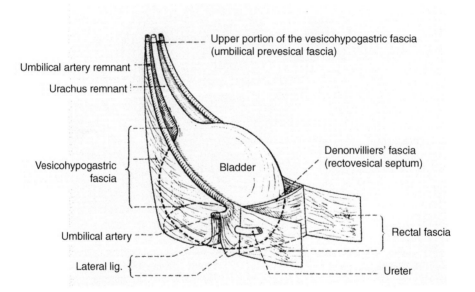

Fig. 2.36 Vesicohypogastric fascia and Denonvilliers fascia. Sato T. Regional anatomy for operative surgery of genitor-urinary organs.18. Urinary bladder and prostate (5) Lymphatics and fascial structures. Japanese Journal of Clinical Urology. 43:1039–1048, 1989

However, the subperitoneal fascia theoretically envelops the entire peritoneum, and Sato's figure describing the pelvic anatomy shows superficial and deep layer of subperitoneal fasciae, with the former corresponding to the posterior lamina of the transversalis fascia (Fig. 2.34).

Sakurai (the author) concurs with Sato's description, but uses nomenclature consistent with an anterior surgical approach, preferring the term "preperitoneal fascia" rather than "subperitoneal fascia" (Figs. 2.33 and 2.37).

It is unclear whether the fascia covering the inferior epigastiric vessels dorsally at the posterior wall of the inguinal canal is the Cooper's posterior lamina of the transversalis fascia [9, 10], or if it is the preperitoneal fascia-membranous layer as described by Fowler [14], but such a fascia clearly exists. The author (Sakurai) believes that the superficial layer of preperitoneal fascia is corresponded with the posterior lamina of the transversalis fascia and as claimed by Sato, the umbilical prevesical fascia is formed by the deep layer of preperitoneal fascia. Furthermore, the bladder is not contained within the umbilical prevesical fascia but sits behind it, as described by Sato [27–29] and Stoppa [15, 16] (Fig. 2.37).

The classical preperitoneal space is divided into three spaces by two layers of preperitoneal fascia (Fig. 2.38). Superficially, the space between the transversalis and superficial layer of

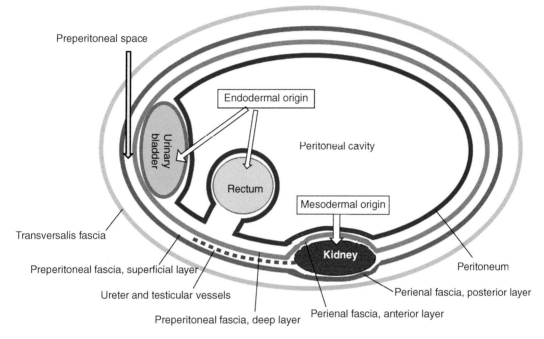

Fig. 2.37 Fascial structures of the abdominal wall drawn by Sakurai. Preperitoneal fasciae enclose entire abdominal cavity. Preperitoneal fascia, superficial layer = Transversalis fascia, posterior lamina, Preperitoneal fascia, deep layer = Umbilical prevesical fascia. Sakurai S. Anatomy of groin. Operation. 69, 4: 491–523, 2015. Fig. 55, p 517

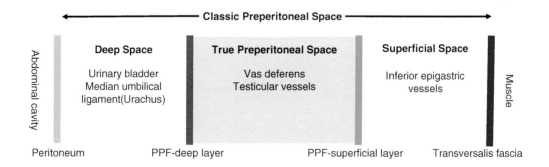

Fig. 2.38 The classic preperitoneal space is separated by two preperitoneal fasciae (PPF) into three subspaces, which are the superficial space, the middle-true preperitoneal space, and the deep space. *PPF* Preperitoneal fascia. Sakurai S. Anatomy of groin. Operation. 69, 4: 491–523, 2015. Fig. 57, p 518

preperitoneal fasciae contains the inferior epigastric vessels behind the posterior wall of the inguinal canal and is the superficial space of the Bogros space [23]. The middle space between the superficial and deep preperitoneal fasciae is the true preperitoneal space, or Retzius space (Figs. 2.31 and 2.38), that contains the kidney, ureter, testicular vessels, vas deferens, preperitoneal fat, and lateral umbilical fold. The deepest space between the deep layer of preperitoneal fascia and peritoneum includes the bladder and median umbilical fold (urachus), and the deep space of the space of Bogros [23] which is exposed by dissection during parietalization of the cord components and the recommended placement of a retroparietal mesh [15, 16].

2.17.1 The Following Points Differ in Western Reports

Stoppa [15, 16] notes that the urogenital membrane does not cover the entire anterior abdominal wall. The umbilico-prevesical fascia is composed of two layers of urogenital fascia. In some cases, tissue that may be the posterior lamina of the transversalis fascia is observed, which is separate from the urogenital fascia. Mirilas and Skandalakis [13, 21] note that since the bladder and lower colon both stem from the mesoderm, they are enveloped by the same fascia. The umbilical prevesical fascia envelops the median umbilical ligament and medial umbilical ligament, and is continuous with the vesical fascia. Those points remain controversial.

2.17.2 Fascial Anatomy of Indirect Inguinal Hernia

In considering the anatomy of indirect inguinal hernia, it is helpful to follow the prenatal descent of the testis [17] (Figs. 2.39 and 2.40). The testes form near the kidneys from around 8 weeks of gestation. At 12–32 weeks the processus vaginalis with surrounding two layers of preperitoneal

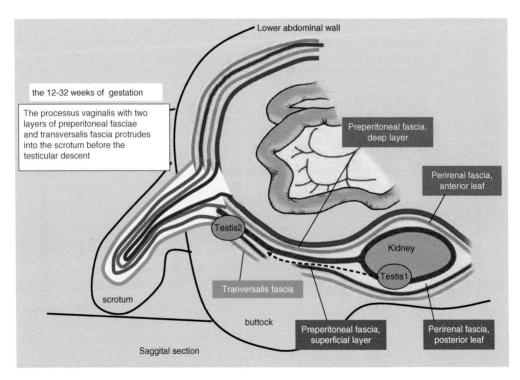

Fig. 2.39 In fetal life, peritoneal evagination to form the processus vaginalis precedes the descent of testis into the scrotum. Sakurai S. Anatomy of groin. Fig. 59-b. In Hernia Surgery, pp 7–35. Edited by Sakurai S, Nankodo, Tokyo, Japan, 2017. Sakurai S. Anatomy of groin. Operation. 69, 4: 491–523, 2015. Fig. 58, p 518

fasciae and transversalis fascia protrudes into the scrotum before the testicular descent (Fig. 2.39). The rim of the protruded transversalis fascia is the internal inguinal ring. Next, the testes are pulled by the gubernaculum testis as the abdominal walls and cavity grow. The organs maintain their relative anatomical positions as the testes descend until they exit the internal inguinal ring and reach the base of the scrotum. Most of adult indirect inguinal hernias arise from the processus vaginalis, with the hernia sac enveloped by the deep layers of preperitoneal fascia. The vas deferens and testicular vessels run between the deep and superficial layers of preperitoneal fasciae, and these fasciae are further enveloped by the internal spermatic fascia, which is continuous with the transversalis fascia (Fig. 2.40).

Indirect inguinal hernia is illustrated in a coronal section anterior to the inguinal canal (Fig. 2.41), as well as in a cross-section of the spermatic cord (Fig. 2.42).

2.18   Inguinal Nerves

There are three nerves in the inguinal area. From cranial to caudal, they are the iliohypogastric nerve (IHN), the ilioinguinal nerve (IIN), and the genital branch of the genitofemoral nerve (GFN-GB) (Figs. 2.6 and 2.7). Anatomical aberrations are not uncommon. The IHN is contained within the superficial interparietal fascia and adheres to the internal oblique muscles (in neural bed). The IIN is contained within the cremasteric fascia and adheres to the cremaster muscle. The GFN-GB is contained within the cremasteric fascia as well.

The IHN is a sensory and motor nerve arising from the Th12 and L1 spinal nerves, running along the anterior surface of the quadratus lumborum muscle in the lower lateral direction. The IHN penetrates the transverse abdominal muscles from the retroperitoneal space about 2 cm medial to the anterior superior iliac spine. It often

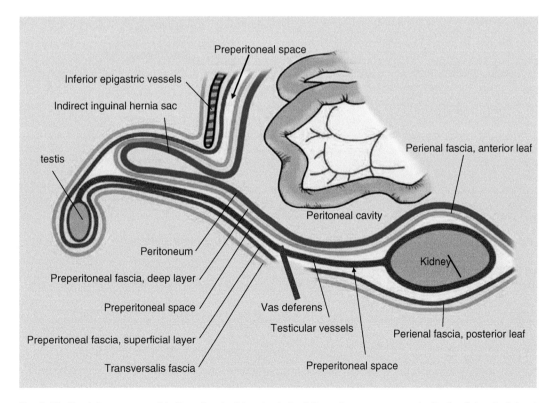

Fig. 2.40 Fascial structures of indirect inguinal hernia derived from the processus vaginalis, by Sakurai. Sakurai S. Anatomy of groin. Operation. 69, 4: 491–523, 2015. Fig. 58, p 518

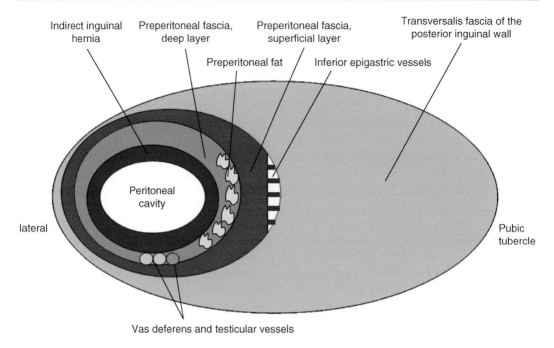

Fig. 2.41 Right indirect inguinal hernia, illustrated in a coronal section anterior to the inguinal canal, by Sakurai. Sakurai S. Anatomy of groin. Operation. 69, 4: 491–523, 2015. Fig. 59, p 518

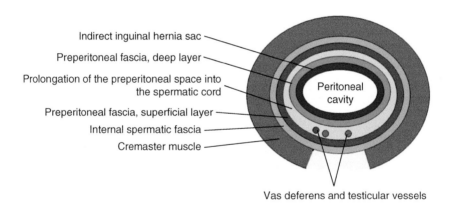

Fig. 2.42 Cross-section of the spermatic cord containing indirect inguinal hernia derived from the processus vaginalis, by Sakurai. Sakurai S. Anatomy of groin. Operation. 69, 4: 491–523, 2015. Fig. 60, p 518

penetrates the internal oblique muscle lateral to the internal inguinal ring, and runs medially along the surface of the internal oblique muscle, covered by the transparent superficial interparietal fascia (Fig. 2.7).

According to Wijsmuller [32], the IHN passes on average 2.4 cm (1.5–4.4 cm) cranial to the internal inguinal ring. It runs anteriorly over the anterior rectus sheath at the lateral edge of the

rectus muscle, penetrating the aponeurosis of the external abdominal oblique muscle, on average 3.8 cm (2.5–5.5 cm) cranial to the external inguinal ring to distribute subcutaneously. In 11% of cases, the nerve is buried within the internal oblique muscle, appearing superficially near the midpoint of the spermatic cord (Fig. 2.43).

Rarely, the nerve takes a subaponeurotic course, passing behind the internal oblique

Internal oblique muscle Anterior rectus sheath

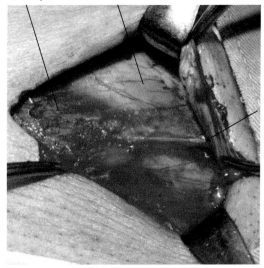

IHN piecing the external oblique aponeurosis to the subcutaneous tissue

Fig. 2.43 Iliohypogastric nerve (IHN) buried within the internal oblique muscle, appearing superficially near the lateral border of the anterior rectus sheath. Sakurai S. Anatomy of groin. Operation. 69, 4: 491–523, 2015. Fig. 61, p 519

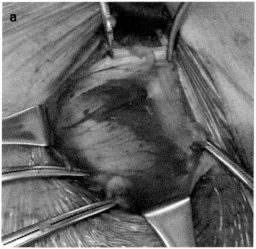 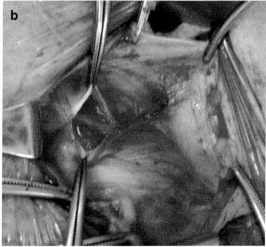

Fig. 2.44 Iliohypogastric nerve (IHN) coursing within the rectus sheath (subaponeurotic course). (**a**) There is no IHN coursing anterior to the anterior rectus sheath. Short segment of IHN penetrating the anterior rectus sheath is identified near the linea alba. (**b**) IHN coursing within the rectus sheath (subaponeurotic course). Sakurai S. Anatomy of groin. Operation. 69, 4: 491–523, 2015. Fig. 62, p 519

muscle as well as the aponeurosis of the internal oblique muscle, running through the rectus sheath, finally appearing through the rectus sheath and aponeurosis of the external oblique muscle near the midline (Fig. 2.44).

The ilioinguinal nerve (IIN) is a sensory and motor nerve arising from the Th12 and L1 spinal nerves. Like the IHN, it penetrates the transversus abdominis and internal oblique muscles. Surrounded by the superficial interparietal fascia, it then runs medially along the surface of the internal oblique muscle. The IIN is often found to be enveloped by the cremasteric fascia and fixed to the anterior surface of the spermatic cord. The

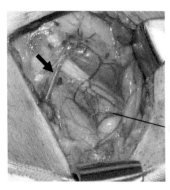

External inguinal ring

Fig. 2.45 The branch of the ilioinguinal nerve pierces the external oblique aponeurosis superolateral aspect of the external inguinal ring and runs toward the thigh. Sakurai S. Anatomy of groin. Operation. 69, 4: 491–523, 2015. Fig. 4, p 492

nerve is sometimes buried within the cremaster muscle. Typically, it exits the external inguinal ring and distributes to the skin of the inguinal region, but it may occasionally exit singularly prior to reaching the external inguinal ring to penetrate the aponeurosis of the external abdominal oblique muscle and to innervate the inner thigh (Fig. 2.45).

The IHN and IIN have many aberrations. Al-dabbagh [33] noted that classic textbook anatomy was only found in 41.8% of cases. Aberrations were seen in 58.2% of cases, and included the following:

1. acute infero-lateral angulation of the IIN at its exit behind the external inguinal ring fibers in 18.2%
2. similar direction of the IIN but in a plane superficial to the external oblique aponeurosis and proximal to the external inguinal ring in 16.4%
3. a single stem for both nerves over the spermatic cord in 21.8%
4. absence of one or both nerves in 7.3%
5. accessory IIN or IHN in 2.7%
6. aberrant origin of the IIN from GFN in 1.8%.

The genitofemoral nerve (GFN) is a sensory and motor nerve containing fibers from L2 and L3. It descends along the surface of the greater psoas muscle, and bifurcates behind the inguinal ligament to form the femoral branch (GFN-FB) which continues femorally, and the genital branch (GFN-GB) which runs dorsally to enter the inguinal canal.

According to Wijsmuller [32], he GFN-GB typically (94%) enters the inguinal canal after passing the caudolateral edge of the internal inguinal ring, but there are rare cases where it directly penetrates the transverse fascia of the posterior wall of the inguinal canal. Amid [34] noted that the GFN-GB runs caudally to the spermatic cord in tandem with the external spermatic vessels within the cremasteric fascia. The external spermatic vein can be visualized intraoperatively as a "blue line" along with its accompanying structures, the spermatic artery and GFN-GB (Figs. 2.10, 2.14, and 2.15).

However, Wijsmuller [32] claimed that the "blue line" could only be visualized in 22% of cases, and further reported that the GFN-GB passes the external inguinal ring and continues to the base of the scrotum in 94% of cases, and does so dorsally (44%), medially (28%), or laterally (22%) in relation to the spermatic cord.

2.19 The Femoral Sheath, the Femoral Ring, and the Femoral Canal (Fig. 2.46)

The external iliac vessels run along the anterior surface of the psoas major muscle, descending within the retroperitoneum to the vascular lacuna bounded by the iliopectineal arch, Cooper's ligament, and iliopubic tract. The external iliac vessels exit the vascular lacuna to become the femoral vessels. The transversalis fascia from the iliopectineal arch, Cooper's ligament, and iliopubic tract form an approximately 4-cm-long sheath surrounding and merging with the adventitia of the femoral vessels. This cylindrical sheath formed by the transversalis fascia is referred to as the femoral sheath. The portion of the femoral

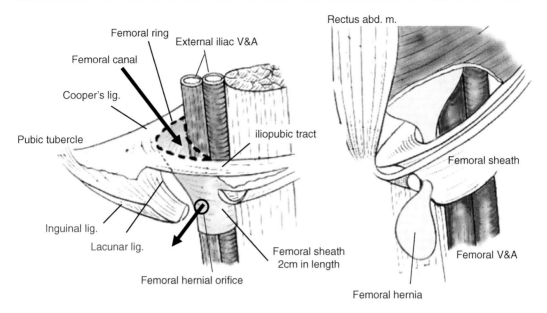

Fig. 2.46 Anatomy of femoral hernia. Black arrows represent the course of femoral hernia protrusion. Sakurai S. Anatomy of groin. Operation. 69, 4: 491–523, 2015. Fig. 64, p 520

sheath extending from Cooper's ligament over the pectineal muscle is the pectineal fascia.

The vascular lacuna are divided into three side-by-side compartments, containing the femoral artery laterally, the femoral vein in the center, and the femoral canal medially. The femoral canal is a conical space about 2 cm in length. Lymph vessels penetrate the tip of the femoral canal, which contains a deep inguinal lymph node (Rosenmuller or Cloquet's node) and preperitoneal adipose tissue [2].

The femoral nerve runs laterally to the femoral sheath along the surface of the iliopsoas muscle.

The femoral ring is the preperitoneal opening of the femoral canal, bounded by the medial wall of the femoral vein, Cooper's ligament, and the iliopubic tract.

Femoral hernias descend through the femoral ring along the femoral canal, stretching the transverse fascia and two layers of preperitoneal fascia at the medial aspect of the femoral sheath to protrude from the oval fossa (saphenous opening). The femoral hernia orifice is where the fem-

oral hernia exits the femoral sheath. The presence of the robust lacunar ligament medial to this orifice makes incarceration and strangulation common at this site.

2.20   Inguinal Anatomy as Seen from the Peritoneal Cavity

Observation of the anterior lower abdominal wall from the peritoneal cavity reveals that the peritoneum has a median fold, as well as additional longitudinal folds—two each on the left and right sides [20, 35] (Fig. 2.47).

1. Median umbilical fold or ligament: located at the midline, it joins the umbilicus and the apex of the bladder. It includes the obliterated urachus which closed in the space between the peritoneum and the deep layer of preperitoneal fascia.
2. Medial umbilical fold or ligament: a pair of folds located lateral to the median fold, running from the umbilicus to the lateral edge of

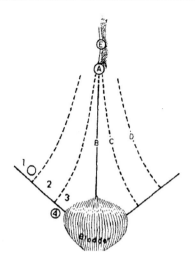

Fig. 2.47 Diagram of the fossae of the anterior abdominal wall and their relation to the sites of groin hernias. (A) Umbilicus; (B) median umbilical lig. (obliterated urachus); (C) medial umbilical lig. (obliterated umbilical aa.); (D) lateralumbilical lig. containing inferior epigastric aa.; (E) falciform lig. Sites of possible hernias: (1) lateral fossa (indirect inguinal hernia); (2) medial fossa (direct inguinal hernia); (3) supravesical fossa (supravesical hernia); (4) femoral ring (femoral hernia). Colborn GL, Skandalakis JE. Laparoscopic cadaveric anatomy of the inguinal area. Prob Gen Surg. 12: 13–20, 1995

the bladder. It includes the obliterated umbilical artery.

3. Lateral umbilical fold or ligament: another pair of folds located lateral to the medial folds, and they include the inferior epigastric vessels.

Three peritoneal fossae are formed on each side between these five folds.

1. Supravesical fossa: between the median and medial folds. This is the site of supravesical hernia.
2. Medial inguinal fossa: between the medial and lateral folds. This is the site of direct inguinal hernia.
3. Lateral inguinal fossa: between the lateral folds and internal inguinal rings. This is where indirect inguinal hernia occurs, including herniation of spermatic cord lipoma.

2.21 Inguinal Anatomy as Seen from the Preperitoneal Space

The anatomy of the abdominal wall following removal of the peritoneum, two layers of preperitoneal fasciae, and preperitoneral fat is shown in Fig. 2.14.

2.22 Three Locations That Require Particular Care During Laparoscopic Surgery [20, 37]

1. Triangle of Doom
   A triangular area with the internal inguinal ring at the apex, bordered medially by the testicular vessels, laterally by the vas deferens, and the peritoneum inferiorly, as dissected during parietalization of the cord components. This area contains the external iliac vessels and the GNF-GB. Damaging the former will result in profuse bleeding along with an unfavorable outcome.
2. Triangle of Pain
   An area under the iliopubic tract, dorsal to the testicular vessels. Contained within this triangle area, medially to laterally, the femoral branch of GFN, the femoral nerve, and the lateral femoral cutaneous nerve, all of which pass under the iliopubic tract. Fixation of a mesh along this portion of the iliopubic tract runs the risk of nerve injury.
3. Circle of Death (Fig. 2.48)
   An aberrant obturator artery may form an arterial ring joining the common iliac artery, internal and external iliac arteries, obturator artery, and inferior epigastric arteries. Inadvertent injury to this arterial ring may result in potentially fatal hemorrhage from both the external and internal iliac arterial supplies. An aberrant obturator vein is actually more prevalent, posing difficulties with hemostasis.

Fig. 2.48 The "Circle of Death". (1) Common iliac artery. (2) Internal iliac artery. (3) Obturator artery. (4) Area of anastomoses of obturator and aberrant obturator artery. (5) Aberrant obturator artery. (6) Inferior epigastric artery. (7) External iliac artery

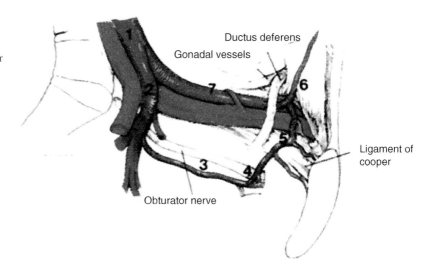

2.23   Summary

The surgical anatomy of the inguinoferoral area is presented with emphasis on anatomic entities related to surgery.

It is very important to know the difference between a fascia and an aponeurosis (tendon), because the precise understanding of fascial structures of the abdominal wall is the key for successful groin hernia repair.

Not only the surgical anatomy for anterior repair but also the posterior or preperitoneal anatomy for laparoscopic or open preperitoneal mesh repair is presented. Admitting the anatomy of the inguinal region yet defies total explication in a form agreeable to all, especially the existence of considerable controversy in the anatomy of preperitonal space, every effort was made to report Western and Japanese perspectives, including those of my own, on the fascial structures and cleavable anatomical spaces located between the transverse fascia and the peritoneum.

References

1. Hureau J. The space of Bogros and interparietoperitoneal spaces. In: Bendavid R, editor. Abdominal wall hernias. New York: Springer; 2001. p. 101–6.
2. Condon RE. Anatomy of the inguinal region and its relation to groin hernia. In: Nyhus LM, Condon RE, editors. Hernia. 4th ed. Philadelphia: J.B. Lippincott; 1995. p. 16–53.
3. McVay CB. Abdominal wall. In: Anson & McVay surgical anatomy. 6th ed. Philadelphia: WB Saunders Co.; 1984. p. 484–584.
4. Fruchaud H. Anatomie Chirurgicale dses Hernies de L'aine. Paris. Doin G. 1956. Surgical anatomy of hernias of groin. Translated and edited by Bendavid R Distributed by Pandemonium Books. www.pandenomonium.ca.
5. Gilbert AI, Graham MF, Voigt WJ. The lateral triangle of the groin. Hernia. 2000;4:234–7.
6. Panagoiotis N, Skandalakin LJ, Gray SW, et al. Supravesical hernia. In: Nyhus LM, Condon RE, editors. Hernia. 4th ed. Philadelphia: J.B. Lippincott; 1995. p. 400–11.
7. Cooper AP. The anatomy and surgical treatment of inguinal and congenital hernia. London: Longman; 1804.
8. Copper AP. The anatomy and surgical treatment of crural and umbilical hernia. London: Longman; 1807.
9. Read RC. Cooper's posterior lamina of transversalis fascia. Surg Gynecol Obstet. 1992;174:426–34.

10. Read RC. Anatomy of abdominal herniation: the pre-peritoneal space. In: Nyhus LM, Baker RJ, Fischer JE, editors. Mastery of surgery. Boston: Little Brown Co.; 1997. p. 1795–806.

11. Tobin CE. The renal fascia and its relation to the transversalis fascia. Anat Rec. 1944;89:295–311.

12. Lytle WJ. Internal inguinal ring. Br J Surg. 1945;32:441–6.

13. Mirilas P, Mentessidou A, Skandalakis JE. Secondary internal inguinal ring and associated surgical planes: surgical anatomy, embryology, applications. J Am Coll Surg. 2008;206:561–70.

14. Fowler R. The applied surgical anatomy of the peritoneal fascia of the groin and the "secondary" internal ring. Aust N Z J Surg. 1975;45:8–14.

15. Stoppa R, Diarra B, Mertl P. The retroparietal spermatic sheath—an anatomical structure of surgical interest. Hernia. 1977;1:55–9.

16. Diarra B, Stoppa R, Verhaeghe P, et al. About prolongations of the urogenital fascia into the pelvis: an anatomic study and general remarks on the interparietal-peritoneal fasciae. Hernia. 1997;1:191–6.

17. Sadler TW. Chapter 16: Urogenital system. In: Langman's medical embryology. 6th ed. Baltimore: Williams & Wilkins; 1990. p. 260–96.

18. Arregui ME. Surgical anatomy of the preperitoneal fasciae and posterior transversalis fasciae in the inguinal region. Hernia. 1997;1:101–10.

19. Bendavid RA. The space of Bogros and the deep inguinal venous circulation. Surg Gynecol Obstet. 1992;174:355–8.

20. Colborn GL, Skandalakis JE. Laparoscopic inguinal anatomy. Hernia. 1998;2:179–91.

21. Mirilas P, Skandalakis JE. Surgical anatomy of the retroperitoneal spaces part 2. The architecture of the retroperitoneal space. Am Surg. 2010;76:33–42.

22. Bogros JA, translation by Bendavid RA. Essay of surgical anatomy of the iliac region and description of a new procedure for the ligation of the epigstric and external iliac arteries. Special issue: the space of Bogros. In: Bendavid RA, editor. Postgraduate general surgery. Vol. 6. 1995. p. 4–14.

23. Stoppa R, Diarra B, Verhaeghe P, et al. Some problems encountered at re-operation following repair of groin hernia with pre-peritoneal prostheses. Hernia. 1998;2:35–8.

24. Retzius AA. Some remarks on the proper design of the semilunar lines of Douglas. Edinb Med J. 1858;3:865–7.

25. Sato T. Fundamental plan of the fascia strata of the body wall. J Clin Exp Med. 1980;114:C168–75.

26. Sato T. Regional anatomy for operative surgery of genitor-urinary organs. 2. I. Kidney B. Renal fascia. Jpn J Clin Urol. 1988;42:689–96.

27. Sato T, Sato K. Regional anatomy for operative surgery of genitor-urinary organs. 13. Fascial structures in the pelvis. Jpn J Clin Urol. 1989;43:576–84.

28. Sato T. Regional anatomy for operative surgery of genitor-urinary organs. 14. Urinary bladder and prostate. Jpn J Clin Urol. 1989;43:669–76.

29. Sato T. Regional anatomy for operative surgery of genitor-urinary organs. 18. Urinary bladder and prostate (5) Lymphatics and fascial structures. Jpn J Clin Urol. 1989;43:1039–48.

30. Sato T. A morphological consideration of the visceral fasciae with special reference to the renal fascia and its differentiation in the pelvic cavity. Jpn Res Soc Clin Anat. 2011;11:82–83.

31. Cahiers D'Anatomie. Petit Bassini I. p. 163. Perlemuter L, Waligora J, et al., translated by Sato T, Central foreign books. Tokyo; 1984.

32. Wijsmuller AR, Lange JFM, Kleinrensink GJ, et al. Nerve-identifying inguinal hernia repair: a surgical anatomical study. World J Surg. 2007;31:414–20.

33. Al-dabbagh AK. Anatomical variations of the inguinal nerves and risks of injury in 110 hernia repairs. Surg Radiol Anat. 2002;24(2):102–7.

34. Amid PK. Lichtenstein tension-free hernioplasty: its inception, evolution, and principles. Hernia. 2004;8:1–7.

35. Colborn GL, Skandalakis JE. Laparoscopic cadaveric anatomy of the inguinal area. Prob Gen Surg. 1995;12:13–20.

36. Nyhus LM. An anatomical reappraisal of the posterior inguinal wall. Surg Clin North Am. 1964;5:1305.

37. Cooper AP. Fig. 5 of PlateXII. In: The anatomy and surgical treatment of abdominal wall hernia. 2nd ed. London: Longman & Co.; 1827.

Abdominal Wall Hernia Classification

Basim Alkhafaji

3.1 Introduction

In literature, many different groin hernia classifications are discussed and quite a lot of them have shortcomings. Most of them are fairly complex and not easily reproduced in clinical practice. The Nyhus classification is one of the most frequently used classification, but is difficult to memorize [1]. Stoppa classification is modified from Nyhus with the addition of aggravating factors [2]. Some other available classifications, like Gilbert classification [3], lack the description of femoral hernias or combined hernias (e.g. pantaloon hernia). Schumpelick et al. [4] described in 1994 the simplest Aachen classification, based on type and size of the hernia defect which was very effective. The European Hernia Society (EHS) has proposed a similar easy and simple classification system and has been promoting its general and systematic use for intraoperative description of the type of hernia to increase the comparison of results available in literature.

B. Alkhafaji (✉)
Head of Surgery Department, Canadian Specialist Hospital, Dubai, UAE

3.2 Groin Hernia Classification

The EHS groin hernia classification [5] resembles largely the Aachen classification with some modifications which make it appropriate for laparoscopic surgery too. In the Aachen classification, 1.5 cm is used as reference for the size of the hernia orifice. The tip of the index finger is mostly around 1.5–2 cm, therefore, it is used as reference marker for open groin hernia procedures. As the EHS classification system is also applicable to laparoscopic surgery, length of the branches of a pair of most laparoscopic graspers, dissectors, or scissors, which comes out to be around 1.5–2 cm as well, is used to measure the orifice size and is taken for reference.

In Table 3.1, the size of the hernia orifice is registered as 1 (1 finger), 2 (1–2 fingers), and 3 (3 fingers). Thus, a hernia orifice of 2.5 cm is depicted as a size 2 hernia.

For anatomic localization, the criteria is as shown in Table 3.1 (L = lateral, M = medial, F = femoral). Different types of hernias can easily be described in the table, and for combined hernia appropriate boxes need to be ticked. In addition, the letter P or R can be encircled to depict, respectively, a primary or a recurrent hernia.

© Springer Nature India Private Limited 2020
P. Chowbey, D. Lomanto (eds.), *Techniques of Abdominal Wall Hernia Repair*,
https://doi.org/10.1007/978-81-322-3944-4_3

Table 3.1 EHS inguino-femoral classification

P = primary hernia
R = recurrent hernia

0 = no hernia detectable
1 = < 1,5 cm (one finger)
2 = < 3   cm (two fingers)
3 = > 3   cm (more than two fingers)
x = not investigated

L = lateral/ indirect hernia
M = medial/ direct hernia
F = Femoral hernia

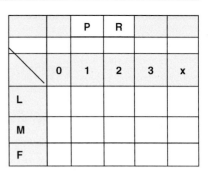

Table 3.2 EHS classification for primary abdominal wall hernias

EHS primary abdominal wall hernia classification		Diameter cm	Small <2 cm	Medium ≤2–4 cm	Large ≤4 cm
Midline	Epigastric				
	Umbilical				
Lateral	Spigelian				
	Lumbar				

3.3 Primary and Incisional Abdominal Wall Hernias Classification

In 2009, EHS classification for both primary and incisional abdominal wall hernias was published [6]. Localization and size of the hernia were used as the two variables for defining and describing the hernia sac.

3.3.1 Classification of Primary Abdominal Wall Hernias

3.3.1.1 Localization of the Hernia
Two midline (epigastric and umbilical) and two lateral hernias (Spigelian and lumbar) are identifiable entities with distinct localizations.

3.3.1.2 Size of the Hernia
Primary abdominal wall hernias are round or oval shaped. Therefore, the size can be described with one measurement. Width and length will be more or less comparable most of the time (Table 3.2).

3.3.2 Classification of Incisional Abdominal Wall Hernias

3.3.2.1 Localization of the Hernia
The abdomen is divided into a medial or midline zone and a lateral zone.

3.3.2.2 Medial and Midline Hernias
The borders of the midline area are defined as (Fig. 3.1):

(a) Cranial: the xiphoid, (b) caudal: the pubic bone, (c) lateral: the lateral margin of the rectal sheath. Thus, all incisional hernias between the lateral margins of both rectus muscle sheaths are classified as midline hernias. In this classification there are 5 M zones from M1 to M5 going from the xiphoid to pubic bone:

1. M1: subxiphoidal (from the xiphoid till 3 cm caudally)
2. M2: epigastric (from 3 cm below the xiphoid till 3 cm above the umbilicus)
3. M3: umbilical (from 3 cm above till 3 cm below the umbilicus)
4. M4: infraumbilical (from 3 cm below the umbilicus till 3 cm above the pubis)

5. M5: suprapubic (from pubic bone till 3 cm cranially).

3.3.2.3 Lateral Hernias

The borders of the lateral area are defined as (Fig. 3.1):

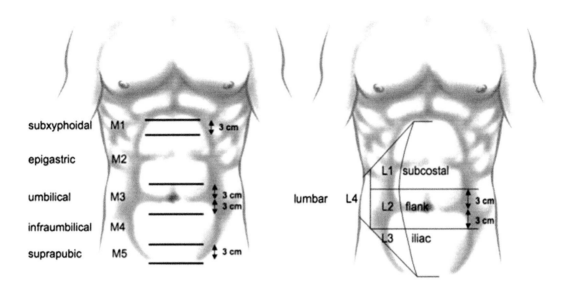

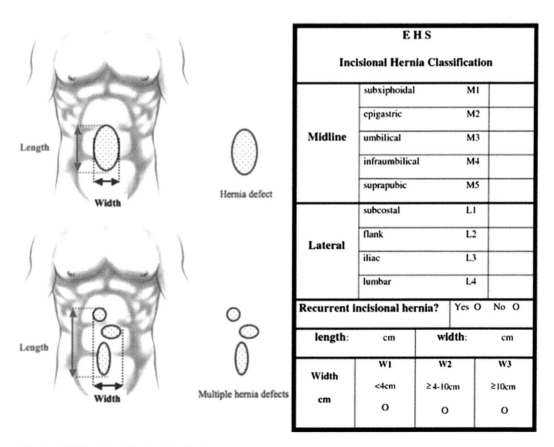

Fig. 3.1 EHS incisional hernia classification

Table 3.3 EHS grid for classification of parastomal hernias

EHS Parastomal Hernia classification		Small ≤5 cm	Large >5 cm
Concomitant incisional hernia?	No	I	III
	Yes	II	IV
		P ☐	R ☐

(a) Cranial: the costal margin, (b) caudal: the inguinal region, (c) medially: the lateral margin of the rectal sheath, (d) laterally: the lumbar region. The four L zones on each side are defined as:

1. L1: subcostal (between the costal margin and a horizontal line 3 cm above the umbilicus)
2. L2: flank (lateral to the rectal sheath in the area 3 cm above and below the umbilicus)
3. L3: iliac (between a horizontal line 3 cm below the umbilicus and the inguinal region)
4. L4: lumbar (latero-dorsal of the anterior axillary line)

3.3.2.4 Size of the Hernia

There was an agreement in EHS that width and length be used to determine size of hernia. The width of the hernia defect was defined as the greatest horizontal distance in cm between the lateral margins of the hernia defect on both sides. In case of multiple hernia defects, the width is measured between the most laterally located margins of the most lateral defect on that side (Fig. 3.1). The length of the hernia defect was defined as the greatest vertical distance in cm between the most cranial and the most caudal margin of the hernia defect. In case of multiple hernia defects from one incision, the length is between the cranial margin of the most cranial defect and the caudal margin of the most caudal defect (Fig. 3.1).

3.4 Parastomal Hernia Classification

In 2014, European Hernia Society classification of parastomal hernias (PH) was published and was based on the defect size of the PH being small ≤5 cm and large >5 cm with the presence of a concomitant incisional hernia (cIH) [7]. In addition, the classification grid includes details about whether the hernia observed is a primary type or has recurred after a previous PH repair. Subclasses of classification were defined as follows (Table 3.3):

- Type I: PH ≤5 cm without cIH.
- Type II: PH ≤5 cm with cIH.
- Type III: PH >5 cm without cIH.
- Type IV: PH >5 cm with cIH.
- P: primary PH.
- R: recurrence after previous PH treatment

References

1. Nyhus LM, Klein MS, Rogers FB. Inguinal hernia. Curr Probl Surg. 1991;28:403–50.
2. Stoppa R. Groin hernias in the adult. In: Chevrel J-P, editor. Hernias and surgery of the abdominal wall. 2nd ed. Berlin: Springer; 1998. p. 175–8.
3. Gilbert AI. An anatomical and functional classification for the diagnosis and treatment of inguinal hernia. Am J Surg. 1989;157:331–3.
4. Schumpelick V, Treutner KH, Arlt G. Classification of inguinal hernias. Chirurg. 1994;65:877–9.
5. Miserez M, et al. The European hernia society groin hernia classification: simple and easy to remember. Hernia. 2007;11(2):113–6.
6. Miserez M, et al. Classification of primary and incisional abdominal wall hernia. Hernia. 2009;13(4):407–14.
7. Śmietański M. European Hernia Society classification of parastomal hernias. Hernia. 2014;18(1):1–6.

Imaging of Abdominal Wall Hernias

4

Rakesh K. Mathur and Nidhi Goyal

4.1 Introduction

Abdominal wall hernias are defects in abdominal wall with protrusion of some part of the abdominal contents through the defect.

Hernias are caused due to laxity of the muscles and persistent increase in intraabdominal pressure due to chronic coughing, straining at stool, and obesity, which leads to weakness of muscles of the abdominal wall. Abdominal trauma and previous surgical procedure are the other common causes.

Abdominal wall hernias are the commonest external hernias, and they pose a surgical problem. There is an incidence of 4–5% of abdominal wall hernias in general population [1].

Hernias are also a common incidental finding in abdominal computed tomography (CT) performed for other clinical problems. Abdominal wall hernias are mostly asymptomatic but can present with acute complications, which require urgent surgical management, like strangulation or incarceration.

Strangulation refers to ischemia due to restricted blood supply and incarceration refers to an irreducible sac. These are common complications in umbilical and paraumbilical hernias [2].

Diagnosis of hernia is commonly made on physical examination. In cases where clinical assessment is difficult due to body habitus or painful condition, imaging studies have assumed importance for diagnosis and to delineate the extent of hernia. Conventional radiographs and Barium studies are no longer used, as multidetector computed tomography (MDCT) is widely available and remains the mainstay for diagnosis, sometimes aided with ultrasound (USG).

Abdominal imaging is usually required for correct diagnosis, precise anatomical details, and diagnosis of complications and to differentiate hernia from other abdominal masses like tumors, hematomas, abscesses, or metastasis.

Imaging studies other than USG and MDCT like magnetic resonance imaging (MRI) are rarely used but can be supportive for problem-solving. CT is fast and acquires volume data permitting multiplanar isotropic reconstruction and 3D volume rendering. MDCT accurately delineates the location, size, type of hernia, and its contents.

The ability of MDCT to delineate clear anatomical details helps to easily detect early signs of strangulation, like mesenteric fat stranding, enhancement of the bowel wall, wall thickening, and fluid or free air in the hernial sac.

This chapter is a comprehensive review of common abdominal wall hernias and their CT appearance, emphasizing the role of multiplanar reformation (MPR) to demonstrate the exquisite anatomical details. MPR images not only aid

R. K. Mathur (✉)
Health Plus Diagnostic and Imaging Center, New Delhi, India

N. Goyal
Department of Radiology and Imaging Sciences, Indraprastha Apollo Hospital, New Delhi, India

© Springer Nature India Private Limited 2020
P. Chowbey, D. Lomanto (eds.), *Techniques of Abdominal Wall Hernia Repair*, https://doi.org/10.1007/978-81-322-3944-4_4

in diagnosis but also facilitate demonstration of findings to the surgeon, which can be helpful in surgical planning.

4.2   MDCT Technique

Several MDCT techniques have been utilized in the evaluation of abdominal wall hernias and almost all of these are acceptable. The routine abdominal CT scan is performed in supine position using positive water-soluble oral and IV contrast. The data set acquired can be reconstructed in multiple other planes without loss of resolution, e.g., a data set if obtained at 5 mm scan thickness can be retrospectively reconstructed at sub millimeter scan thickness which permits exquisite multiplanar reconstruction with isotropic resolution. Some hernial orifices/defects are better appreciated in oblique planes.

In those cases where the hernias are clinically silent or are suspected, various maneuvers which create an increase in intraabdominal pressure like straining/Valsalva maneuver can help precipitate those hernias which manifest only on increase in intraabdominal pressure.

Contrast-enhanced CT scan, especially arterial phase, is necessary for establishing the integrity of the vascular supply of the bowel wall. Oral contrast is essential in evaluating all types of hernia as it delineates the bowel loop and enables tracking of the movement of contents through the bowel.

Real-time MPR images provide useful information supplementing those provided by axial images and in delineating the size and shape of the hernial orifice and its associated complications, if any. Displaying the images in multiple anatomical planes increases the understanding of imaging findings by the surgeon.

4.2.1   Abdominal Wall Anatomy (Fig. 4.1)

Anterior abdominal wall extends superiorly from the xiphoid process of sternum and costal cartilage to the iliac crest and pubic bones of the pelvis inferiorly. Anterior abdominal wall has multiple layers including skin, subcutaneous fat, fascia (superficial and deep), muscles, fascia transversalis, and parietal peritoneum. Muscle layer includes the external oblique muscle, internal oblique muscle,

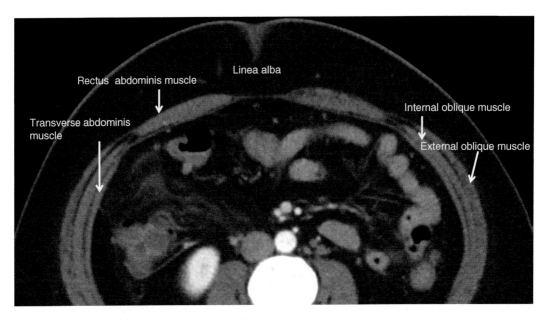

Fig. 4.1 CT anatomy of the anterior abdominal wall

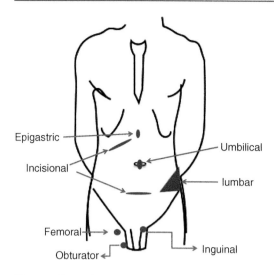

Fig. 4.2 Pictorial presentation of sites of various abdominal wall hernias

Table 4.1 Types of hernia

Groin hernias	Inguinal	Femoral
	Direct	
	Indirect	
Ventral hernias	Anterior	Lateral
	Umbilical	Spigelian
	Paraumbilical	
	Epigastric	
	Hypogastric	
Lumbar		
Incisional		
Rare	Abdominal	Pelvic
	Interparietal	Sciatic
	Richter	Obturator
	Littre	Perineal
Traumatic		

transverse abdominis muscle antero-laterally, and rectus abdominis muscle anteriorly. The fascia surrounding the anterolateral muscles fuse anteriorly and attaches to rectus abdominis muscle at the linea semilunaris. CT images clearly depict the anterior abdominal wall anatomy, precisely delineating the layers of anterior abdominal wall, abdominal wall muscles and peritoneal cavity.

4.3 Types of Abdominal Wall Hernias (Fig. 4.2)

Hernias may be congenital or acquired and occur in various anatomical sites of the abdominal wall. Hernias are primarily classified by the location and content, majority being inguinal hernias (75%), followed by femoral hernias (15%) and umbilical hernias (8%) [1] (Table 4.1).

4.4 Groin Hernias

Inguinal hernias: Inguinal hernias are the most common type of abdominal wall hernias. Two types of inguinal hernias are indirect and direct.

Indirect inguinal hernias are more common in children. In adults both direct and indirect hernias are seen with equal frequency.

Indirect hernias pass through the inguinal canal into the scrotal sac lateral to inferior epigastric vessels and occur due to failure of obliteration of processus vaginalis. It is a peritoneal extension along the spermatic cord up to the testis [3]. Inguinal hernias are more common in male population irrespective of the age. Direct inguinal hernias are medial to inferior epigastric vessel and result from acquired defect in transversalis fascia of the Hesselbach triangle. These are commonly seen in the age group of 30–40 years and are often bilateral [3] (Fig. 4.3).

Femoral hernia: Femoral hernias are less frequent than inguinal hernias and are more common in females. Anatomically these hernias pass through the femoral canal, medial to femoral vein and posterior to the inguinal ligament [3, 4]. These hernias are more common on the right side [5] (Fig. 4.4).

The femoral artery and inferior epigastric artery form the basis for differentiation between inguinal and femoral hernia (Fig. 4.5). Radiologically it is difficult to differentiate between these two hernias, and femoral hernias have a higher tendency to incarcerate [5, 6].

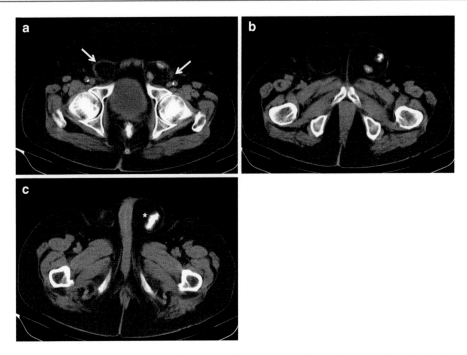

Fig. 4.3 Inguinal hernia; axial images (arrow) depicting bilateral inguinal hernia (arrows) with right-sided herniation of fat and left-sided herniation of bowel loops (∗) as hernial contents

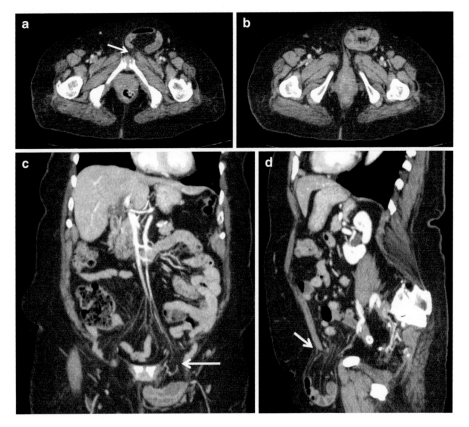

Fig. 4.4 Femoral hernia; Axial (**a**, **b**), MPR coronal (**c**), and sagittal images (**d**) hernial orifice (arrow) with bowel in hernial contents

Fig. 4.5
Differentiation of
femoral from direct
and indirect inguinal
hernia

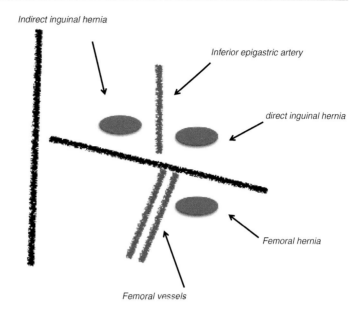

Indirect inguinal hernia

Inferior epigastric artery

direct inguinal hernia

Femoral hernia

Femoral vessels

4.5   Ventral Hernias

Ventral hernias occur in anterior and lateral abdominal wall. Midline ventral hernias include umbilical, paraumbilical, epigastric, and hypogastric hernias. Amongst these, umbilical hernias are the most common.

Umbilical Hernia: Umbilical hernias are usually small, seen more commonly in women, and are the most common type of ventral hernia. Umbilical hernia occurring in children is due to failure of closure of umbilical ring. During the embryonic period, there is physiological herniation of intestinal loops through the umbilicus, which returns to abdominal cavity by the 12th week of gestation. In the middle-aged and elderly they occur due to increased intraabdominal pressure secondary to ascites, obesity, and sometimes large intraabdominal masses. Umbilical hernias are usually small and run a higher risk of incarceration (Fig. 4.6). Hernial contents are either omental fat or bowel loops (Fig. 4.7).

Paraumbilical Hernia: Paraumbilical hernias are abdominal wall defects, through the linea alba adjacent to the umbilicus, and are due to diastasis of the rectus abdominis muscle [7] (Fig. 4.8). Paraumbilical hernias superior to umbilicus are called epigastric hernias and inferior to umbilicus are called hypogastric hernias. Epigastric hernias, like umbilical hernias, contain fat, vessels, and sometimes abdominal viscera. These hernias

are usually clinically occult and become apparent only after onset of complications like incarceration and strangulation.

Paramedian Hernia: Paramedian hernias are defects lateral to the midline and usually have omentum and small bowel as hernial contents. These are relatively less common; however, the risk of incarceration is high.

Spigelian Hernia: Spigelian hernia occurs through the defect in anterior abdominal wall adjacent to the linea semilunaris and is also known as spontaneous lateral ventral hernia. The hernial defect is located in Spigelian fascia between the lateral border of rectus abdominis muscle and linea semilunaris. Linea semilunaris is the curved tendinous intersection on either side of rectus abdominis muscle and extends from the cartilage of ninth rib to the pubic tubercle and is formed by aponeurosis of internal oblique muscle, reinforced laterally by external oblique muscle and posteriorly by transversus abdominis muscle.

Spigelian hernia is usually is seen at the site of deficient posterior sheath and it is interparietal with herniation occurring through the aponeurosis of transverse and internal oblique muscles. It is contained within the intact aponeurosis of external oblique muscle i.e. between the muscles of abdominal wall. Incidence is about 1.5% of all the abdominal wall hernias. The contents are usually omentum and small bowel loops [8] (Fig. 4.9).

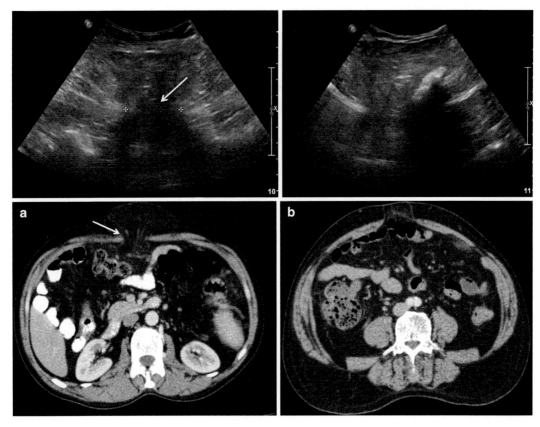

Fig. 4.6 USG reveals anterior abdominal wall defect marked as (+). There is herniation of omentum and bowel in the hernial sac (arrow). (**a**) Umbilical hernia; CT showing midline anterior abdominal wall defect with her-niation of omentum through it. (**b**) Small umbilical hernia showing separation of rectus abdominis muscle and her-niation of omental fat limited to subcutaneous fat

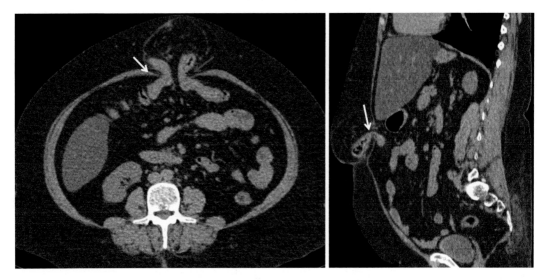

Fig. 4.7 Afferent and efferent loops in anterior abdomi-nal wall hernia. White arrow depicts afferent loop and red arrow depicts efferent loop. Herniated bowel is normal in caliber with normal attenuation of omentum suggesting nonobstructed hernia

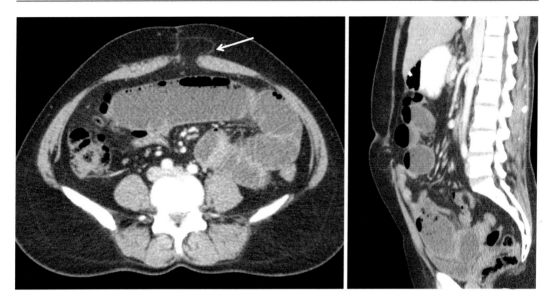

Fig. 4.8   Paraumbilical hernia containing omental fat and no vessels (arrow)

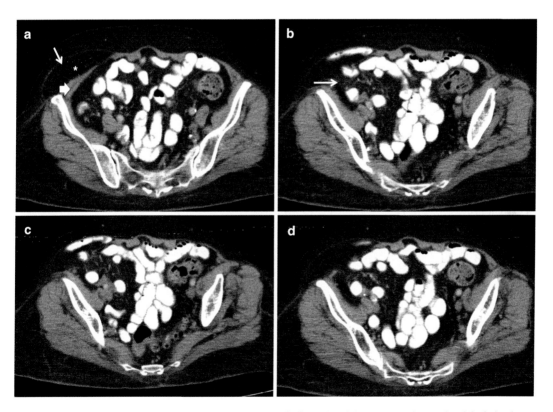

Fig. 4.9   Spigelian hernia. (**a**, **b**, **c** and **d**) Contiguous axial sections through lower abdomen showing herniation of bowel and omentum through the spigelian fascia with white arrow depicting intact external oblique muscle, (∗) depicting hernial contents and arrow head depicting internal oblique and transverse abdominis muscles. (**b**) Arrow in figure (**b**) depicts the hernial defect

4.6   Lumbar Hernias

Lumbar hernias are less common than groin or anterior abdominal wall hernias. These hernias occur posteriorly through the defects in lumbar muscle. Lumbar hernia generally occurs through the posterior fascia below the 12th rib, bounded by the erector spinae muscle medially and external oblique muscle laterally and iliac crest inferiorly.

Lumbar hernia can be of two types, occurring through superior or inferior lumbar triangle. The hernia through superior lumbar triangle is called Grynflett-Lesshaft and is bounded by internal oblique muscle anteriorly, 12th rib superiorly and spinal muscles posteriorly [9]. The inferior lumbar hernia called Petit is bounded by external oblique muscle anteriorly, iliac crest inferiorly, and lattisimus dorsi posteriorly [9] (Fig. 4.10).

Lumbar hernias are usually a sequel to surgery or previous trauma [9]. They occur more commonly in males with age ranging from 50 to 70 years. Contents of lumbar hernia vary from bowel loops, retroperitoneal fat, and kidneys with strangulation being a common complication [8] (Fig. 4.11).

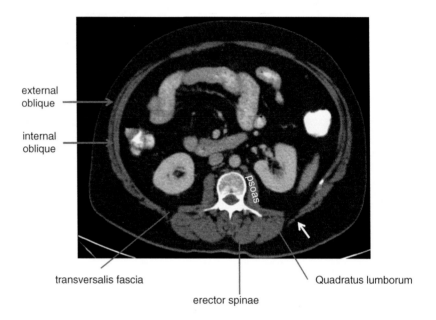

Fig. 4.10 Normal anatomy of the posterior abdominal wall muscle depicting site of lumbar hernia (arrow)

external oblique

internal oblique

psoas

transversalis fascia

erector spinae

Quadratus lumborum

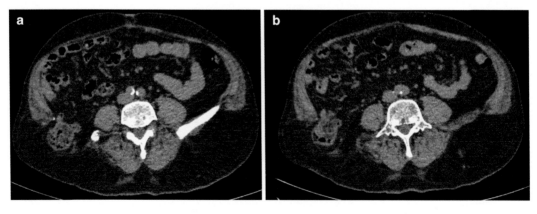

Fig. 4.11 Lumbar hernia: defect along the lumbar triangle (**a, b**) reveals herniation of large bowel through the wall defect. (**c, d**) Sagittal and coronal MPR images reveal the hernia through lumbar muscles

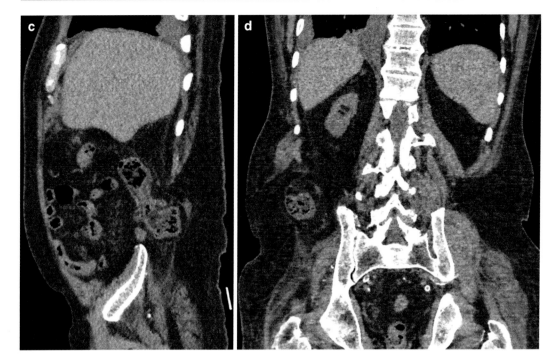

Fig. 4.11 (continued)

4.7 Incisional Hernias

Incisional hernias occur as complications of prior abdominal surgery due to breakdown of fascia. More commonly seen with vertical incisions compared to transverse incision with a high prevalence in obese patients, and chronic smokers [3, 10]. These hernias occur in first the few months following abdominal surgery and the incidence ranges from 0.5 to 13.9% [10]. Incidence of incisional hernias is reported to be as high as 41% following surgery for aortic abnormalities [10, 11]. 5–10% of incisional hernias remain dormant for up to 5 years [10].

Parastomal hernias are a subtype of incisional hernias. They occur adjacent to a stoma and are therefore difficult to detect clinically. CT shows bowel loops herniating through the opening of stomal site.

4.7.1 Other Rare Hernias of the Abdominal Wall

Interparietal: Interparietal hernias are also called interstitial hernias. The hernial sac is limited between the abdominal wall muscles without extension into the subcutaneous tissue.

Richter: Richter hernia refers to the herniation of antimesentric wall of bowel without involving the entire wall circumferentially. It can occur through any of the abdominal wall hernial orifices described above. It usually does not lead to bowel obstruction.

Litter: It is a type of inguinal hernia which contains Meckel's diverticulum.

Complications, as in other types of hernias, are incarceration and strangulation.

4.7.2 Other Hernias of the Pelvic Floor

Pelvic hernias occur mainly in elderly women and are acquired due to a weakness in muscles of the pelvic floor.

Obturator hernias pass through the obturator foramen between the pectineus and obturator muscles, and are more commonly seen on the right side [9].

Sciatic hernias pass through the greater and lesser sciatic foramina. Contents of the obturator and sciatic hernia are usually small bowel loops or rarely ureter or urinary bladder [9].

Perineal hernias are not common and seen mainly in elderly females occurring in gluteal region, adjacent to labia majora and anus [9, 12].

4.8   Traumatic Hernias

Blunt traumas resulting from high-velocity motor vehicle accidents lead to sudden increase in intraabdominal pressure resulting in disruption of abdominal wall musculature and herniation of abdominal contents. These defects can range from small to large depending upon the severity of the injury and due to the degree of compression on impact [13].

The common sites of posttraumatic hernias are through the areas of relative anatomic weakness, which are lumbar region and the lower abdomen [13]. Abdominal contents can herniate into the chest through a diaphragmatic rupture. These hernias are also associated with other intraabdominal injuries in about 60% of cases [13].

4.9   Complications of Abdominal Wall Hernias

Bowel obstruction, incarceration, and strangulation are the most common complications of abdominal wall hernias [14]. Common presenting symptoms of complications of hernia are abdominal pain and distention.

Clinical evaluation will usually be difficult if complications are present, because of pain and tenderness. However, it may reveal an abdominal mass, which is tender, firm, and irreducible.

Further complications will lead to peritoneal signs, which will present as dehydration, discoloration of skin, and derangements of systemic vital signs [15].

Imaging studies are necessary to differentiate hernia from other causes of abdominal mass and abdominal pain, when symptoms or clinical assessment is confusing [6]. Imaging studies also help to evaluate the complications of hernia and associated systemic manifestations, improving

patient outcome [16]. Accurate and timely diagnosis is mandatory for early diagnosis and appropriate management of complications.

4.9.1   Bowel Obstruction

Abdominal wall hernias are the second most common cause of small bowel obstruction with an incidence of about 10–15% [17].

Bowel obstruction occurs after the strangulation or incarceration of the hernia with the transition point at the hernial orifice or within the hernial sac.

The commonest content in abdominal wall hernia is the omentum and bowel loops. If it contains bowel then there is an afferent and an efferent loop. The proximal segment of bowel herniating through the defect is afferent loop and the distal segment of bowel entering back in abdominal cavity through the defect is the efferent loop (Fig. 4.7). The obstruction usually occurs at either the entry point of afferent loop or exit point of efferent loop, and sometimes within the herniated loop due to a twist.

CT findings will reveal dilatation of bowel loops proximal to the site of obstructed hernia and normal or collapsed bowel distal to the obstruction (Fig. 4.12). The bowel loops within the hernial sac may or may not be dilated. The dilatation will depend on whether the obstruction is occurring at the point of entry or at the point of exit. There will be narrowing of the afferent or efferent limbs at the hernial orifice.

The extent of dilatation of the proximal bowel loop indicates the degree of obstruction, and if it is acute or subacute, complete or incomplete. One finding of obstructions is "Fecal sign" which is identified by presence of particulate material mixed with gas within the lumen of obstructed dilated bowel loops.

4.9.2   Incarceration

Incarceration refers to the clinical diagnosis of an irreducible hernia, when the hernial contents cannot be reduced or pushed back into the peritoneal

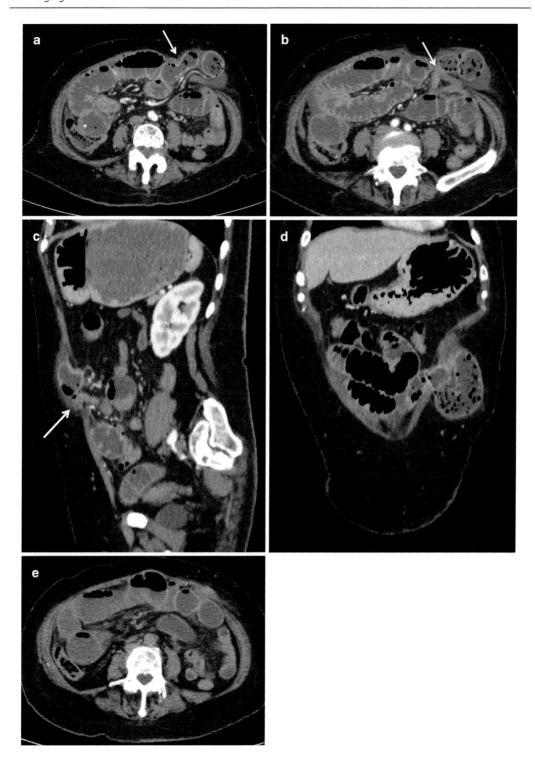

Fig. 4.12 Obstructed anterior abdominal wall hernia: (**a**) arrow showing afferent loop which is dilated (**b**) Arrow showing collapsed efferent loop. The site of obstruction is at the entry point of bowel. There is marked dilatation of bowel loop proximal to efferent loop in the abdomen and there is fluid in hernial sac due to mesenteric congestion. (**c**, **d**) MPR images in sagittal and coronal planes depicting the hernia. (**e**) Conservative management of hernia with manual reduction of hernia and no bowel loops are seen in the hernial sac

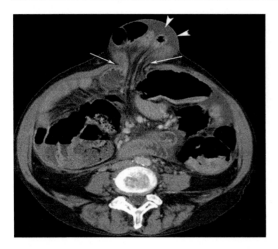

Fig. 4.13 Midline abdominal wall hernia with obstruction (arrows): there is herniation of bowel and fluid in the hernial sac (arrow heads), a sign of incarceration

cavity manually. Incarceration occurs when the herniation of the contents has occurred through a small defect due to a narrow neck of the hernial sac which predisposes the bowel to inflammation, obstruction, and ischemia. The role of imaging is to assess the complications secondary to incarceration (Fig. 4.13). Isotropic imaging with MPR images helps better visualization of hernial defect and its contents [9].

Hernias, which contain only omentum, can also show signs of incarceration evident as fat stranding and free fluid in the hernia sac.

Some hernias may show signs of impending strangulation. Suspicion arises with presence of free fluid in the hernial sac, dilatation of bowel loops, bowel wall thickening and persistent contrast enhancement of the bowel wall [6, 18]. These signs indicate the requirement for urgent surgical decompression to prevent bowel necrosis [6].

4.9.3 Strangulation

Strangulation is an uncommon complication of anterior abdominal wall hernias, and if it occurs, has a high surgical mortality ranging from 6 to 23% [19]. Strangulation is the compromised blood supply to the herniated bowel leading to ischemia. It occurs secondary to obstruction at both afferent and efferent loops resulting in a closed-loop obstruction of the herniated bowel.

MDCT will reveal closed-loop obstruction seen as dilated fluid-filled herniated bowel loops with narrowing at both the afferent and efferent sites [16]. This will result in dilatation of the proximal bowel loops. The signs of ischemia will be manifested as bowel wall thickening secondary to mural edema, altered attenuation of bowel wall ranging from hypo-attenuation in plain scans to hyper-enhancement in post-contrast scans. There may be intramural hemorrhage seen as hyper-attenuation in plain scans. Other findings are mesenteric fat stranding, engorgement of mesenteric vessel, and free fluid in the hernia sac. There is a "serrated beak" appearance of the afferent and efferent limbs at the transition point (Fig. 4.14).

Strangulated hernia is a clinical emergency and needs prompt surgical management.

4.9.4 Trauma

Trauma in a patient with preexisting abdominal wall hernia should be evaluated both clinically and radiologically for injury to hernial sac and contents. Radiologically, presence of free fluid in hernia sac, bowel wall thickening and abnormal enhancement of bowel wall, and mesenteric vessel engorgement with mesenteric fat stranding in and around hernia should raise the suspicion of trauma to the hernial contents. This also requires immediate surgical management.

4.9.5 Other Uncommon Complications

Less common complications include herniation of intraabdominal viscera, which can be either solid (e.g., liver, kidneys) or hollow (e.g., stomach, bladder).

Herniation of bladder in inguinal hernia is not a common phenomenon and carries a high risk of bladder injury (Fig. 4.15). Unusual cases of complicated urinary bladder herniation with strangulation are also encountered seen as thickening of bladder wall with differential enhancement representing impending ischemia (Fig. 4.16).

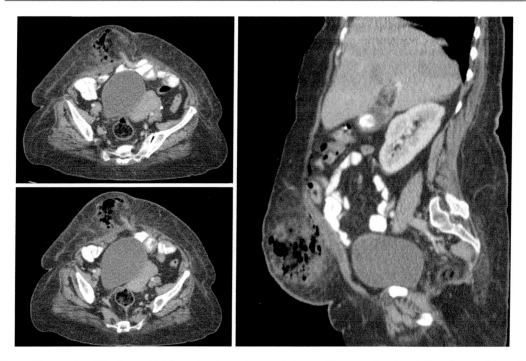

Fig. 4.14 Anterior abdominal wall defect with signs of strangulations and incarceration: herniation of omental fat and vessels, increased fat stranding with air pockets within the herniated contents, a definitive sign of ischemia

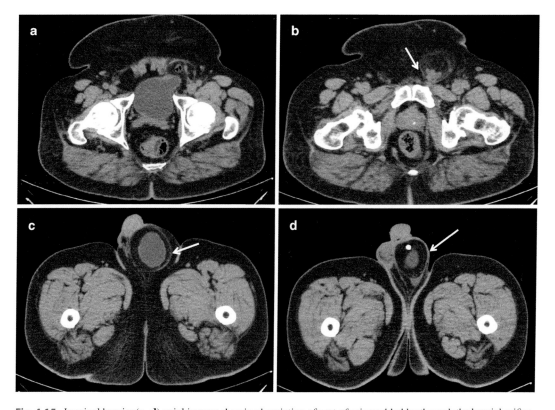

Fig. 4.15 Inguinal hernia: (**a–d**) axial images showing herniation of part of urinary bladder through the hernial orifice. (**e, f**) MPR: Inguinal hernia with herniation of part of urinary bladder through it

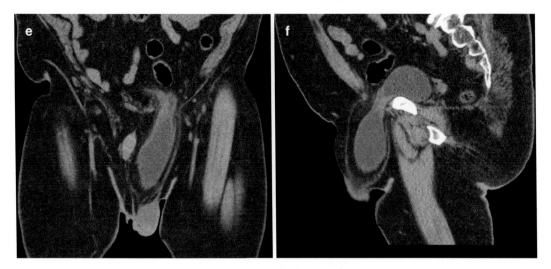

Fig. 4.15 (continued)

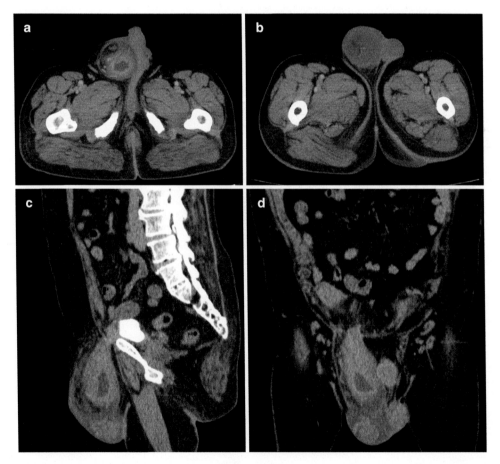

Fig. 4.16 (**a**, **b**) Axial images herniation of bladder through inguinal orifice: There is thickening of wall of herniated urinary bladder, with differential enhancement of the wall and free fluid in the hernial sac which are signs of strangulation. (**c**, **d**) Are MPR in coronal and sagittal planes showing the hernial defect and signs of obstruction with impending ischemia. This patient presented with pain and hematuria

In rare cases, intraabdominal tumors or chronic infectious diseases may herniate through the abdominal wall or may be a part of the hernial sac. The extension of intraabdominal inflammatory conditions like tuberculosis and inflammatory bowel disease into the hernia sac may exacerbate mild symptoms (Figs. 4.17 and 4.18).

4.9.6   Postoperative Hernial Mesh Appearance

A normal hernial mesh is also visualized following surgical repair and it is important to recognize these implants and be familiar with their radiological appearance (Fig. 4.19).

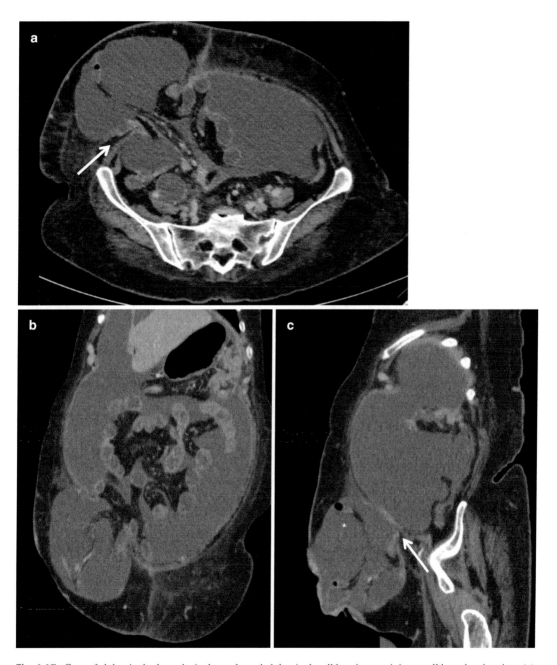

Fig. 4.17 Case of abdominal tuberculosis: lower lateral abdominal wall hernia containing small bowel and ascites. (**a**) Axial (**b, c**) sagittal and coronal MPR images

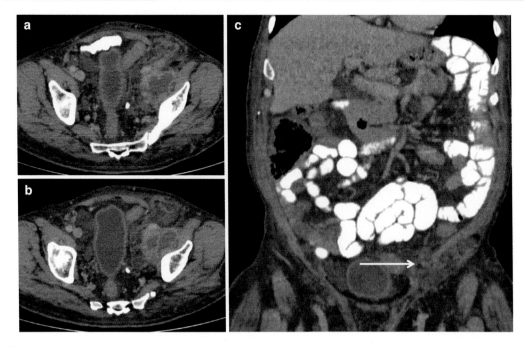

Fig. 4.18 In a case of omental metastasis there is herniation of metastatic deposits through the left lateral abdominal wall (arrow) seen in CT axial (**a**, **b**) and coronal (**c**) images

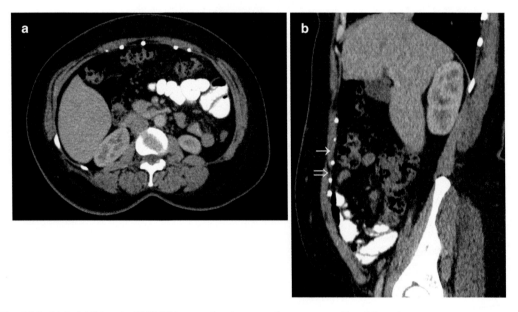

Fig. 4.19 (**a**) Axial (**b**) sagittal MDCT images showing normal appearance of hernial mesh

4.10   Postsurgical Complications

Complications following surgical hernia repair are not uncommon with an incidence of 50% depending upon the preoperative hernial sac contents and integrity of the vasculature and the operative technique adopted. Accurate detection of complications by MDCT helps in planning appropriate treatment [8, 20, 21].

4.10.1 Fluid Collections

Fluid collection is an immediate postoperative complication of hernial repair. It occurs in about 17% of cases depending upon the surgical technique and type of hernial mesh used [19]. Fluid collection may be serous fluid (seroma) or blood (haematoma) (Fig. 4.20).

Imaging studies reveal fluid collection at postoperative site superficial or deep to the anterior abdominal wall. This fluid collection may be loculated, multiloculated, or tubular, with or without enhancement of the wall. Fluid levels if present generally indicates presence of infection. MDCT helps to differentiate between localized fluid collection and recurrence.

Most seromas resolve spontaneously within 4 weeks. However, if the collection persists beyond 6 weeks, or if there is an increase in size of collection, or the patient becomes symptomatic secondary to superimposed infection, aspiration is indicated [19, 21]. USG/CT-guided aspiration/drainage is preferred, and an oblique approach should be adopted, and a small diameter catheter should be used to avoid resistance from folds of the mesh.

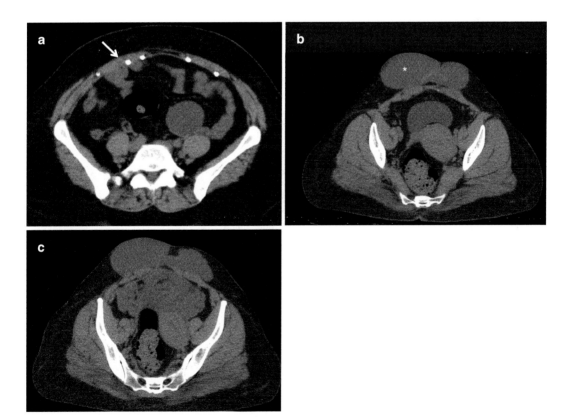

Fig. 4.20 Axial (**a**, **b** and **c**) images showing hernial mesh (arrow) and fluid collections in subcutaneous tissue depicted by * represents seroma formation, post hernial repair

4.10.2 Hernial Recurrence

Recurrence post hernia repair constitutes the most common complication and is related to weakening of muscles and aging of tissues. The prevalence of recurrence of hernia depends upon the type of repair. With open surgical repair without mesh placement there is up to 30% chance of recurrence. If mesh is used for hernial repair there is a 10% chance of recurrence and in up to 7.5% cases after laparoscopic repair [19, 21]. Recurrence usually occurs after 2–3 years and may happen even after 5 or more years in some cases [19, 20].

MDCT plays a crucial role in evaluation as clinical evaluation is limited by presence of mesh, accompanying fibrosis, obesity and abdominal distention. Imaging findings will clearly depict the site, size, recurrence and contents of hernia.

4.10.3 Infection

Infections in postoperative fluid collections occurs in about 1–5% of cases, if surgery is delayed and depending on the surgical technique [20]. Such complications occur more frequently in older female patients, and if the surgical repair is done on a strangulated or incarcerated hernia [19]. Infection manifests early in the postoperative period (within 2 weeks after surgery) and there is high chance of recurrence in such cases [22].

Infected fluid collections may be subcutaneous or deep to the mesh. The differentiation between the two is important because superficial infections are managed conservatively, whereas deep infections are managed with percutaneous drainage or even removal of the mesh.

Diagnosis is by clinical examination and presence of pain, fever, or leukocytosis. Imaging is used to confirm the presence, delineate the location and volume of infected collection.

Imaging findings indicating infection in fluid collection includes the presence of gas or thick septations in the collection. Post contrast peripheral enhancing rim or inflammatory fat stranding in surrounding tissues are other findings. Sometimes imaging findings alone are not specific to assess the nature of a fluid collection, and guided aspiration becomes necessary (Fig. 4.21).

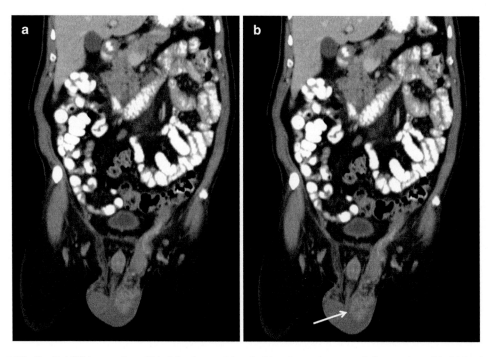

Fig. 4.21 Sagittal CT images (**a** and **b**): Infection post inguinal hernia repair seen as inflammation with thickening of spermatic cord (∗) and free fluid in hernial orifice and scrotum (arrow)

4.10.4 Mesh-Related Complications

Inflammatory changes after hernial repair may lead to fibrosis in tissues adjacent to the mesh and is seen as an irregular shape of the mesh at CT and in rare cases there is a chance of mesh shrinkage [19].

Intraperitoneal adhesions predispose to small bowel obstruction. Occasionally, the mesh may detach and migrate within the abdominal wall [22].

4.10.5 Other Complications

Postoperative complications in inguinal hernias include ischemia with testicular atrophy and thickening of the spermatic cord [22]. Transection or disruption of the vas deferens, hydrocele, osteitis pubis, and thrombosis of adjacent vessels are other uncommon complications [19, 23].

4.11   Differential Diagnosis

Several other abdominal wall diseases may pose a diagnostic dilemma at physical examination and some may be difficult to differentiate from hernia. MDCT helps in differentiating these conditions as CT findings are usually specific for hernia.

Benign abdominal wall tumors like lipomas, fibromas, hemangiomas, and less-frequently malignant tumors and metastases can be confused with hernias. Primary sarcomas may also present as abdominal wall distension or lump and mimic hernia on clinical examination.

Metastases to abdominal wall are either a direct invasion by intraabdominal lesions or occur secondary to vascular spread. Lung tumors and pancreatic tumors are the most common primary tumors that metastasize to the abdominal wall. CT reveals solid nodules in the abdominal wall and should arouse suspicion leading to a search for an occult primary [24].

Desmoid tumors (musculoaponeurotic fibromatoses) are locally invasive dysplastic soft tissue masses of mesoderm that involve skeletal muscle and fascial layers. These tumors occasionally arise in surgical scars or in the mesentery, and they occur in women during or following pregnancy. A familial form of desmoid tumor is associated with Gardner syndrome [25, 26]. These tumors are large solid enhancing soft tissue masses and can be easily differentiated from hernia on imaging.

Rectus sheath hematomas may occur as a result of trauma to the abdominal wall or following a sudden violent episode of coughing. These may be secondary to disorders of coagulation or blood dyscrasias. CT demonstrates high attenuating spindle or lens-shaped lesion/collection on noncontrast computed tomography (NCCT) within abdominal wall (Fig. 4.22). Hematomas are treated conserva-

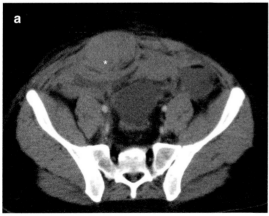 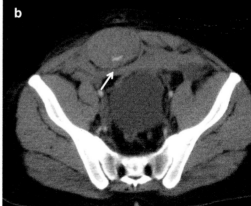

Fig. 4.22 Clinical mimickers of anterior abdominal wall hernia; Axial plain (**a**) and post contrast (**b**) images showing abdominal wall hematoma (∗) is difficult to differentiate from an obstructed hernia of the abdominal wall. CT depicts lenticular high attenuation collection representing blood (**a**). White arrow shows site of active bleed in a post contrast scans (**b**)

tively with gradual regression of size but a residual mass may persist for several weeks. Rectus sheath hematomas are not difficult to differentiate from hernias at MDCT. High attenuation of hemorrhage on unenhanced images with lack of enhancement, and gradual resolution on follow-up studies helps differentiating hematoma from hernia [27, 28].

4.12   Conclusion

Abdominal wall hernias are one of the most common indications for surgery. There may be occult hernias incidentally detected on imaging or clinically detectable hernias with or without complications. MDCT allows precise detection and delineation of abdominal wall anatomy and the site, size and contents of hernia and postoperative complications if any. Multiplanar reformations provides detailed images for better understanding by surgeons which helps them in surgical planning.

References

1. Digestive diseases in the United States: epidemiology and impact. NIH Publication No. 94-1447. Bethesda: NIDDK; 1994.
2. Stabile Ianora AA, Midiri M, Vinci R, Rotondo A, Angelelli G. Abdominal wall hernias: imaging with spiral CT. Eur Radiol. 2000;10:914–9.
3. Harrison LA, Keesling CA, Martin NL, Lee KR, Wetzel LH. Abdominal wall hernias: review of herniography and correlation with cross sectional imaging. Radiographics. 1995;15:315–32.
4. Shadbolt CL, Heinze SB, Dietrich RB. Imaging of groin masses: inguinal anatomy and pathologic conditions revisited. Radiographics. 2001;21 Spec No:S261–71.
5. Zarvan NP, Lee FT Jr, Yandow DR, Unger JS. Abdominal hernias: CT findings. AJR. 1995;164:1391–5.
6. Rettenbacher T, Hollerweger A, Macheiner P, et al. Abdominal wall hernias: cross sectional imaging signs of incarceration determined with sonography. AJR. 2001;177:1061–6.
7. Lee GH, Cohen AJ. CT imaging of abdominal hernias. AJR. 1993;161:1209–13.
8. Miller PA, Mezwa DG, Feczko PJ, Jafri ZH, Madrazo BL. Imaging of abdominal hernias. Radiographics. 1995;15:333–47.
9. Aguirre DA, Casola G, Sirlin C. Abdominal wall hernias: MDCT findings. AJR Am J Roentgenol. 2004;183:681–90.
10. Ghahremani GG, Jimenez MA, Rosenfeld M, Rochester D. CT diagnosis of occult incisional hernias. AJR Am J Roentgenol. 1987;148:139–42.
11. Raffetto JD, Cheung Y, Fisher JB, et al. Incision and abdominal wall hernias in patients with aneurysm or occlusive aortic disease. J Vasc Surg. 2003;37:1150–4.
12. Lassandro F, Iasiello F, Pizza NL, Valente T, et al. Abdominal hernias: radiological features. World J Gastrointest Endosc. 2011;3(6):110–7.
13. Killeen KL, Girard S, DeMeo JH, Shanmuganathan K, Mirvis SE. Using CT to diagnose traumatic lumbar hernia. AJR Am J Roentgenol. 2000;174:1413–141.
14. Aguirre DA, Santosa AC, Casola G, Sirlin CB. Abdominal wall hernias: imaging features, complications, and diagnostic pitfalls at multi-detector row CT. Radiographics. 2005;25:1501–20.
15. Neblett WW 3rd, Pietsch JB, Holcomb GW Jr. Acute abdominal conditions in children and adolescents. Surg Clin North Am. 1988;68:415–30.
16. Yu CY, Lin CC, Yu JC, Liu CH, Shyu RY, Chen CY. Strangulated transmesosigmoid hernia: CT diagnosis. Abdom Imaging. 2004;29:158–60.
17. Macari M, Megibow A. Imaging of suspected acute small bowel obstruction. Semin Roentgenol. 2001;36:108–17.
18. Astarcioglu H, Sokmen S, Atila K, Karademir S. Incarcerated inferior lumbar (Petit's) hernia. Hernia. 2003;7:158–60.
19. Bendavid R. Complications of groin hernia surgery. Surg Clin North Am. 1998;78:1089–103.
20. Abrahamson J. Etiology and pathophysiology of primary and recurrent groin hernia formation. Surg Clin North Am. 1998;78:953–72, vi.
21. Gossios K, Zikou A, Vazakas P, et al. Value of CT after laparoscopic repair of postsurgical ventral hernia. Abdom Imaging. 2003;28:99–102.
22. Parra JA, Revuelta S, Gallego T, Bueno J, Berrio JI, Farinas MC. Prosthetic mesh used for inguinal and ventral hernia repair: normal appearance and complications in ultrasound and CT. Br J Radiol. 2004;77:261–5.
23. Courtney CA, Lee AC, Wilson C, O'Dwyer PJ. Ventral hernia repair: a study of current practice. Hernia. 2003;7:44–6.
24. Stojadinovic A, Hoos A, Karpoff HM, et al. Soft tissue tumors of the abdominal wall: analysis of disease patterns and treatment. Arch Surg. 2001;136:70–9.
25. Kaplan DB, Levine EA. Desmoid tumor arising in a laparoscopic trocar site. Am Surg. 1998;64:388–90.
26. Overhaus M, Decker P, Fischer HP, Textor HJ, Hirner A. Desmoid tumors of the abdominal wall: a case report. World J Surg Oncol. 2003;1:11.
27. Fukuda T, Sakamoto I, Kohzaki S, et al. Spontaneous rectus sheath hematomas: clinical and radiological features. Abdom Imaging. 1996;21:58–61.
28. Moreno Gallego A, Aguayo JL, Flores B, et al. Ultrasonography and computed tomography reduce unnecessary surgery in abdominal rectus sheath haematoma. Br J Surg. 1997;84:1295–7.

Part II

Groin Hernia

Biomaterials for Inguinal Hernia Repair

5

Rolf Ulrich Hartung

5.1 Introduction

Biomaterial has been used for hernia repair since the beginning of hernia treatment. The idea to implant a material with high biocompatibility was already in the mind of surgeons since Billroth: "If we could artificially produce tissues of the density and toughness of the fascia and tendon, the secret of radical cure of hernia can be discovered". Injection of gold particles and transplantation of autografts such as the lata fascia and dura patches have been used to deal with the defect in the abdominal wall. Pre-fabricated prosthetics made from tantalum gauze and silver-coated wire meshes were abandoned due to high complication rates. Francis Usher implanted the first synthetic mesh made of polypropylene and published his first experimental series of hernia repairs with Marlex mesh in 1959 [1]. Since then the development of meshes has exploded and resulted in biophysical and clinical research in order to find the ideal mesh. Today more than 500 different meshes are on the market offering meshes of different material, size, composition, coating, density and weight, pore-size, structure, flexibility, tensile strength and durability, pre-formed anatomical shape, self-fixing surface and visibility in imaging techniques. The tremendous choices challenge surgeons and patients on which mesh to choose for the repair of an individual hernia. Detailed knowledge of available biomaterials became therefore a necessary requirement for every hernia surgeon.

5.2 Biomaterial and Biocompatibility of Meshes for Hernia Repair

A biomaterial is either a natural or a synthetic or a combined material that is suitable for introduction into living tissue especially as a part of a medical device that treats, augments, or replaces any tissue, organ, or function of the body; especially, material suitable for use in prostheses that will be in contact with living tissue [2]. Synthetic material might be any material including mesh, patch, sutures, staples, glue, plastic and metal. Transplanted material can be an autograft, allograft or xenograft. Modern medical devices and prostheses are often made of more than one material alone. Although biomaterials have been used for hernia repair since the beginning of surgery, the science of biomaterials is less than 60 years old. The commonly used biomaterial for inguinal hernia repair is a mesh. The material and characteristics of the prosthetic mesh used determine integration, durability, functionality, incorporation and comfort.

R. U. Hartung (✉)
Medical Director, Mediclinic City Hospital—Dubai
Healthcare City, Dubai, UAE

© Springer Nature India Private Limited 2020
P. Chowbey, D. Lomanto (eds.), *Techniques of Abdominal Wall Hernia Repair*,
https://doi.org/10.1007/978-81-322-3944-4_5

Biocompatibility is related to the behavior of biomaterials in various contexts. The term refers to the ability of a material to perform with an appropriate host response in a specific situation [3]. As modern medical devices and prostheses are often made of more than one material it might not always be sufficient to talk about the biocompatibility of one specific material alone. The biocompatibility of a long-term implantable medical device (non-absorbable mesh) refers to the ability of the device to perform its intended function, with the desired degree of incorporation in the host, without eliciting any undesirable local or systemic effects in that host. The biocompatibility of a scaffold or matrix for a tissue-engineering product (biologic mesh) refers to the ability to perform as a substrate that will support the appropriate cellular activity, including the facilitation of molecular and mechanical signaling systems, in order to optimize tissue regeneration, without eliciting any undesirable effects in those cells, or inducing any undesirable local or systemic responses in the eventual host.

5.3   Foreign Body Reaction

Any biomaterial will trigger a foreign body reaction starting at the very moment of its introduction into the host [4]. Proteins will adhere to the prosthetic material only seconds after its implantation, followed by the invasion of platelets releasing a variety of cytokines that will attract white blood cells, macrophages and fibroblasts [5, 6]. Within hours the implant will be covered by an inflammatory infiltrate and fibroblasts, leading to the formation of a fibrotic capsule around each and every filament or part of the prosthetic implant. New vessels will invade 7–14 days after the onset of the reaction thus forming a foreign body granuloma. Different biomaterials have more or less accentuated foreign body reactions. Thicker the granuloma grows over each filament more likely it will cause excessive scar formation and the risk of bridging from one filament to the next thus transforming the flexible mesh into a stiff scar and finally a solid plate. The functionality and biophysical outcome of the prosthetic implant depend in major parts on the degree of this foreign reaction. Excessive scar formation and shrinkage of the prosthetic implant are the main reasons for a poor outcome after surgery possibly causing recurrence, discomfort and pain.

5.4   The Material

Different biomaterials have been developed for the construction of meshes; synthetic non-absorbable material such as polypropylene being the most commonly used substance. Polyvinylidene fluoride (PVDF), polyester (PET), polyamide (nylon) and polytetrafluoroethylene (PTFE) are further synthetics used as either patches or knitted filaments for the production of non-absorbable meshes [7–9]. Polyglactin 910 and polyglycolic acid are commonly used for absorbable implants (Table 5.1). Composite meshes are fabricated out of different materials most commonly with a permanent and an absorbable component. Biologic implants have been developed for the production of scaffolds made from human, porcine or bovine origin with the aim to address the problem of chronic inflammation and foreign body reaction. The donor tissue is processed to acellular, porous matrix scaffolds of collagen and elastin. The porous structure allows cells to enter the mesh and to adhere. A process of degradation of the biologic mesh and regeneration of the collagen scaffold will lead to a replacement of the mesh by host tissue (Table 5.2). Surgeons hoped that there will be less risk of bacterial invasion of the implant leading to the final necessity of explantation of the biomaterial as the scaffold will disappear by time.

Once the mesh is knitted or woven it can be coated to avoid adhesions, minimize the risk of infection or reduce the foreign body reaction. Different materials will shrink more or less once implanted, polypropylene having the highest shrinkage rate [7]. The material is either hydrophobic (polypropylene) or hydrophilic (polyester), the latter being less durable as hydrolysis can cause degradation of the filaments. PTFE is com-

Table 5.1 Examples of synthetic meshes used for inguinal hernia repair including absorbable meshes

Brand name	Company	Material	Structure	Pore size	Weight	Absorbable
3DMax	Bard	Polypropylene	Monofilament/3D	Small	Heavy	No
3D Max Light	Bard	Polypropylene	Monofilament/3D	Large	Light	No
Dexon	Syneture	Polyglycolic acid	Multifilament	Medium	Medium	Yes, entirely 60–90 days
Dynamesh Endolap 3D	FEG	PVDF	Monofilament/3D	Large	Light	No
Goretex Dualmesh	Gore	ePTFE	Composite	Small	Heavy	No
Marlex (historic)	Bard	Polypropylene	Monofilament	Small	Heavy	No
Optilene	B. Braun	Polypropylene	Monofilament	Large	Light	No
Parietex Hydrophilic	Medtronic/Covidien	Polyester	Multifilament	Large	Light	No
Parietex Lightweight	Medtronic/Covidien	Polyester	Monofilament	Large	Light	No
ProGrip	Medtronic/Covidien	PET/PLA microgrips	Monofilament	Large	Light	Partially, PLA 18 months
Prolene	Ethicon J&J	Polypropylene	Monofilament	Medium	Heavy	No
Ultrapro Advanced	Ethicon J&J	Polypropylene/polyglecapron	Monofilament	Large	Light	Partially
Versatex	Medtronic/Covidien	Polyester	Monofilament	Large	Light	No
Vicryl	Ethicon J&J	Polyglactin 910	Monofilament	Small	Medium	Yes, entirely 60–90 days

Table 5.2 List of biologic meshes

Brand name	Company	Type	Origin	Cross-linked	Sterilized
Alloderm	LifeCell	Dermis	Human	No	No
Allomax	CR Bard	Dermis	Human	No	Yes
Collamend	CR Bard	Dermis	Porcine	Yes	Yes
Flex HD	MTF	Dermis	Human	No	No
Periguard	Synovis	Pericardium	Bovine	Yes	Yes
Permacol	Covidien	Dermis	Porcine	Yes	Yes
Strattice	LifeCell	Dermis	Porcine	No	Yes
Surgimend	TEI	Dermis	Bovine	No	Yes
Surgisis	Cook	Intestine	Porcine	No	Yes
Tutopatch	Tutogen	Pericardium	Bovine	No	Yes
Veritas	Synovis	Pericardium	Bovine	No	Yes
XenMatrix	CR Bard	Dermis	Porcine	No	Yes
BioA	WL Gore	Synthetic absorbable	Synthetic	N/A	Yes
TIGR	Novus Scientific	Synthetic absorbable	Synthetic	N/A	Yes

pletely inert and will be rather incapsulated than integrated. Not only the material itself matters when it comes to durability and risk of infection but also the characteristics of the mesh, how it is knitted or woven, whether mono- or polyfilaments are used. Accordingly some meshes can be cut into shape while others cannot be. Last but not least, the production of the raw material itself matters. Not every polypropylene mesh has the same characteristics in density, weight and porosity thus influencing the biocompatibility and performance in the individual host. The mechanical strength and density of meshes have been thoroughly investigated in experimental studies to determine weight and strength of reduced material, the ideal pore size and consequently the flexibility and shrinkage rate [10]. Light-weight meshes have a weight of around 30 g/m^2 while heavy meshes weigh up to 100 g/m^2. The effective difference for a 10 × 15 cm mesh is 1 g (heavy weight 1.5 g versus light weight 0.5 g). Large pores measure more than 1 mm (1–3 mm). Pores less than 75 μm in size will not allow macrophages to enter and hereby significantly decrease the resistance to infection (PTFE). Even the lightest meshes available on the market withstand twice the maximum intra-abdominal pressure peeks of 170 mmHg during coughing and jumping. Different coatings shall not only minimize the tendency of adhesions but also prevent infection and possibly make meshes visible by imaging such as ultrasound and MRI investigations. Experimental and clinical studies with iron nanoparticle coating have resulted in information about displacement and long-term shrinkage rates of different mesh types. 3D meshes aim to preform the anatomical shape of the inguinal region and might allow future onsite production of a precisely fitting 3D printed mesh for an individual patient.

5.5   The Choice of Mesh

Ideally a mesh should be chemically inert, non-toxic, non-allergenic and non-carcinogenic, sterilizable, easy to be fabricated and formed, and easy to be handled and implanted. There should be no or very little foreign body reaction and no risk of adhesions. It should resist infection and seroma formation, have a sufficient mechanical strength and durability, and enough flexibility to allow normal body movements. The mesh should be incorporated such as autologous tissue and guarantee a lifelong repair of the hernia without recurrence and pain.

However the success and long-term outcome of an inguinal hernia repair are not only dependent on the mesh itself but also on the condition of the individual patient, the size of the defect, the presence of infection or contamination. Large defects will need to be covered by larger and stronger meshes in order to avoid mesh migration and herniation into the defect. The discussion whether to implant a synthetic or a biologic mesh or no mesh at all in presence of contamination and infection is still ongoing. Human acellular dermal matrix (HADM) and animal skin and intestine from pigs (porcine) and cows (bovine) are commonly used biologic materials for hernia repair with own risks and side effects [11]. Cultural, religious and personal factors influence the decision on the choice of biologic meshes. All biologic implants are considered to be temporary scaffolds, absorbable implants aiming to improve patients own repair mechanisms by forming durable scars. However the knowledge about deficient collagen in acquired hernias limits the expectations of this ideal appearing concept. Furthermore the three-fold higher costs of biologic meshes are not in favour of the routine use of those implants.

When it comes to the decision about the choice of mesh for hernia repair, the surgeon will consider the ease of handling and fixation of the implant. Introduction and deployment have to be guaranteed without damaging the structure or surface of the mesh. Self-fixing meshes might apparently have less risk of displacement; however, the intracorporal handling requires more advanced skills and precision of the surgeon. Once the mesh is correctly placed, many surgeons prefer to fix the mesh at least in one or two areas of reference, in inguinal hernia repair typically at Cooper's ligament. All the available fixation devices are equally made of biomaterial, permanent or absorbable, whether sutures, tacks or glue are used. Every single component of the entire biomaterials used during inguinal hernia repair will influence the outcome and possible side effects of the procedure. As in all different open and laparoscopic surgical techniques of inguinal hernia repair the mesh will be placed in the pre- or extraperitoneal space, the mesh will not need to have an anti-adhesive coating. When it comes to the size of the mesh 10 × 15 cm meshes are recommended for laparoscopic inguinal hernia repair and larger meshes are available to ensure a sufficient preferably 5 cm overlap to all sides. Plugs placed inside the opening are not favoured anymore. For most cases of inguinal hernia repair a monofilament synthetic mesh (polypropylene, polyester, PVDF) with large pores and low density will be the right choice [12, 13].

5.6 Clinical Outcome

Since the development of meshes for inguinal hernia repair the direct suture repair techniques have decreased significantly. Only in pediatric hernias the suture repair is still the method of choice. Whether open Lichtenstein procedure is performed or laparoscopic techniques such as TEP and TAPP in all cases a mesh will be implanted. Long-term studies and analysis of hernia registries have shown that the tension free repair with mesh resulted in lower recurrence rates and less pain after surgery in comparison to direct suture repair techniques such as Shouldice and Bassini repair representing less than 10% of all inguinal hernia repairs today. All international guidelines have therefore recommended the use of mesh for inguinal hernia repair over the direct suture repair based on level 1A evidence that mesh repair results in less recurrences when compared to techniques without the use of mesh. With level 1B evidence material-reduced meshes with large pores are favoured for the open inguinal hernia repair due to less long-term discomfort and foreign body sensation [14].

5.7 Summary

Nowadays the commonly used biomaterial for inguinal hernia repair is a mesh. Ninety percent of all inguinal hernia repairs are performed by implantation of synthetic meshes. The advantage of a tension-free repair over the suture repair with tension has resulted in lower recurrence rates and less pain. All international guidelines recommend the use of synthetic non-absorbable or composite mesh with a non-absorbable component based on Level 1A evidence. The development of material-reduced lightweight meshes with large pores has contributed to better long-term results with less discomfort for the patient. The implantation of biological meshes has not resulted in better outcomes but contributed to higher costs only.

References

1. Skandalakis JE, Colborn GL, Skandalakis LJ, McClusky DA. Historic aspects of groin hernia repair. In: Fitzgibbons RJ, Greenburg AG, editors. Nyhus and Condon's hernia. 5th ed. Philadelphia: Lippincott, Williams & Wilkins; 2002. p. 39.
2. Williams DF, editor. Definitions in biomaterials, Proceedings of a Consensus Conference of the European Society for Biomaterials. Amsterdam: Elsevier; 2004.
3. Williams DF. On the mechanisms of biocompatibility. Biomaterials. 2008;29(20):2941–53.
4. Klosterhalfen B, Hermanns B, Rosch R. Biological response to mesh. Eur Surg. 2003;35:16–20.
5. Pereira-Lucena CG, Artigiani-Neto R, Lopes-Filho GJ, Frazao CV, Goldenberg A, Matos D, et al. Experimental study comparing meshes made of polypropylene, polypropylene + polyglactin and polypropylene + titanium: inflammatory cytokines, histological changes and morphometric analysis of collagen. Hernia. 2010;14:299–304.
6. Klosterhalfen B, Junge K, Klinge U. The lightweight and large porous mesh concept for hernia repair. Expert Rev Med Devices. 2005;2:103–17.
7. Klosterhalfen B, Klinge U, Schumpelick V. Polymers in hernia repair-common polyester vs. polypropylene surgical meshes. J Mat Sci. 2000;35:4769–76.
8. Deeken CR, Abdo MS, Frisella MM, Matthews BD. Physicomechanical evaluation of polypropylene, polyester, and polytetrafluoroethylene meshes for inguinal hernia repair. J Am Coll Surg. 2011;212:68–79.
9. Gonzalez R, Ramshaw BJ. Comparison of tissue integration between polyester and polypropylene prostheses in the preperitoneal space. Am Surg. 2003;69:471–6, discussion 476–7.
10. Agarwal BB, Agarwal KA, Mahajan KC. Prospective double-blind randomized controlled study comparing heavy- and lightweight polypropylene mesh in totally extraperitoneal repair of inguinal hernia: early results. Surg Endosc. 2009;23:242–7.
11. Harth KC, Rosen MJ. Major complications associated with xenograft biologic mesh implantation in abdominal wall reconstruction. Surg Innov. 2009;16(4):324–9.
12. Bilsel Y, Abci I. The search for ideal hernia repair; mesh, materials and types. Int J Surg. 2012;10(6):317–21.
13. Brown CN, Finch JG. Which mesh for hernia repair. Ann R Coll Surg Engl. 2010;92(4):272–8.
14. Simons MP, Aufenacker T, Bay-Nielsen M, Bouillot JL, Campanelli G, Conze J, De Lange D, Fortelny R, Heikkinen T, Kingsnorth A, Kukleta J, Morales-Conde S, Nordin P, Schumpelick V, Smedberg S, Smietanski M, Weber G, Miserez M. European Hernia Society guidelines on the treatment of inguinal hernia in adult patients. Hernia. 2009;13(4):343–403.

Anaesthesia for Laparoscopic Abdominal Wall Hernia Repair

6

Aparna Sinha and Lakshmi Jayaraman

6.1 Anaesthesia for Laparoscopic Abdominal Wall Hernia Repair

Abdominal wall hernia is a very common surgical problem. In the last two decades laparoscopic/endoscopic approach has become the preferred surgical option for management of the same. Laparoscopic techniques have become popular due to the major advantages they offer. These include minimal incision size, minimal postoperative discomfort, earlier discharge readiness, lesser postoperative pain, enhanced recovery and lesser incidence of postoperative wound infections. These factors further contribute to lesser hospital stay and minimal perioperative morbidity.

The advancements in the surgical techniques of endohernia repair have led to innovations and refinement in the anaesthetic management of the same. The repair endohernia is one of the most commonly performed surgeries today.

The endoscopic hernia repair includes management of myriad of conditions including, totally extra-peritoneal (TEP), transabdominal preperitoneal (TAPP) repair of inguinal hernia and intraperitoneal onlay mesh (IPOM) repair of ventral hernia. Laparoscopy allows identification of contralateral hernia and its safe repair by avoiding cord structures and regional nerves.

- Totally extra-peritoneal repair (TEP): In this technique there is the placement of mesh into the preperitoneal space.
- Trans-abdominal (TAPP): Placement of mesh over peritoneal defects in the abdominal wall.
- Laparoscopic intraperitoneal onlay mesh (IPOM).

The TEP is preferred in simple unilateral, bilateral or recurrent hernia, whereas TAPP allows the surgeon to approach large scrotal, incarcerated and complex recurrent hernias, with greater ease. This also allows a concomitant diagnostic laparoscopy. However, laparoscopy is not without its associated problems and complications. Moreover, based on the type of hernia the repair may involve placing the patient in extremes of position, which brings its own challenges. A thorough understanding of anesthetic implications of endoscopic hernia repair is mandatory for safe execution of anaesthesia.

Thorough preoperative evaluation, preparation, protocols to troubleshoot consequences of raised intra-abdominal pressure (IAP) and effective pain management are keys to safe anaesthesia practice.

A. Sinha (✉) · L. Jayaraman
Institute of Minimal Access, Metabolic and Bariatric
Surgery, Max Super Speciality Hospital,
New Delhi, India

© Springer Nature India Private Limited 2020
P. Chowbey, D. Lomanto (eds.), *Techniques of Abdominal Wall Hernia Repair*,
https://doi.org/10.1007/978-81-322-3944-4_6

6.1.1 Pathophysiological Changes During Endoscopic Hernia Repair

Though laparoscopy offers advantages to both patients and surgeons, it can impose significant alteration in respiratory and cardiovascular homeostasis and should never be regarded as another minor intervention. During laparoscopic procedures, the major barriers to normal homeostasis are patient positioning, introduction of several liters of gas (CO_2) into the extraperitoneal space (TEP) or abdominal cavity (as in TAPP and IPOM) to produce carboperitoneum and the raised intra-abdominal pressure (IAP) that ensues from it. All these produce several pathophysiological changes, some of which are unique to laparoscopy (Tables 6.1 and 6.2).

6.1.2 Positioning and Associated Pathophysiologic Problems

Initial introduction of the Verees needle may require the patient to be placed in the Trendelenburg position (15°–20°) for most her-

Table 6.1 Hemodynamic effects of carboperitoneum

- Hypertension, tachycardia: Increased myocardial oxygen demand
- Increased noradrenaline levels: Increased SVR (and decreased Q)
- Hypercarbia and acidosis
- Reduced urine output and increased plasma renin activity (PRA)
  - Increased intra-abdominal pressure (IAP)
  - Local compression of renal vessels
- Intra-abdominal distension: Decrease in pulmonary dynamic compliance
- Low compliance plus increased minute volume of ventilation: Raised peak airway pressures

Table 6.2 Respiratory effects in endo-hernia repair

- Carboperitoneum ventilatory and respiratory changes
- Thoracopulmonary compliance ↓ (30–50%)
- $PaCO_2$ 15–20% ↓ (CO_2 absorption from peritoneal cavity)
- $PEtCO_2$ plateaus in 30 min
- Increase $PEtCO_2$ > 25% in<30 min suggestive of subcutaneous emphysema

nia repairs to allow introduction of carbon dioxide.

This displaces the abdominal viscera and thus prevents visceral injury during trocar insertion. It increases venous return (VR), right atrial pressure (RAP), central blood volume and cardiac output [1, 2]. Respiratory mechanics are also affected, due to cephalad displacement of diaphragm [1–3].

This augments development of atelectasis especially in obese, elderly and debilitated patients. In ASA I and II patients no major changes are seen [4].

The same IPOM procedure's reverse Trendelenburg position (20°–30°) is adopted, this improves diaphragmatic functions and is more favourable for respiration; however, compromises on the central blood volume and cardiac output [5]. The pathophysiological changes may vary in extra-peritoneal repairs (Fig. 6.1).

The steepness of the tilt and duration of surgery ultimately decide the magnitude of these changes. Deleterious effects can occur in patients with cardiovascular dysfunction [4]. The reduced pressures due to Trendelenburg position reduce blood loss from the pelvic viscera, but increase the risk of gas embolism [4, 6].

Nerve injuries have been potential complications of head low position. Caution must be exercised to prevent them particularly the brachial plexus injuries. This can be prevented by placing the arms of the patient by the side and applying shoulder supports (Figs. 6.2 and 6.3).

6.1.3 Insufflation of Exogenous Gas

Choice of an optimal insufflating gas to create pneumoperitoneum remains a significant issue in laparoscopy. Various gasses have been used for creating pneumo-peritonium in laparoscopy including oxygen, air, nitrous oxide (N_2O), nitrogen (N_2), carbon di oxide (CO_2), Argon and Helium. Carbon dioxide (CO_2) has remained the insufflation gas of choice. It is relatively inert, readily absorbed, and does not support combustion and hence permits the use of electrocautery [7].

Fig. 6.1 Effects of position and carboperitoneum

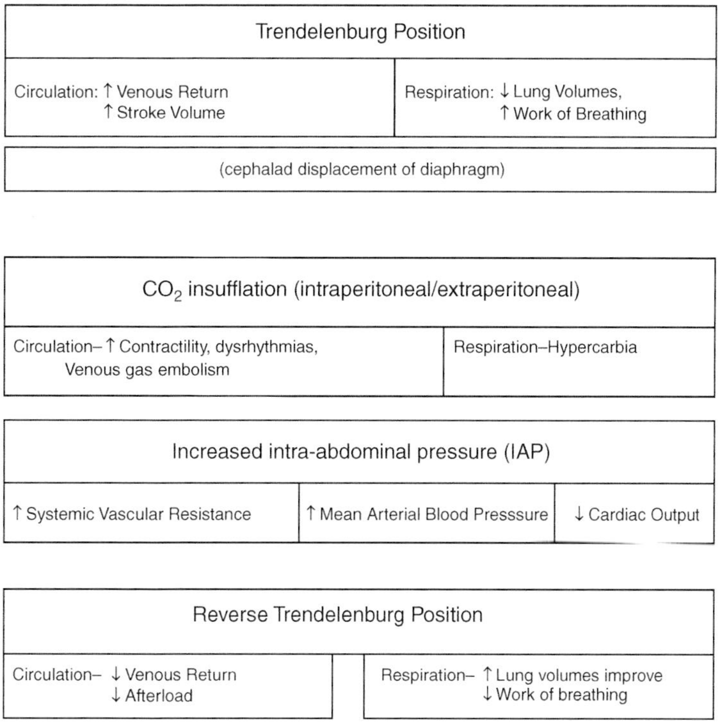

Trendelenburg Position	
Circulation: ↑ Venous Return ↑ Stroke Volume	Respiration: ↓ Lung Volumes, ↑ Work of Breathing

(cephalad displacement of diaphragm)

CO_2 insufflation (intraperitoneal/extraperitoneal)	
Circulation– ↑ Contractility, dysrhythmias, Venous gas embolism	Respiration–Hypercarbia

Increased intra-abdominal pressure (IAP)		
↑ Systemic Vascular Resistance	↑ Mean Arterial Blood Presssure	↓ Cardiac Output

Reverse Trendelenburg Position	
Circulation– ↓ Venous Return ↓ Afterload	Respiration– ↑ Lung volumes improve ↓ Work of breathing

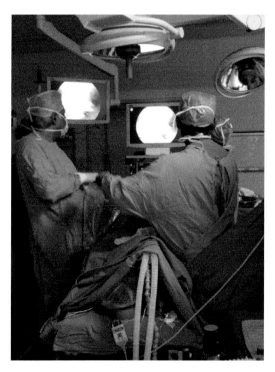

Fig. 6.2 Shows position of OT table, monitors and surgeons during TEP

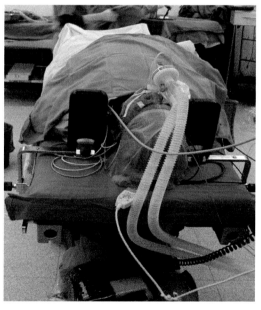

Fig. 6.3 Patient in Trendelenburg position, both arms by the side and shoulder supports in place to prevent sliding of patient during extremes of position

It is very highly soluble in blood (solubility coefficient = 0.49) at 37 °C and has a linear and steep dissociation curve. If $PaCO_2$ ranges between 45 and 50 mmHg, the absorption of CO_2 during carboperitoneum has minimal impact on hemodynamics. Whereas, if the $PaCO_2$ ranges between 51 and 60 mmHg, it causes sympathetic response and alters the cardiovascular response. The elevation in catecholamines and the pathophysiological changes of laparoscopy have been largely attributed to the increase in IAP rather than rise in CO_2.

In healthy patients (ASA I and II), the rise in pCO_2 and the resulting acidemia is clinically insignificant because of the buffering systems and rapid elimination by lungs. The rise in CO_2 elimination is not due to hyper metabolism, as suggested by increase in CO_2 elimination but unchanged O_2 consumption. The initial rise in intracranial pressure is due to mechanical effects of raised IAP, whereas the delayed rise seen in prolonged surgeries is due to vasodilatation induced by hypercapnia. Caution needs to be exercised in patients of chronic obstructive pulmonary disease, who have elevated baseline $PaCO_2$. These patients may show signs and symptoms of raised CSF pressure in the form of headache, blurring of vision and papilledema.

Central pipeline or cylinders may be used to supply carbon dioxide.

N_2O is not a part of acid-base buffer system and has only weak hemodynamic effects. This is not a preferred agent due to its property to support combustion. Nitrous oxide (N_2O) is better as an insufflating gas when the procedure is to be conducted under regional anaesthesia, since it produces minimal irritation of the peritoneal cavity [8]. However; caution needs to be exercised with use of cautery.

Helium insufflation is a reasonable alternative in patients at risk for CO_2 retention or has significant cardiopulmonary compromise [9]. Its low water and plasma solubility makes it unsuitable in the event of gas embolism.

Argon is yet another alternative, which is odorless, colorless gas, with no effect on acid-base status. It has poor solubility in blood makes it dangerous in case embolism happens.

Table 6.3 Properties of an ideal insufflating gas

- Readily available
- Nontoxic and colorless
- Relatively inert
- Non-combustible
- Inexpensive
- High Ostwald blood/gas partition coefficient (0.48) (readily soluble and easily ventilated through lungs)

Carbon dioxide possesses most of the desirable characteristics hence the term carboperitoneum is used synonymously with pneumoperitoneum [8–10] (Table 6.3).

6.1.3.1 Carboperitoneum and Increased Intra-abdominal Pressure

With the rise in IAP, the perfusion of viscera particularly that of the renal and hepatic perfusion is significantly compromised and is a major concern in patients with existing disease. Duration of carboperitoneum can have significant implications on the outcomes.

The renal effects of carboperitoneum are recognized as independent cause of acute kidney injury. The mechanism for this is secondary to the combined effect of reduced renal afferent flow due to impaired cardiac output and reduced efferent flow in view of raised renal venous pressure.

Increase in the intra-abdominal pressure contributes to circulatory instability during laparoscopy [11]. Since TEP is performed without establishing carboperitoneum, the adverse effects of a raised IAP are not seen, unlike in TAPP and IPOM, which necessitate the establishment of carboperitoneum [12].

Since the resorptive surface area is much larger in extra-peritoneal repairs, the rise in $EtCO_2$ is much greater [10, 13, 14]. The absorption of CO_2 steadily increases in TEP repair, while it tends to reach a plateau in TAPP [15]. Disruption of the microvascular and lymphatic channels in TEP, facilitates direct intravascular uptake of CO_2 [16].

The absorption of gases from the peritoneum is less at the commonly used pressure of 14–18 mmHg (for TAPP, IPOM repair) and increases as the pressure is lowered to 12–15 mmHg (used for TEP repair), due to a reduced capillary blood flow [17].

Long-standing IAPs over 20 mmHg impede the perfusion of abdominal viscera by up to 40% resulting in progressive tissue acidosis, which is directly related to rising pressures. This further lowers the threshold for arrhythmias. However, hemodynamic alterations occur only when the $PaCO_2$ is increased by 30% above the normal limit [10].

In view of the adverse effects described above, it is advisable to maintain intra-abdominal pressure around 12 mmHg, as much as a good exposure would allow. Each laparoscopic procedure needs to be individualised. Any single value of IAP for all cases cannot be ascertained.

6.1.3.2 Gasless Laparoscopy

In patients with cardio-respiratory compromise several surgeons may be suggested and tempted to perform the procedure in gas-less mode. Wherein, the procedure is performed at an IAP of 6–8 mmHg. However, this is associated with poor surgical exposure and greater technical difficulty, and no greater benefit in postoperative discomfort or return to normal activity. Due to the poor field exposure and longer duration, its feasibility may be of questionable value for high risk patients. Though there are conflicting reports on its benefits in laparoscopic cholecystectomy, for execution of mesh placement following hernia repair it may be really challenging [18, 19].

6.1.3.3 Preanaesthetic Assessment

A thorough preanaesthetic assessment with optimisation of the cardiac and pulmonary status is essential. Absolute anaesthetic contraindications to laparoscopy are rare. However, caution needs to be exercised in patients with raised intracranial pressure and hypovolemia. Laparoscopy is safe in patients with ventricular peritoneal shunt and peritoneojugular shunt as they are protected by unidirectional valves. In patients with glaucoma, the effects on intraocular pressure are not significant [20].

Patients with co-existing ventricular dysfunction, with severe congestive heart failure and ter-minal valvular insufficiency are more prone to develop cardiac complications induced by carbo-peritoneum and change of patient position than patients with coronary heart disease.

6.1.3.4 Premedication

Pre-emptive analgesia may be achieved with non-steroidal anti-inflammatory drugs (NSAIDs). Routine administration of anxiolytics and antiemetic like proton pump inhibitors and H2-receptor antagonists are beneficial in reducing postoperative nausea and vomiting (PONV), as well as the volume and pH of gastric secretions [21].

6.1.3.5 Anaesthetic Techniques

Anaesthetic techniques that have been successfully used for laparoscopic surgeries include general, local and regional anaesthesia.

6.1.3.6 General Anaesthesia

Conventionally general anaesthesia with controlled ventilation and endotracheal intubation has been the gold standard for laparosco-endoscopic repair of hernia (esp TEP). This allows good muscle relaxation and ability to control hypercarbia, protection from aspiration of gastric contents. The third-generation supraglottic devices, particularly ProSeal™ have gained popularity [22–25].

Ventilation should be adjusted to maintain $PECO_2$ between 35 and 40 mmHg. This can be achieved by 15–25% increase of minute ventilation. In case of subcutaneous emphysema develop it may become difficult to maintain the levels.

Cardiac patients may need infusion of vasodilating drugs/vasopressors to minimise the hemodynamic response [25–28].

In our experience, a mixture of oxygen, air with total intravenous anaesthesia or inhalational agents in the form of sevoflurane or desflurane is used for the maintenance of anaesthesia. Inclusion of air in place of nitrous oxide improves surgical conditions of intestines and the space available for hernia repair [29]. These agents are cardio stable and ensure rapid recovery with minimal PONV [23]. Intra-operative administration of intravenous dexamethasone, ondansetron, metoclopramide, droperidol before completion of surgery prevents PONV [30]. Laparoscopy has the potential for reflex increases of vagal tone, hence atropine should be readily available. All patients should be monitored for postoperative hypoxemia and hypercapnia, they should receive supplemental oxygen till they are fully awake [31–38].

6.1.3.7 Role of Regional Anaesthesia

Some anaesthesia providers may prefer to use regional techniques in certain patient conditions [39–41]. Epidural anaesthesia, combined epidural and spinal anaesthesia and nerve blocks provide excellent postoperative analgesia, lower incidence of PONV and no sequalae of general anaesthesia such as sore throat, muscle pain and airway trauma.

However, practice of regional anaesthesia as a sole technique should be reserved for ASA I and II patients only. Laparoscopic procedures under regional anaesthesia can potentiate the development of vagal stimulation due to sympathetic block.

Any requirement for sedation is achieved with midazolam, fentanyl or propofol infusion (4–6 mL/kg/h). This may further decrease the sensitivity of CO_2 to hypoxia; these patients may be unable to deal effectively with hypercarbia. The carboperitoneum and sedation can together lead to arterial oxygen desaturation [42].

Patient may experience discomfort during manipulation of the contents of the hernial sac, hence a very gentle surgical technique is advisable. Since TEP is an entirely extra peritoneal procedure, it can be successfully accomplished under regional anaesthesia.

However, local anaesthesia alone may not allow for technically optimal herniorrhaphy in anxious patients. A relaxed, cooperative patient is essential for the procedure to be conducted successfully under local anaesthesia [43, 44].

6.1.3.8 Local Anaesthesia

Repair of a small, direct inguinal hernia (TEP) can be performed under local (inguinal) block. Ilioinguinal and iliohypogastric block can be used for inguinal herniorrhaphy with supplementation with a genitofemoral block. Surgeon needs to be very gentle to improve patient compliance [45–48]. However, local anaesthesia alone may

not allow for technically optimal herniorrhaphy in anxious patients [49].

Disadvantages of Regional Anaesthesia for Laparoscopy
- Enhanced vagal reflexes
- Increased requirement for sedation
- Inability to compensate for hypercarbia
- Risk of patient disorientation and cooperation
- Increased chances of desaturation

Keys to Successful Management for High-Risk Patients
- Slow insufflation
- Low intra-abdominal pressure
- Hemodynamic optimisation before carboperitoneum
- Adjustment of ventilatory settings to maintain normocarbia
- Patient tilt after insufflation
- Normocarbia prior to extubation
- Experienced surgeon

Requirements for the Success of Laparoscopy Under Regional Anaesthesia
- Contraindication to general anaesthesia
- Patient cooperation
- Skilled laparoscopic
- Low intra-abdominal pressure
- Low degree of tilt of the operating table

6.2 Pain Management in Abdominal Wall Hernias

Pain management remains the hallmark of perioperative anaesthetic care and single most important determinant of patient safety. Laparoscopic surgery can be associated with moderate to severe pain, and effective analgesia is essential to enhance postoperative recovery.

Pain after laparoscopy is multifactorial and is mostly parietal. Multimodal approach seems to give maximum benefits. Goal of perioperative analgesia should be to provide pain relief with short-acting opioids so as to have enhanced recovery with minimal or none residual effects. This can be achieved by appropriate inclusion of paracetamol, NSAIDS, local anaesthetics in the form of port site infiltration, neuraxial blocks, loco-regional blocks, intraperitoneal instillation; with minimal opioids and careful evacuation of residual CO_2.

Several miscellaneous agents like, ketorolac, magnesium, lignocaine, alpha-2 agonists and hydrocortisone have been used in various combinations to bring down the requirement of opioids. These modalities together reduce the requirements for opioids, expedite recovery and are especially useful under day care settings. In our experience pre-emptive port site infiltration makes a remarkable difference in intra- and postoperative opioid requirement and in allowing early ambulation. Several practitioners are routinely performing transversus abdominis plane (TAP) block for postoperative pain relief, following laparoscopic hernia surgeries [46, 49].

The transversus abdominis plane (TAP) block and its variants are locoregional techniques that have emerged as a very promising option for pain management in laparoscopic abdominal hernia surgeries.

It provides analgesia to the parietal peritoneum as well as the skin and muscles of the anterior abdominal wall hence the abdominal field blocks such as TAP block, rectus sheath block and its variants can be used in various combinations, based on site of ports.

6.2.1 Localizing the Transversus Abdominis Plane

It is vital for the anaesthesiologists to identify the correct plane and to have the local anaesthetic deposited there. Failing which optimum results may not be achieved. The same can be achieved by one of the following ways:

- Blind technique (double pop technique or the loss of resistance technique)
- US-guided localisation
- Peripheral nerve stimulator guided (involves the double pop technique with PNS)

The technique as described by Rafi, involves identification of Petit's triangle. This is a triangle formed by medial margin of lattisimus dorsi, iliac crest and lateral border of eternal oblique muscles. This lumbar triangle of Petit is easily identifiable, fixed and palpable landmark and is located dorsal to the mid-axillary line. The transversus abdominis neuro-fascial plane can be easily accessed via this triangle, and local anaesthetic deposited into this plane, using the loss of resistance technique.

It is a myocutaneous sensory block and covers the skin, subcutaneous tissue, muscles and parietal peritoneum involving T6 to L1.

One can use a blunted tip needle as a Touhy needle or a pencil tip needle like the Sonoplex and after skin puncture gently advance it towards the midline. During USG blocks one must keep the needle tip in the view. Normal saline can initially be used for hydrodissection to identify the correct plane. Safe dose of the agent must be kept in mind while maintaining adequate volume. Though there are no guidelines so far to suggest correct volume. In our practice at 20 mL of the anaesthetic must be instilled on either side to produce the desired effect. Some studies have suggested that the effects of TAP block above T10 are less reliable. Higher incisions may require incorporation of a variant such as rectus sheath block or sub-costal block (Figs. 6.4, 6.5, and 6.6).

6.2.2 Sub-costal TAP

Recently, another variant of the conventional technique, better known as the sub-costal block has been described. The aim of subcostal block is to provide analgesia for incisions above the umbilicus. Better accomplished under US guidance, here the local anaesthetic is deposited around the same nerves but aiming for a more cephalad injection.

When the point of injection of the local anaesthetic into the TAP is midway between the costal margin and the iliac crest it is called posterior TAP block and has been found to be more suitable for surgeries below the level of the umbilicus. However, when the surgical incision is above the level of T10, it has been found that a variant of TAP, known as sub-costal TAP is more suitable. Here the TAP plane immediately lateral to the linea-semilunaris and parallel to the costal margin is used.

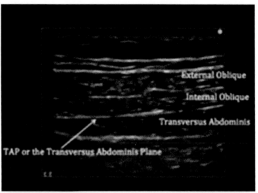

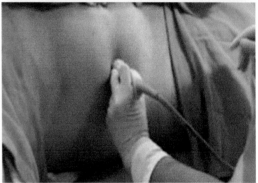

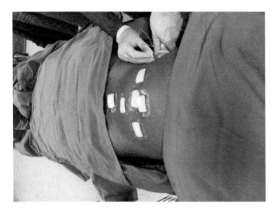

Fig. 6.4 Ultrasound-guided transversus abdominis plane block. The choice of abdominal field blocks is determined by the position of ports. Supra-umbilical ports usually need a combination of rectus sheath block and subcostal block. Surgeries involving infra-umbilical ports benefit the most with posterior TAP block

Fig. 6.5 Depicting the appearance of the sono-anatomy of muscle layers and the probe location for posterior TAP block

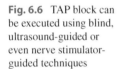

Fig. 6.6 TAP block can be executed using blind, ultrasound-guided or even nerve stimulator-guided techniques

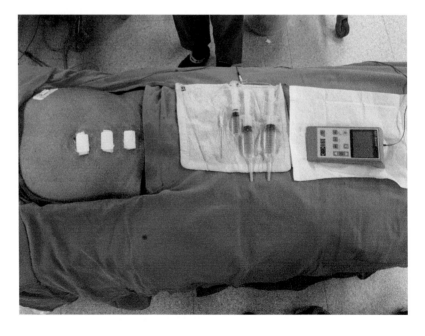

Further to this, if the injecting needle is directed medial to the linea-semilunaris and is directed towards the iliac crest (along a line referred to as oblique sub costal line). This block has been referred to as oblique sub costal block. This aims to cover both above and below T10 level incisions.

6.3 Ultrasound-Guided Techniques

These should be considered wherever available, for guiding the needle (Figs. 6.4 and 6.5). It allows the option of choosing the point of injection depending on the site of incision. The choice is between posterior, subcostal and oblique subcostal.

For achieving sensory block below the umbilicus it is preferable to choose the posterior block and position the probe laterally above the iliac crest. However, for achieving analgesia in and around the umbilicus, subcostal block is preferable. Here the probe is positioned in the subcostal margin lateral to the rectus muscle.

6.3.1 Subcutaneous Emphysema and USG Blocks

Presence of subcutaneous emphysema may interfere with the visualisation of muscle layers and blind technique might be preferred in such conditions.

6.4 Surgeon-Assisted Approach to TAP Block

Several practitioners have demonstrated that surgeons can help to facilitate these blocks. Herein, the laparoscopic camera can be used to visualise the peritoneal bulge while the TAP injection is being given based on anatomical landmarks.

6.5 Monitoring

Major hernia repairs particularly the revisional surgeries may last several hours and have significant pathophysiological disturbances.

It is mandatory to monitor all the patients intra- and postoperatively. The standard monitoring includes pulse oximetry, electrocardiography, non-invasive blood pressure, $EtCO_2$, the insufflation pressure and airway pressure. Most healthy patients need only capnography and pulse oximetry to monitor $PaCO_2$ and arterial oxygen saturation in the absence of acute intraoperative disturbances. Capnography and pulse oximetry, can assess only the effects on respiratory system, which are further complimented by information on airway pressures, lung volumes, and observing dynamic flow-volume loops in modern anaesthesia workstations [48, 49].

The mean gradient (Δa-ETCO$_2$) between $PaCO_2$ and the end-tidal carbon dioxide tension (PETCO$_2$) does not change significantly during peritoneal insufflation of CO_2 in ASA I patients. Whereas [49] the $PaCO_2$ and Δa-ETCO$_2$ increase more in ASA class II and III patients. These findings hold good even in patients with chronic obstructive pulmonary disease (COPD) and in children with cyanotic congenital heart disease [50]. As a result, hypercapnia can develop, even in the absence of abnormal PECO$_2$. Postoperative intra-abdominal CO_2 retention results can result in postoperative respiratory distress in patients breathing spontaneously.

Patients with cardiovascular co-morbidities may benefit with the use of invasive monitoring during prolonged surgery.

Due to the effects of IAP on the intrathoracic and cardiac filling pressures assessment of preload may be challenging, and pressure-based indices of preload such as central venous pressure may be misleading in presence of carboperitoneum.

However, devices such as the oesophageal Doppler monitor and lithium dilution (which utilise dilution cardiac output method) provide more accurate assessments of preload in these situations. In revisional hernia surgeries and complex cases that may last several hours and may involve frequent change of positions, it may be desirable to utilise invasive monitoring methods (Table 6.4).

6.5.1 Complications

Besides the complications commonly observed in any laparoscopic procedure the following are more commonly observed after endohernia repair.

Table 6.4 Interpreting the monitors

Capnography	Rising $EtCO_2$			Dropping $EtCO_2$	
	No	Yes	Yes	Yes	Yes
Pulse oximetry	Drop in SpO_2	No change	Drop in SpO_2	Drop in SpO_2	Drop in SpO_2
Airway pressure	Rise	No change	Rise	Rise	No change
Clinical examination					
Air entry	Reduced	Normal	Reduced	Reduced	Murmur
Hyper resonance	No	No	Yes	Yes	Hypotension
Swelling and crepitus	No	Yes	May be	May be	ECG changes
Presumptive diagnosis	Endobronchial intubation	Subcutaneous emphysema	Capnothorax	Pneumothorax	CO_2 embolism

6.6 Subcutaneous Emphysema

One of the commonest respiratory complications of extra peritoneal CO_2 insufflation and may also occur due to extra peritoneal leakage of carbon dioxide. Any rise in $PECO_2$ levels after it has plateaued is suggestive of this complication. There is a sudden rise in $PECO_2$ without hemodynamic instability or a change in the peak inspiratory pressure or oxygen saturation [51].

If it becomes difficult to control hypercapnia by adjustment of ventilation, the procedure should be temporarily discontinued till the hypercapnia settles to acceptable levels and then surgery can be resumed at lower IAP.

The extent of emphysema is seen to be directly related to the rise in CO_2, this readily resolves at end of the procedure when the further insufflation ceases. Even the cervical extent of the emphysema does not contraindicate tracheal extubation. However, caution needs to be exercised while planning extubation in COPD patients. Management is essentially conservative [52].

These patients may need extended monitoring in the PACU.

6.7 Pneumothorax

This is a rare but serious complication; may lead to respiratory and hemodynamic disturbances. Movement of CO_2 during creation of pneumoperitoneum may lead to development of capnothorax, capnomediastinum and even capnocardium. This can occur across embryonic remnants, which can become potential channels of communication, and open up particularly at high intraperitoneal pressures [53, 54]. It has also been reported after even 35 min of surgery when the insufflation pressure is kept at 12 mmHg [54]. Any weak areas in the aortic or esophageal hiatus may allow passage of gasses. Opening of peritoneopleural ducts is associated with mainly right-sided pneumothoraces.

Capnothorax (CO_2 causing a pneumothorax) reduces thoracopulmonary compliance and increases airway pressures. There is increase in both $PaCO_2$, and $PECO_2$ due to an increase in the absorption surface of CO_2, (more from the pleural cavity than from the peritoneal cavity). However, in pneumothorax secondary to alveolar rupture, the $PECO_2$ decreases because of fall in the cardiac output. Diagnosis of tension pneumothorax is guided by hemodynamic changes and oxygen desaturation. The surgeon may observe abnormal motion of one hemidiaphragm when a tension pneumothorax has occurred. Cervical and upper thoracic subcutaneous emphysema can develop in the absence of pneumothorax.

Capnothorax is treated with positive end expiratory pressure, and conservatively in the postoperative period, with continuous monitoring of oxygen saturation (SpO_2). It resolves without the placement of a chest tube. Contrastingly, thoracocentesis is mandatory if the pneumothorax is secondary to rupture of preexisting bullae, PEEP is contraindicated [53].

6.8 Endobronchial Intubation

The cephalad displacement of diaphragm can displace the carina leading to endobronchial intubation especially in procedures like TEP repairs, which are conducted in Trendelenburg position. This may result in decrease in the oxygen saturation associated with an increase in plateau airway pressure. We rarely encounter this in our center due to the widespread use of supraglottic devices in laparoscopic endohernia repairs (Table 6.5).

6.9 Air Embolism

This rare but most dreaded complication of laparoscopy can occur following direct needle or trocar placement into a vessel or insufflation into an abdominal organ [55, 56]. Most commonly occurs during induction of carboperitoneum. Carbon dioxide remains the most common choice due to its higher solubility than air, oxygen or N_2O, hence faster elimination in the event of any intra vascular injection (the lethal dose of CO_2 is five times higher than other air).

Slow insufflation, lower pressures and adequate preloading can minimise the effects of gas embolism. Routine use of invasive or expensive monitors to detect embolisation of small quantities of gas is not recommended due its very low incidence. Signs of embolism and electrocardiographic changes of right-sided heart strain usually appear when embolus is about 2 mL/kg of air. Capnometry and capnography are more valuable than pulse oximetry in providing early diagnosis of gas embolism.

The management includes immediate cessation of insufflation, release of pneumoperitoneum, steep head down and left lateral decubitus position to displace the embolised gas laterally and caudally. Nitrous oxide should be discontinued and 100% oxygen should be administered. Central venous catheter or pulmonary artery catheter can be introduced to aspirate the gas. External cardiac massage can help in defragmenting the CO_2 bubbles.

Conclusion: Details to anaesthetic technique remains an indispensable and significant part of patient outcome and safety following laparoscopic abdominal wall hernia repair. It is imperative for the anaesthesiologist to be mindful of ventilatory and hemodynamic changes following various types of laparoscopic abdominal hernia repairs. The role of multimodal analgesia and abdominal field blocks go a long way in achieving enhanced recovery and patient satisfaction.

Clinical Pearls
Recommendations for patient undergoing TEP [57]
- Maintain insufflation pressure <12 mmHg
- Limit operating time to less than 60 min
- Adjust ventilation to achieve desired $PECO_2$
- Intermittently examine abdominal and chest wall to detect subcutaneous emphysema
- Exclude causes of subcutaneous emphysema and acute hypercarbia

Road to Safety
- Slow insufflation
- Low intra-abdominal pressure
- Hemodynamic optimisation before carboperitoneum
- Patient tilt after insufflation

Table 6.5 Complications of carboperitoneum
- Pain in abdomen (peritoneal irritation)
- Shoulder pain (carbonic acid)
- Lowers threshold for arrhythmias with halogenated hydrocarbons
- Venous gas embolism
- Promotion of port site tumor growth

References

1. Cunningham AJ, Brull SJ. Laparoscopic cholecystectomy. Anaesthetic implications. Anesth Analg. 1993;76:1120–33.
2. Safran DB, Orlando R. Physiological effects of pneumoperitoneum. Am J Surg. 1994;167:281.
3. Makinen MT, Yli-Hankala A. Respiratory compliance during laparoscopic hiatal and inguinal hernia repair. Can J Anaesth. 1998;45:865.

4. Wilcox S, Vandam LD. Alas, poor Trendelenburg and his position! A critique of its uses and effectiveness. Anesth Analg. 1988;67:574.

5. Joris JL, Noirot DP, Legrand MJ, Jacquet NJ, Lamy ML. Hemodynamic changes during laparoscopic cholecystectomy. Anesth Analg. 1993;76:1067–71.

6. Bazin JE, Gillart T, Rasson P, et al. Haemodynamic conditions enhancing gas embolism after venous injury during laparoscopy: a study in pigs. Br J Anaesth. 1997;78:570.

7. Uhlich GA. Laparoscopy. The question of the proper gas. Gastrointest Endosc. 1982;28:212–3.

8. Ferzli GS, Dysarz FA. Extraperitoneal endoscopic inguinal herniorrhaphy performed without carbon dioxide insufflation. J Laparoendosc Surg. 1994;4:301–4.

9. Fitzgerald SD, Andrus CH, Baudendistal LJ, Dahms TE, Kaminski DL. Hypercarbia during carbon dioxide pneumoperitoneum. Am J Surg. 1992;163:186–9.

10. Magno R, Medegard A, Bengtsson R, Tronstad SE. Acid–base balance during laparoscopy. Acta Obstet Gynecol Scand. 1979;58:81.

11. Ishizaki Y, Bandai Y, Shimomura K, Abe H, Ohtomo Y, Idezuki Y. Changes in splanchnic blood flow and cardiovascular effects following peritoneal insufflation of carbon dioxide. Surg Endosc. 1993;7:420–3.

12. Andrus CH, Naunheim KS, Wittgen CM. Anaesthetic considerations. In: MacFadyen Jr BV, editor. Operative laparoscopy and thoracoscopy. Philadelphia: Lippincott-Raven and Ponsky JL Publishers; 1996. p. 18–20.

13. Mullet CE, Viale JP, Sagnard PE, Miallet CC, Ruynat LG, Counioux HC. Pulmonary CO2 elimination during surgical procedures using intra- or extraperitoneal CO2 insufflation. Anesth Analg. 1993;76:622–6.

14. Wolf JS Jr, Monk TG, McDougall EM, McClennan BL, Clayman RV. The extra-peritoneal approach and subcutaneous emphysema are associated with greater absorption of carbon dioxide during laparoscopic renal surgery. J Urol. 1995;154:959–63.

15. Sumpf E, Crozier TA, Ahrens D, Brauer A, Neufang T, Braun U. Carbon dioxide absorption during extra-peritoneal and transperitoneal endoscopic hernioplasty. Anesth Analg. 2000;91:589–95.

16. Glascock JM, Winfield HN, Lund GO, Donovan JF, Ping ST, Griffiths DL. Carbon dioxide homeostasis during transperitoneal or extraperitoneal laparoscopic pelvic lymphadenectomy. J Endourol. 1996;10:319–23.

17. Blobner M, Bogdanski R, Jelen Esselborn S. Visceral absorption of intra-abdominal insufflated carbon dioxide in swine. Anaesthesiol Intensivmed Notfallmed Schmerzther. 1999;34:94–9.

18. Koivusalo AM, Kellokumpu I, Lindgren L. Gasless laparoscopic cholecystectomy: comparison of post-operative recovery with conventional technique. Br J Anesth. 1996;77:576–80.

19. Ge B, Zhao H, Chen Q, Jin W, Liu L, Huang Q. A randomized comparison of gasless laparoscopic appendectomy and conventional laparoscopic appendectomy. World J Emerg Surg. 2014;9:3.

20. Lentschener C, Fredi-Reygrobellet D, Bouaziz H, et al. Effect of Co2 pneumoperitoneum on early cellular markers of retinal ischemia in rabbits with alpha-chymotrypsin-induced glaucoma. Surg Endosc. 1997;11:376.

21. Chui PT, Oh TE. Anaesthesia for laparoscopic general surgery. Anaesth Intensive Care. 1993;21:163.

22. Brichant JF. Anaesthesia for minimally invasive abdominal surgery. In: Adams AP, Cashman JN, editors. Recent advances in anaesthesia and analgesia, vol. 19. London: Churchill Livingstone; 1995. p. 33–49.

23. Harris MNE, Plantevin OM, Crowther A. Cardiac arrhythmias during anaesthesia for laparoscopy. Br J Anaesth. 1984;56:1213–7.

24. Maltby JR, Beriault MT, Watson NC, Leipert DJ, Fick GH. LMA–Classic and LM–ProSeal are effective alternatives to endotracheal intubation for gynaecological laparoscopy. Can J Anaesth. 2003;50:71–7.

25. Joris JL, Chiche JD, Canivet JL, et al. Hemodynamic changes induced by laparoscopy and their endocrine correlates: effects of clonidine. J Am Coll Cardiol. 1998;32:1389.

26. Laisalmi M, Koivusalo AM, Valta P, et al. Clonidine provides opioid-sparing effect, stable hemodynamics, and renal integrity during laparoscopic cholecystectomy. Surg Endosc. 2001;15:1331.

27. Aho M, Lehtinen AM, Laatikainen T, et al. Effects of intra muscular clonidine on hemodynamic responses to gynecologic laparoscopy. Anesthesiology. 1990;72:797.

28. Aho M, Scheinin M, Lehtinen AM, et al. Intramuscularly administered dexmedetomidine attenuates hemodynamic and stress hormone responses to gynecologic laparoscopy. Anesth Analg. 1992;75:932.

29. Akca O, Lenhardt R, Fleischmann E, et al. Nitrous oxide increases the incidence of bowel distension in patients undergoing elective colon resection. Acta Anaesthesiol Scand. 2004;48:894.

30. Raphael JH, Norton AC. Antiemetic efficacy of prophylactic ondansetron in laparoscopic surgery: randomized double-blind comparison with metoclopramide. Br J Anaesth. 1993;71:845.

31. Vegfors M, Cederholm I, Lenmarken C, Lofstrom JB. Should oxygen be administered after laparoscopy in healthy patients? Acta Anaesthesiol Scand. 1988;32:350–2.

32. de Grood PM, Harbers JB, van Egmond J, et al. Anaesthesia for laparoscopy: a comparison of five techniques including propofol, etomidate, thiopentone and isoflurane. Anaesthesia. 1987;42:815.

33. Bailie R, Craig G, Restall J. Total intravenous anaesthesia for laparoscopy. Anaesthesia. 1989;44:60.

34. Marshall CA, Jones RM, Bajorek PK, et al. Recovery characteristics using isoflurane or propofol for maintenance of anaesthesia: a double–blind controlled trial. Anaesthesia. 1992;47:461.

35. Rothenberg DM, McCarthy RJ, Peng CC, Normoyle DA. Nausea and vomiting after dexamethasone versus droperidol following outpatient laparoscopy with a propofol-based general anesthetic. Acta Anaesthesiol Scand. 1998;42(6):637–42.

36. Hohlrieder M, Brimacombe J, Eschertzhuber S, et al. A study of airway management using the ProSeal laryngeal mask airway compared with the tracheal tube on postoperative analgesia requirements following gynaecological laparoscopic surgery. Anaesthesia. 2007;62:913.

37. Miller DM, Camporota L. Advantages of ProSeal and SLIPA airways over tracheal tubes for gynaecologic laparoscopies. Can J Anaesth. 2006;53:188.

38. Sinha A, Sharma B, Sood J. ProSeal as an alternative to endotracheal intubation in pediatric laparoscopy. Pediatr Anesth. 2007;17:327–32.

39. Pursnani KG. Laparoscopic cholecystectomy under epidural anaesthesia in patients with chronic respiratory disease. Surg Endosc. 1998;12:1082–4.

40. Chowbey PK, Sood J, Vashistha A, Sharma A, Khullar R, Soni V, et al. Extraperitoneal endoscopic groin hernia repair under epidural anesthesia. Surg Laparosc Endosc Percutan Tech. 2003;13:185–90.

41. Ciofolo MJ, Clergue F, Seebacher J, Lefebvre G, Viars P. Ventilatory effects of laparoscopy under epidural anaesthesia. Anesth Analg. 1990;70:357–61.

42. Brady CE, Harkleroad LE, Pierson WP. Alteration in oxygen saturation and ventilation after IV sedation for peritoneoscopy. Arch Intern Med. 1989;149:1029.

43. Ferzli GS, Massad A, Albert P. Extraperitoneal endoscopic inguinal hernia repair. J Laparoendosc Surg. 1992;2:281–6.

44. Collins LM, Vaghadia H. Regional anaesthesia for laparoscopy. Anesthesiol Clin North Am. 2001;19(1):44–7. WB Saunders Company.

45. Michaloliakou C, Chung F, Sharma S. Preoperative multimodal analgesia facilitates recovery after ambulatory laparoscopic cholecystectomy. Anesth Analg. 1996;82:44.

46. Mixter CG 3rd, Hackett TR. Preemptive analgesia in the laparoscopic patient. Surg Endosc. 1997;11:351.

47. Bisgaard T. Analgesic treatment after laparoscopic cholecystectomy: a critical assessment of the evidence. Anesthesiology. 2006;104:835.

48. McDonnell JG, Curley G, Carney J, Benton A, Costello J, Maharaj CH, Laffey JG. The analgesic efficacy of transversus abdominis plane block after abdominal surgery: a prospective randomized controlled trial. Anesth Analg. 2008;106:186–91.

49. Chetwood A, Agrawal S, Hrouda D, Doyle P. Laparoscopic assisted transversus abdominis plane block: a novel insertion technique during laparoscopic nephrectomy. Anaesthesia. 2011;66(4):317–8.

50. Nyarwaya J, Manoit J, Samii K. Are pulse oximetry and end-tidal carbon di oxide tension monitoring reliable during laparoscopic surgery? Anaesthesia. 1994;49:775.

51. Baraka A, Jabbour S, Hammoud R, et al. End-tidal carbon dioxide tension during laparoscopic cholecystectomy: correlation with the baseline value prior to carbon dioxide insufflation. Anaesthesia. 1994;49:304.

52. Klopfenstein CE, Mamie C, Forster A. Laparoscopic extraperitoneal inguinal hernia complicated by subcutaneous emphysema. Can J Anaesth. 1995;42:523–5.

53. Chien GL, Soifer BE. Pharyngeal emphysema with airway obstruction as a consequence of laparoscopic inguinal herniorrhaphy. Anesth Analg. 1995;80:201–3.

54. Ferzli GS, Kiel T, Hurwitz JB, Davidson P, Piperno B, Fiorillo MA, et al. Pneumothorax as a complication of laparoscopic inguinal hernia repair. Surg Endosc. 1997;11:152–3.

55. Toyoshima Y, Tsuchida H, Namiki A. Pneumothorax during extraperitoneal herniorrhaphy. Anaesthesiology. 1998;89:4.

56. Joris JL, Chiche JD, Lamy ML. Pneumothorax during laparoscopic fundoplication: diagnosis and treatment with positive end expiratory pressure. Anesth Analg. 1995;81:993.

57. Bures E, Fusciardi J, Lanquetot H, et al. Ventilatory effects of laparoscopic cholecystectomy. Acta Anaesthesiol Scand. 1996;40:566.

Surgical Techniques for Inguinal Hernia Repair: Open Techniques—Tissue Repairs

7

Rey Melchor F. Santos

7.1 Introduction

The pathophysiology of inguinal hernia is based primarily on a defect in the myopectineal orifice of Fruchaud (Fig. 7.1), which may be repaired by approximation of tissues together to close the defect (tissue repair) or bridging the defect with a mesh to create a tension-free repair (mesh repair). The rapid development in technology has revolutionized the treatment of hernia repair with the development of the mesh and endoscopic instrumentations which made the posterior approach to the inguinal area accessible, and highly effective in treating the hernia defect. Despite these advances, tissue repair still remains to be an acceptable procedure for some inguinal hernias, particularly in cases where the local condition in the inguinal area is contaminated or potentially contaminated, which contraindicates the use of a foreign material, like the mesh. Besides, some tissue repairs, like the Shouldice repair, have been shown by studies to have a recurrence rate of 1% [1] and that could be comparable to the tension-free or mesh repair, whether done with the anterior or posterior approach. Based on the guidelines of the European Hernia Society, Shouldice repair is the best non-mesh repair for inguinal hernias [2].

A 2012 meta-analysis from the Cochrane Database demonstrated significantly lower rates of hernia recurrence (OR 0.62, CI 0.45–0.85) in patients undergoing Shouldice operations when compared with other open tissue-based methods [3]. *In a study of McGuillicuddy et al., Shouldice repair can compare with Lichtenstein technique in terms of effectivity. However, in the long-term basis Lichtenstein technique has a shorter learning curve, easier to learn, and could be done also under local anesthesia, with lesser recurrences* [4].

The Shouldice repair is a four-layer repair of the posterior inguinal floor that was popularized by Earl Shouldice at the Shouldice Clinic in Toronto, Canada. It is likewise a well-established operation for both primary and recurrent inguinal hernias [5]. Its three crucial components that contribute to its safety, efficacy, and cost-effectiveness are local anesthesia, technical aspects of the repair, and early ambulation [6].

The other types of tissue repairs, which have commonly been used before includes Bassini's and Mc Vay's. The Bassini's repair, developed by Eduardo Bassini in 1884, has been the gold standard in hernia repair for most of the twentieth century [7]; however, it has been shown by studies to have a recurrence rate as high as 32–33% [8], This procedure served, however, as the foundation for the development of Shouldice repair.

The Mc Vay's Repair, or Coppers Ligament Repair involves the suturing of the conjoined tendon to the Cooper's Ligament in an attempt to close the

R. M. F. Santos (✉)
Department of Surgery, Veterans Memorial Medical Center, Quezon City, Philippines

Department of Surgery, FEU-NRMF Medical Center, Quezon City, Philippines

© Springer Nature India Private Limited 2020
P. Chowbey, D. Lomanto (eds.), *Techniques of Abdominal Wall Hernia Repair*,
https://doi.org/10.1007/978-81-322-3944-4_7

Fig. 7.1 The Myopectineal Orifice of Fruchaud is seen depicting the locations of the different types of inguinal hernias. The direct inguinal hernia is seen medial to the inferior epigastric artery while the indirect hernia is seen lateral to the vessel. The femoral hernia is seen below the inguinal ligament at the femoral ring

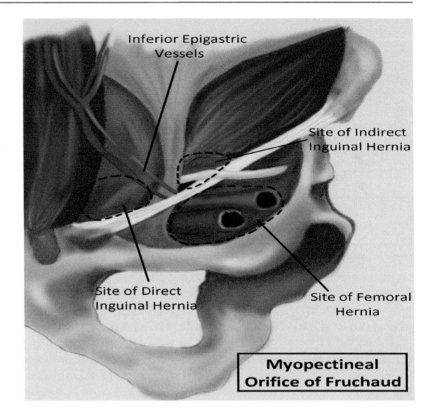

hernia defect. However, tension is generated because of the approximation of structures located at different planes, necessitating the need for a relaxing incision to diffuse the tension. Its primary indication then was for the repair of femoral hernias.

These two procedures, however, have not been used recently because of the relatively high recurrence rates compared to Shouldice and the other types of mesh repairs. In a multicenter French study involving 1647 hernias over 5 years with a median follow-up of more than 5 years, actuarial recurrence at 8 years was 6.1% after a Shouldice, 8.6% after Bassini's and 11.2% after Cooper's ligament technique [9]. The recurrence rate for Shouldice is, however, very much higher compared to the recurrence rate at the Shouldice Clinic in Toronto, Canada, whose reported recurrence rate is 1% [1], which has never been replicated in other institutions. This indicates therefore the need for surgical expertise to attain the low recurrence rate of the Shouldice clinic.

7.2 Indications

Tissue repairs are indicated principally in situations like strangulated inguinal hernias where the local conditions in the inguinal floor is contaminated/infected or potentially contaminated/infected, and the use of foreign materials like mesh to bridge the defect is contraindicated because of the high incidence of infection.

7.3 Contraindications

Tissue repairs are contraindicated in situations where tissues are too attenuated or thinned out particularly in patients with huge hernia defects or collagen diseases. It is also contraindicated in cases where tissues for approximation are too scarred making repair very difficult.

7.4 Preoperative Care

A complete history and physical examination should be done to identify clinical findings compatible with an inguinal hernia. Possible precipitating conditions like Benign Prostatic Hypertrophy, COPD, and ascites should be identified and treated first prior to the hernia repair to prevent recurrence. Risk assessments should be made to determine whether the patient is physically and psychologically prepared for the surgery. The procedure and possible complications and outcome should be explained to the patient well, including the choice of anesthesia, whether general, regional, or local. Preoperatively, patient is placed on NPO and urinary bladder decompressed, without using a foley catheter, if patient is able to urinate prior to surgery. Antibiotic prophylaxis is generally not indicated unless you have a very high-risk patient because of comorbidities.

7.5 Surgical Technique

7.5.1 Initial Skin Incision

1. Through an imaginary line drawn from the anterior superior iliac spine to the pubic tubercle, a 4–5 cm skin incision is made 2 cm above and parallel to the inguinal crease towards the pubic tubercle (Fig. 7.2).
2. The subcutaneous tissue is incised and two consistent branches of the superficial epigastric veins are isolated and ligated or cauterized.
3. Incision is carried through the Scarpa's fascia until the external oblique aponeurosis (EOA) and superficial inguinal ring are exposed.

7.5.2 Division and Dissection of the External Oblique Muscle

4. External oblique aponeurosis (EOA) is then incised along its fibers cutting to the superior portion of the external inguinal ring. Generally, the EOA is divided 3–4 cm above the inguinal ligament to allow enough EOA left to close over the spermatic cord during final closure.
5. The superior medial leaf of the EOA is then dissected from the cord and the internal oblique muscle up to the lateral anterior rectus sheath, taking care not to injure the iliohypogastric nerve, which lies on the internal oblique muscle superior and parallel to the

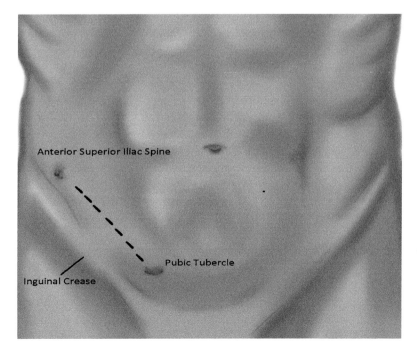

Fig. 7.2 Through an imaginary line drawn from the anterior superior iliac spine to the pubic tubercle, a 4–5 cm skin incision is made 2 cm above and parallel to the inguinal crease towards the pubic tubercle

Anterior Superior Iliac Spine

Pubic Tubercle

Inguinal Crease

Fig. 7.3 The superior medial leaf of the external oblique aponeurosis is then dissected from the cord and the internal oblique muscle up to the lateral anterior rectus sheath, taking care not to injure the iliohypogastric nerve, which lies on the internal oblique muscle superior and parallel to the cord, and the ilioinguinal nerve, which lies anterior to the spermatic cord

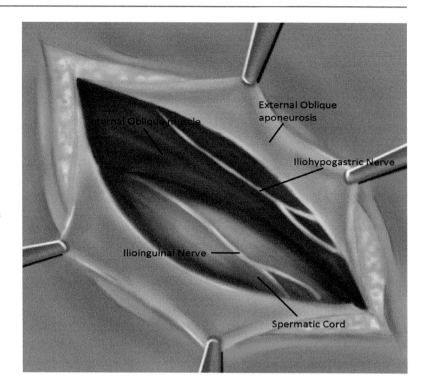

cord, and the ilioinguinal nerve, which lies anterior to the spermatic cord (Fig. 7.3).

6. The inferior lateral leaf is likewise dissected from the cord until the shelving portion of the inguinal ligament is fully exposed.

7.5.3 Isolation of the Spermatic Cord

7. The spermatic cord is then separated from the posterior inguinal floor by dissecting bluntly at the area of the pubic tubercle, taking care not to injure the genitofemoral nerve at the lateral aspect of the cremasteric muscle, using the "blue line" corresponding to the spermatic vessels as a landmark (Fig. 7.4). Once isolated, apply an umbilical tape or penrose drain to apply traction on the cord to expose fully the posterior inguinal floor. Avoid an en masse isolation of the spermatic cord using your finger at the area of the pubic tubercle, to avoid bleeding and injury to the genitofemoral nerve.

7.5.4 Isolation and Handling of the Sac

8. The cremasteric muscle is divided anteriorly into a medial and lateral leaf to expose the anterolateral portion of the cord where the indirect sac could be identified as a glistening white surface. It is then sharply dissected from the spermatic vessels and vas deferens until the level of the preperitoneal fat, where a thickened peritoneal white line is identified when the sac is opened. All structures inside the sac are then reduced back into the peritoneal cavity. A purse string suture is then applied to ligate and transect the sac (Fig. 7.5). After which, the stump spontaneously retracts behind the transversus abdominis aponeurotic arch. The sac may also be pushed back inside the deep internal ring into the preperitoneal space without being ligated. At this point, any lipoma of the cord should be removed and ligated. If the sac extends up to the scrotal area, then it is transected at the middle of the inguinal canal, keeping the distal end open to

Fig. 7.4 The spermatic cord is then separated from the posterior inguinal floor by dissecting bluntly at the area of the pubic tubercle, taking care not to injure the genitofemoral nerve at the lateral aspect of the cremasteric muscle, using the "blue line" corresponding to the spermatic vessels as a landmark

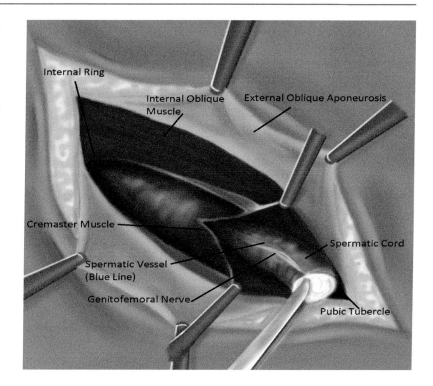

Fig. 7.5 The cremasteric muscle is divided anteriorly into a medial and lateral leaf exposing the anterolateral portion of the cord where the indirect sac could be identified as a glistening white surface. It is then sharply dissected from the spermatic vessels and vas deferens until the level of the preperitoneal fat where a thickened peritoneal white line is identified when the sac is opened. A purse string suture is then applied to ligate and transect the sac after reducing its contents

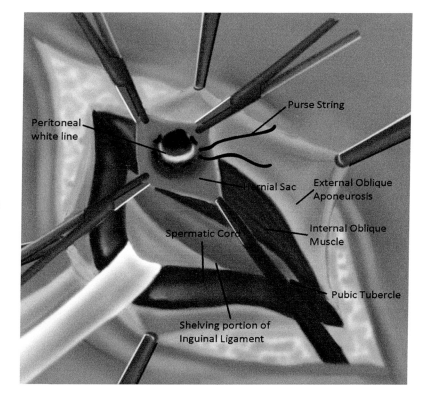

prevent formation of hydrocele. Make sure, however, that bleeding in the sac edges is controlled by ligature or cautery. If the defect is a direct sac with a broad base, then the sac may just be buried with a purse string suture around the sac, to flatten the inguinal floor. If it is a big narrow-based direct sac, then you may opt to open the sac, dissect it, remove excess preperitoneal fat, and close it with a purse string suture after transecting the excess sac.

9. The cord is then completely dissected around the deep inguinal ring cutting through attachments of the cremasteric muscles and the condensed medial margin of the ring, in preparation for the repair of the inguinal floor.

7.5.5 Repair of the Floor

10. The floor is then repaired depending upon the preferred type of tissue repair whether Shouldice, Bassini's, or Mc Vay's.

7.6 Shouldice Repair

(a) The transversalis fascia is incised parallel to the inguinal ligament starting at the medial portion of the deep inguinal ring up to pubic tubercle, taking care not to injure the deep epigastric vessel medial to the ring and below the transversalis fascia (Fig. 7.6). The superior medial leaf is then dissected bluntly away from the preperitoneal fat up to the lateral anterior rectus sheath. The Inferior lateral leaf is likewise dissected from the preperitoneal fat up to the iliopubic tract. The cribriformis fascia below the inguinal ligament on the upper and anterior aspect of the groin is incised from the level of the femoral vessel and the pubis, to allow further mobilization of the EOA later in the repair. With this area opened, exploration of the femoral canal for a coexisting hernia should be done to prevent a missed femoral hernia.

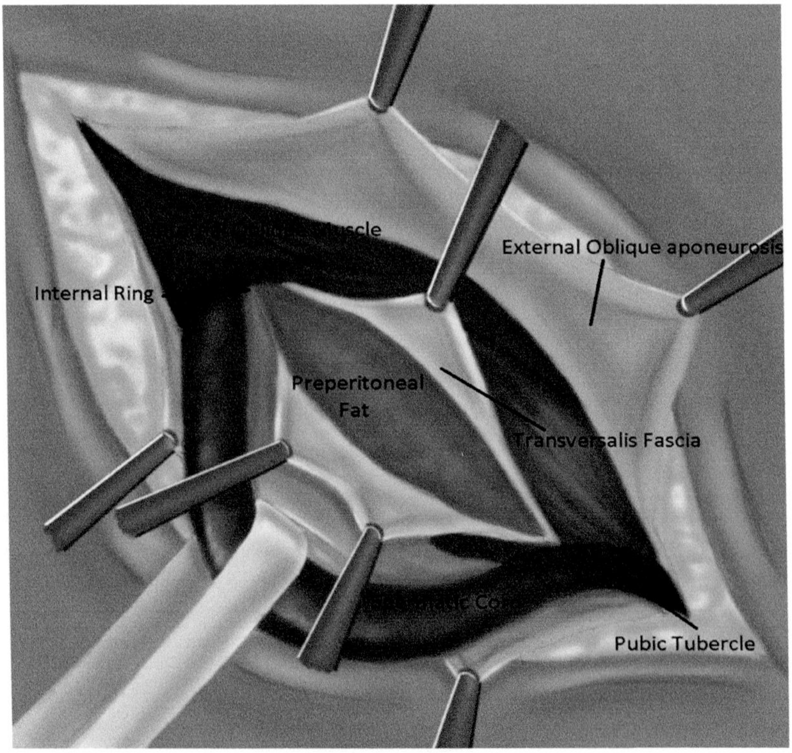

Fig. 7.6 The transversalis fascia is incised parallel to the inguinal ligament starting at the medial portion of the deep inguinal ring up to pubic tubercle, taking care not to injure the deep epigastric vessel medial to the ring and below the transversalis fascia

(b) The first suture line is started at the area of the pubic tubercle by suturing, using a monofilament non absorbable suture, the end of the lateral leaf to the condensed and thickened area of the transversalis fascia, and the transversus abdominis and internal oblique muscles (triple layer) at the undersurface of the medial leaf, making a continuous suture with different depths to prevent tearing up the transversalis fascia and distributing the tension evenly. This is carried up to the medial portion of the internal ring, taking the stump of the lateral cremasteric muscle as it crosses over to the opposite side, suturing the triple layer, in effect creating a new internal ring. Make sure that the ring is being narrowed to accept only the tip of a finger (Fig. 7.7).

(c) The second line of suture starts from the internal ring, as a continuation of the first suture, by suturing the end of the medial leaf to the shelving portion of the inguinal ligament up to the pubic tubercle, where the suture is tied (Fig. 7.8).

(d) The third line of suture starts from the internal ring by suturing the internal oblique and transversus abdominis muscles to the external oblique aponeurosis just above the shelving portion of the inguinal ligament. This is carried up to the pubic tubercle (Fig. 7.9).

(e) The fourth line of suture begins as the previous suture is continued by suturing again the internal oblique and transversus abdominis muscles to the external oblique aponeurosis above the previous suture line and carried up to the internal ring where the suture is finally tied (Fig. 7.10).

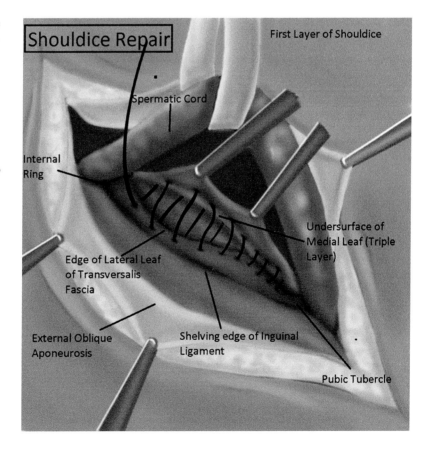

Fig. 7.7 The first suture line is started at the area of the pubic tubercle by suturing the end of the lateral leaf to the condensed area of the triple layer at the undersurface of the medial leaf, making a continuous suture to distribute the tension evenly. This is carried up to the medial portion of the internal ring, taking the stump of the lateral cremasteric muscle as it crosses over to the opposite side, suturing the triple layer, in effect creating a new internal ring

Fig. 7.8 The second line of suture starts from the internal ring, as a continuation of the first suture, by suturing the end of the medial leaf to the shelving portion of the inguinal ligament up to the pubic tubercle, where the suture is tied

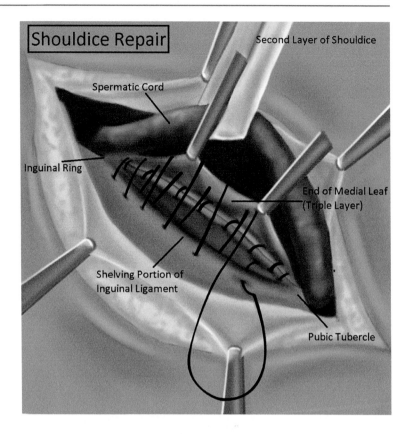

Fig. 7.9 The third line of suture starts from the internal ring by suturing the internal oblique and transversus abdominis muscles to the external oblique aponeurosis just above the shelving portion of the inguinal ligament. This is carried up to the pubic tubercle

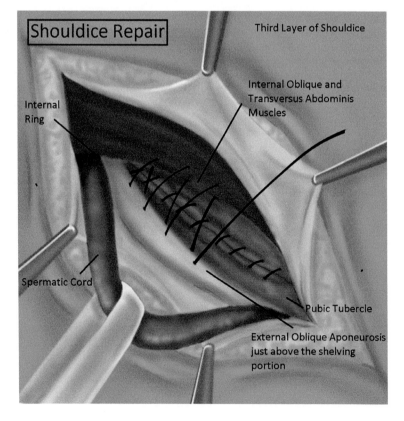

Fig. 7.10 The fourth line of suture begins as the previous suture is continued by suturing again the internal oblique and transversus abdominis muscles to the external oblique aponeurosis above the previous suture line and carried up to the internal ring where the suture is finally tied

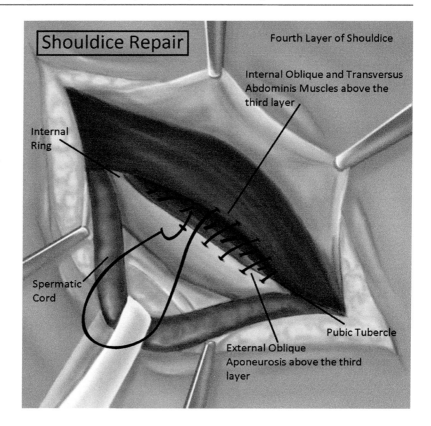

7.7 Bassini's Repair

(a) In the original Bassini's repair, the transversalis fascia is divided from the deep internal ring to the pubic tubercle, and then the superior medial flap of the transversalis fascia is dissected bluntly away from the preperitoneal fat. This allows exposure of the triple layer of the transversalis fascia, the internal oblique and transversus abdominis muscles. The inferior flap of the transversalis fascia is likewise dissected from the preperitoneal fat up to the iliopubic tract. This also facilitates the exploration of the femoral canal to rule out a femoral hernia (Fig. 7.6).

(b) The first stitch in the repair of the posterior inguinal floor using nonabsorbable suture is placed superiorly and medially encompassing the triple layer and part of the anterior rectus sheath and the shelving portion of the inguinal or Poupart's ligament at the area of the pubic tubercle. Interrupted stitches using also nonabsorbable sutures are then applied laterally encompassing the triple layer and the shelving portion of the inguinal ligament until the medial portion of the deep inguinal ring, narrowing it to admit only the tip of a finger. The sutures are then tied but should not be too tight to avoid ischemia or cutting through tissues (Fig. 7.11).

Fig. 7.11 The first stitch in the repair of the posterior inguinal floor is placed superiorly and medially encompassing the triple layer and part of the anterior rectus sheath and the shelving portion of the inguinal ligament at the area of the pubic tubercle. Interrupted stitches are then applied laterally encompassing the triple layer and the shelving portion of the inguinal ligament until the medial portion of the deep inguinal ring, narrowing it to admit only the tip of a finger

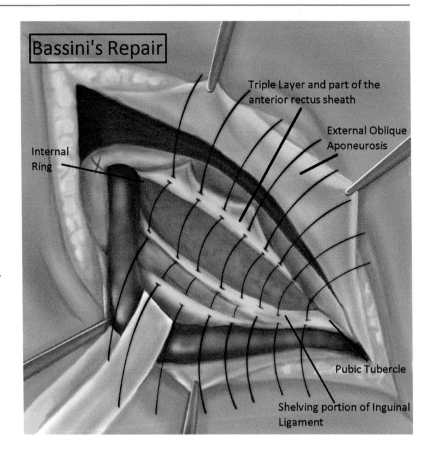

7.8   Mc Vay's Repair

(a) The transversalis fascia is divided from the internal ring to the pubic tubercle, taking care not to damage the inferior epigastric vessel located deep and medial to the internal ring. The preperitoneal space is bluntly dissected to expose the Cooper's or Iliopectineal ligament, taking care not to damage the corona mortis or anastomotic vessels between the obturator and epigastric arteries located usually anterior to the Cooper's ligament. The femoral canal is then explored to look for a femoral hernia. If a femoral sac is noted, then an attempt to reduce it is done. If the sac could not be reduced, then the inguinal ligament above the sac could be transected to allow reduction and inspection of the contents to assess viability of organs within, since a femoral hernia is prone to strangulation.

(b) Repair of the floor is initiated by suturing with multiple interrupted nonabsorbable sutures the triple layer of transversalis fascia,

transversus abdominis and internal oblique muscles to the Cooper's ligament from the pubic tubercle to the femoral vein as it crosses the Cooper's ligament laterally (Fig. 7.12).

(c) 2–3 interrupted transition sutures using nonabsorbable sutures are then placed encompassing the triple layer, the anterior femoral sheath and the shelving portion of the inguinal ligament (Fig. 7.12).

(d) Additional interrupted monofilament nonabsorbable sutures are then placed to approximate the triple layer to the shelving portion of the inguinal ligament proceeding laterally up to the deep internal ring, which must admit only the tip of a finger.

(e) Before the sutures are tied, a relaxing incision on the anterior rectus sheath, which may extend from the deep inguinal ring to the pubic tubercle, must be made to decrease the tension brought about by the approximation of structures not on the same plane (Fig. 7.13).

Fig. 7.12 Repair of the floor is initiated by suturing with multiple interrupted sutures the triple layer to the Cooper's ligament from the pubic tubercle to the femoral vein as it crosses the Cooper's ligament laterally. About 2–3 interrupted transition sutures are then placed encompassing the triple layer, the anterior femoral sheath, and the shelving portion of the inguinal ligament

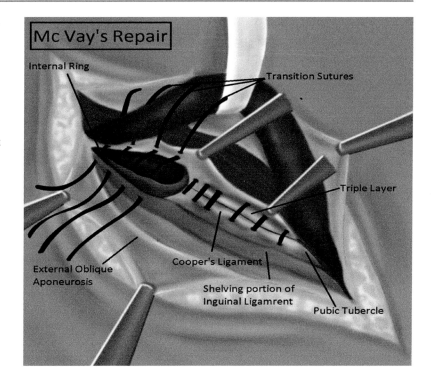

Fig. 7.13 Before the sutures are tied, a relaxing incision on the anterior rectus sheath, which may extend from the deep inguinal ring to the pubic tubercle, must be made to decrease the tension brought about by the approximation of structures not on the same plane

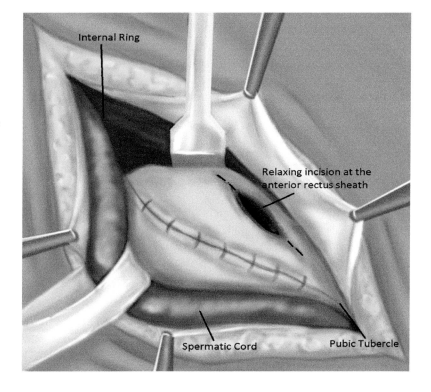

7.8.1 Reconstruction of the External Oblique Aponeurosis and the Superficial Inguinal Ring

11. After repair of the inguinal floor, the spermatic cord is repositioned on the inguinal floor and the external oblique aponeurosis is closed over it with a continuous suturing using a nonabsorbable suture, taking care to reconstruct the external inguinal ring medially without constricting the exiting spermatic cord.

7.8.2 Closure of the Incision

12. The subcutaneous tissue is then apposed with interrupted absorbable sutures, just enough to obliterate any dead space.
13. The skin is finally closed subcuticularly using absorbable sutures.

7.9 Postoperative Care

The patient is encouraged to ambulate during the first 24 h but advised to refrain from heavy activities for 4–6 weeks. Diet is resumed once fully awake and analgesics may be given to alleviate pain and encourage early ambulation.

7.10 Complications

The common complications specific to hernia repair are usually recurrence, chronic inguinal and pubic pain, and injury to the spermatic cord and testis. Most tissue repairs are associated with a high recurrence. The only tissue repair that has an acceptable and relatively low recurrence rate comparable to mesh tension-free repairs is the Shouldice repair. The chronic inguinal pain is usually due to nerve entrapment by sutures, and the pubic pain is due to a pubic osteitis, which develops when sutures are applied directly to the periosteum of the pubic tubercle [10]. A report from the SMIL Study group by Berndsen F. et al., showed

that in terms of chronic discomfort or pain, there is no significant difference when laparoscopic TAPP is compared to Shouldice repair even for a period of 5 years. The presence, however, of mild discomfort or pain on the first postoperative week after Shouldice repair can be predictive of a late discomfort or pain for patients undergoing this type of repair [11]. A meta-analysis done by Bittner et al., showed that endoscopic techniques like TAPP and TEP showed less morbidity in terms of hematoma, nerve injury and chronic groin pain when compared to Shouldice and other open non-mesh or tissue repairs. On the other hand, Shouldice technique showed a shorter operative time due to ease of operation and less incidence of seroma compared to the endoscopic techniques. The Shouldice technique also showed no significant difference in terms of recurrences, surgical site or wound infections, or testicular atrophy when compared to the endoscopic techniques. In general, open non-mesh or tissue repairs other than Shouldice technique showed higher chance of recurrences and surgical site or wound infections when compared to endoscopic techniques like TAPP and TEP [12].

Injury to the cord usually involves direct injury to the vas deferens or as a result of fibrosis encroaching over it. Testicular injury is often times a result of devascularization of the pampiniform plexus of veins during dissection of the sac. Other common complications are bleeding, seroma, wound infection, urinary retention, and ileus.

Acknowledgement I would like to thank and acknowledge my artist illustrator Dr. Frank Joseph Viray for providing the illustrations in my discussion of the various open techniques of tissue repairs for inguinal hernias.

References

1. Glassgow F. The Shouldice Hospital technique. Int Surg. 1986;71:148–53.
2. Simons MP, Aufenacker T, Bay-Nielsen M, Bouillot JL, et al. European Hernia Society guidelines on the treatment of inguinal hernia in adult patients. Hernia. 2009;13:343–403.
3. Amato B, Panico S, et al. Shouldice technique versus other open techniques for inguinal hernia repair. Cochrane Database Syst Rev. 2012;4:CD001543.

4. McGillicuddy JE. Prospective randomized comparison of the Shouldice and Lichtenstein hernia repair procedures. Arch Surg. 1998;133(9):974–8.

5. Obney N, Chan CK. Repair of multiple time recurrent inguinal hernias with reference to common causes of recurrences. Contemp Surg. 1984;25:25–32.

6. Bendavid R. Symposium on the management of inguinal hernias: The Shouldice technique: a canon in hernia repair. Can J Surg. 1997;40(3):199–205.

7. Fitzgibbons R, Richards A. Open hernia repair. ACS surgery principles and practice; 2003. p. 668.

8. Beets G, Oosterhuis KJ, et al. Long term follow up (12-15 years) of a randomized controlled trial comparing Bassini-Stetten, Shouldice and high ligation with narrowing of the internal ring for primary inguinal hernia repair. J Am Coll Surg. 1997;185(4):352–7.

9. Hay JM, Boudet MJ, Fingerhut A, Poucher J, Hennet H, Habib E, et al. Shouldice inguinal hernia repair in the male adult: the gold standard? A multicenter controlled trial in 1578 patients. Ann Surg. 1995;222(6):719–27.

10. Wagner J, Brunicardi FC, Parviz A, Chen D. Inguinal hernia, Swartz's principles of surgery. 10th ed. New York: McGraw Hill Education; 2015. p. 1514.

11. SMIL Study Group, Berndsen F, Petersson U, Arvidsson D, Leijonmarck C-E, et al. Discomfort five years after laparoscopic and Shouldice Inguinal hernia repair: a randomized trial with 867 patients. A report from the SMIL study group. Hernia. 2007;11(4):307–13.

12. Bitner R, Sauerland S, Schedt C-G. Comparison of endoscopic techniques vs Shouldice and other nonmesh techniques for inguinal hernia repair: a meta-analysis for randomized controlled trials. Surg Endosc. 2005;19(5):605–15.

Surgical Techniques for Inguinal Hernia Repair: Open Tension-Free Repairs

8

Ching-Shui Huang

Various mesh materials are now available for open tension-free repair (TFR) for groin hernias, and these materials fall into three categories, namely polyethylene, polypropylene, and absorbable biological mesh, numerous commercial mesh products and mesh devices are derived from these materials. On the other hand, open TFR that utilizes mesh can be classified according to the site of mesh placement (Table 8.1). At present, the most commonly used open TFR are Lichtenstein onlay patch repair (plain flat mesh, for more than 30 years) [1], the PerFix–L® (Bard, Cranston, RI) plug and patch repair (for 23 years), the Modified Kugel® (Bard, Cranston, RI) posterior and anterior patch (for 20 years) and PHS/UHS® (Ethicon, Somerville, NJ) bilayer mesh device repair (for 19 years), and all of these procedures can be performed under local, regional, epidural, spinal, or general anesthesia [2–5].

Table 8.1 Classification of commonly used tension-free groin hernia repair in terms of site of mesh placement

Anterior mesh repair
    Lichtenstein onlay patch (polypropylene, polyethelene, ProGrip, Surgisis/BioDesign)
    Plug and patch (PerFix-Light)
Posterior mesh repair
    GPRVS, Stoppa-Rives (polypropylene, polyethylene), hernia patch with memory ring (Kugel, Ventrio ST)
Anterior and posterior mesh repair
    Modified Kugel with onlay
    Bilayer patches (PHS/UHS)
    Millikan modification of plug and patch (PerFix-Light)

8.1 Lichtenstein Repair

During Lichtenstein repair for direct hernia, the posterior wall is invaginated; for indirect hernia, after the peritoneal sac is inverted or transected, the internal ring is narrowed (like Marcy repair), a piece of prosthetic mesh is sutured as an onlay patch to the transverses arch superiorly, the inguinal ligament inferiorly, and the pubis medially. The mesh tails are crossed laterally across the cord and fixed to the inguinal ligament lateral to the internal ring [6]. This technique does not require opening the posterior wall, and after the prosthetic patch was incorporated with posterior wall, it acts like a reinforcing barrier. Dr. Lichtenstein popularized this technique to become the most frequently

C.-S. Huang (✉)
Department of Surgery, Cathay General Hospital, Taipei, Taiwan

Taipei Medical University, Taipei, Taiwan
e-mail: cshuang@cgh.org.tw

© Springer Nature India Private Limited 2020
P. Chowbey, D. Lomanto (eds.), *Techniques of Abdominal Wall Hernia Repair*,
https://doi.org/10.1007/978-81-322-3944-4_8

performed hernia repair procedures in the United States and possibly worldwide. Dr. Chastan modified this technique by using a self-gripping onlay mesh, Progrip® (Covidien, Dublin, Ireland) [7], reducing the number of fixation stitches.

8.2 The Plug and Patch Repair (Millikan Modification)

After the indirect sac is inverted, the PerFix® Plug is placed beneath the internal ring, the outer layer of the cone-shaped plug is wide open, lying against the under surface of transversalis fascia, the central leaflets were fixed with two sutures to surrounding tissues of the internal ring (Fig. 8.1). When a direct hernia is present, the attenuated transversalis fascia is circumcised, the direct preperitoneal space is entered, with a larger PerFix® Plug placed behind the transversalis fascia, and 4–6 sutures are used to fix the plug (Fig. 8.2) [8]. In addition to the plug, an onlay patch is provided, which can be placed over the posterior wall and around the spermatic cord lateral to the internal ring; the only patch looks like a Lichtenstein repair [9].

8.3 The Modified Kugel Patch

The underlay mesh is a polypropylene, oblong-shaped mesh with a thickened polypropylene thread (coil-spring loaded) thus encourages the mesh to be flatted. An indirect sac is dissected free from the cord, mobilized from the adhesions at hernia neck and retracted or transected, the preperitoneal space of Bogros can be approached through internal ring (indirect hernia), the preperitoneal space of Retzius through a posterior wall defect created by excision of the attenuated transversalis fascia (direct hernia). The vas and internal spermatic vessels are parietalized with blunt and sharp dissection. After all the preperitoneal space of the indirect, direct, and femoral spaces is developed (Fig. 8.3), the prosthesis is inserted to cover the triple triangles, the two leaflets are fixed with sutures to inguinal ligament and aponeurotic internal oblique muscle, this underlay mesh will be further held in place by intraabdominal pressure (Pascal's principle) from behind (Fig. 8.4) [10]. In this procedure, the additional onlay mesh is optional. This approach is designed to protect the internal ring and posterior inguinal floor as well as the femoral canal [11].

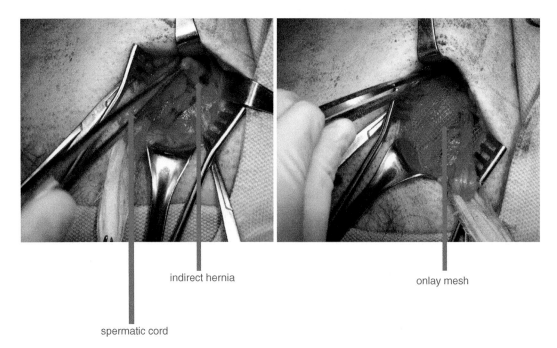

indirect hernia

onlay mesh

spermatic cord

Fig. 8.1 Lt type II, use PerFix-L-L repair

plug at direct preperitoneal space   onlay mesh

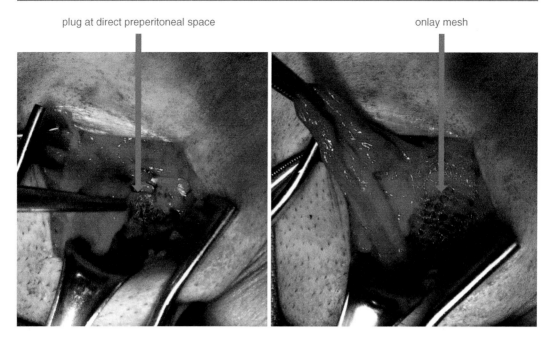

Fig. 8.2 Lt rec type V post Shouldice repair, post and ant repair with PerFix-L-L

Cooper's ligament

Ventrio-ST

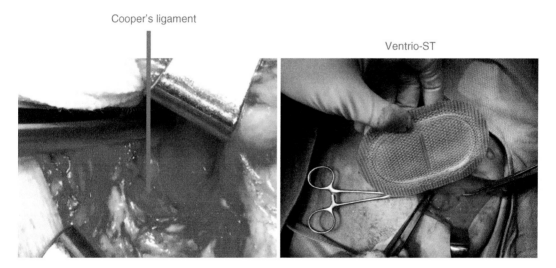

Fig. 8.3 Rt type IV hernia, always expose Cooper's bone during posterior repair

8.4   The Bilayer Patch Devices

The bilayer patch devices (PHS/UHS®) combine an onlay graft (like the Lichtenstein repair) and underlay graft (like the Stoppa or Kugel patch); these two grafts are held together by a connector (like a plug). The external oblique aponeurosis is opened through a 5-cm groin incision, the sper-matic cord is elevated, and an anterior space is created for the placement of the onlay compo-nent of the device. If an indirect hernia sac is present, it is dissected free from the cord, with the direction of dissection from the hernia head through neck, then to hernia shoulders. The her-nia sac is invaginated at the neck, along this tis-sue plane the peritoneum is separated from the

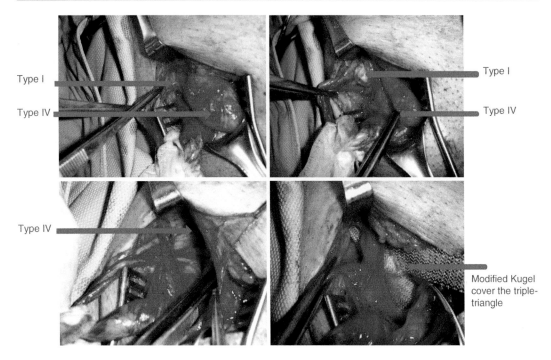

Fig. 8.4 Rt type VI (IV+ rudimentary I), severe weak post wall, use Kugel 8 × 12 + onlay

transversalis fascia (shoulder), the vas and internal spermatic vessels are parietalized as well. If a direct hernia is present, the attenuated transversalis fascia is circumscribed. In either case, the preperitoneal space (space of Bogros and Retzius) is dissected free with a 4 × 4 sponge. The entire device of PHS/UHS® is inserted through the posterior wall defect or internal ring, the underlay component is deployed to cover the direct and indirect space, with the lateral portion of the underlay graft descends caudally to the Cooper's ligament, thereby protecting the femoral canal (Fig. 8.5) [12, 13]. The onlay graft is extracted and placed against the posterior wall into the anterior space beneath the external oblique aponeurosis and laid against the transverses arch down to and over the pubic tubercle. A few sutures are placed in the onlay graft. At minimum, one is placed at the pubic tubercle, one at the mid portion of the transverses arch, and one at the mid portion of the inguinal ligament (Fig. 8.6). The spermatic cord is accommodated with a central or lateral slit in the onlay component [14–16].

8.5 Tailored Open TFR: Cathay General Hospital Experiences

TFR has replaced Shouldice repair for adult groin hernias in our institution since 2001, and we use a tailored approach with selective usage of four types of mesh devices (onlay mesh, plug and patch, bilayer mesh devices, and Kugel/Modified Kugel) based on each patient's myopectineal orifice (MPO) pathology and comorbidity burden. The selection criteria are: localized defect with healthy surrounding post wall tissues (Gilbert type 1, 2, 5, and 7) use anterior mesh repair with plug and patch or Lichtenstein repair using Progrip®, Biodesign® (Cook, Bloomington, IN) under local or intravenous general anesthesia. The anterior mesh repairs are also preferred for females, young adults, very old patients, or patients with severe comorbidity. For patients with moderate destruction of internal ring, or posterior wall with Gilbert type 3, 4, and 6 defects, using bilayer PHS/UHS® or Modified Kugel® under epidural or local anesthesia is suggested.

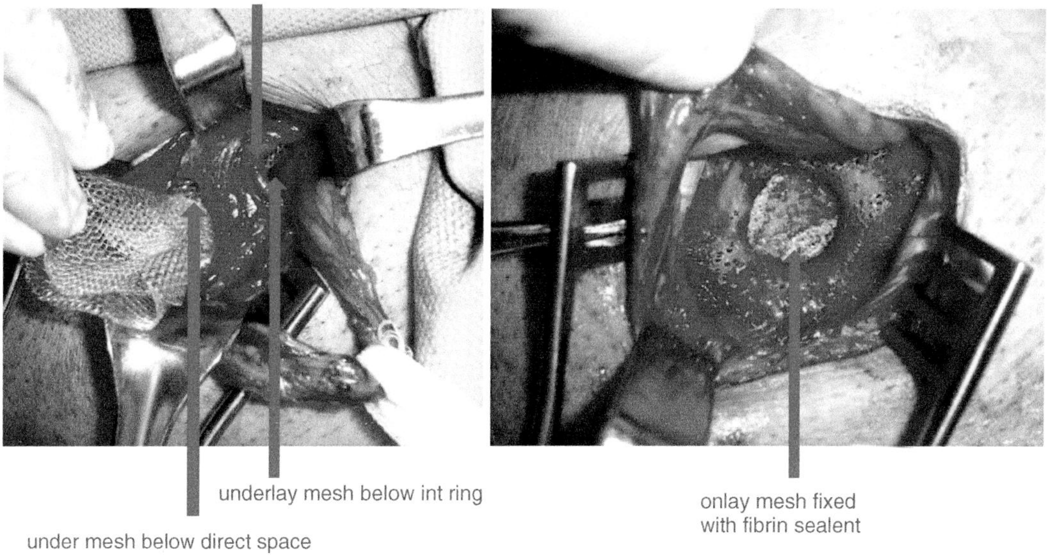

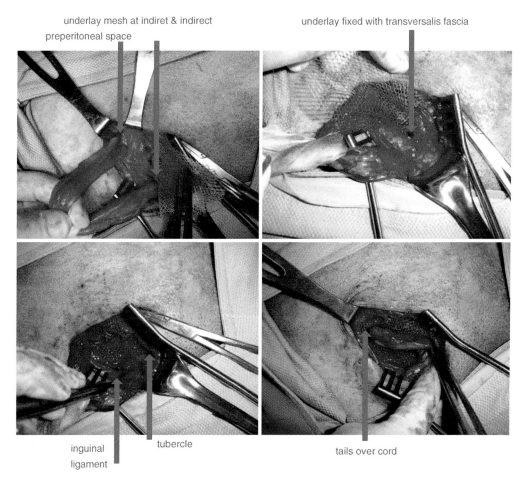

deep inferior epigastric artery

underlay mesh below int ring

under mesh below direct space

onlay mesh fixed
with fibrin sealent

Fig. 8.5 Lt type 6, use PHS/UHS-L repair, fixation with fibrin sealent

underlay mesh at indiret & indirect
preperitoneal space

underlay fixed with transversalis fascia

inguinal
ligament

tubercle

tails over cord

Fig. 8.6 Rt rec type VI (IV and I), UHS-L repair

Patients with severe destruction of internal ring, or posterior wall tissue with Gilbert type 3, 4, and 6 hernias, posterior mesh repairs using Kugel® or Modified Kugel® (Mini-Stoppa procedure)/ Ventrio ST® (Bard, Cranston, RI) under epidural or general anesthesia is preferred (Fig. 8.7). From Feb 2001 to Nov 2015, 3299 consecutive patients with 3850 sides of TFR of groin hernias included onlay mesh (124), plug and patch (1105), bilayer mesh devices (1727), Kugel or Modified Kugel® mesh (894) were performed (Table 8.2). Among 3850 repairs, 499 were for recurrent groin hernias. The long-term follow-up revealed 6.9% of the patients had chronic inguinal discomfort (severe pain: 0.8%), 0.4% of patients had recurrences (2.0% for the recurrent hernias) (Table 8.3).

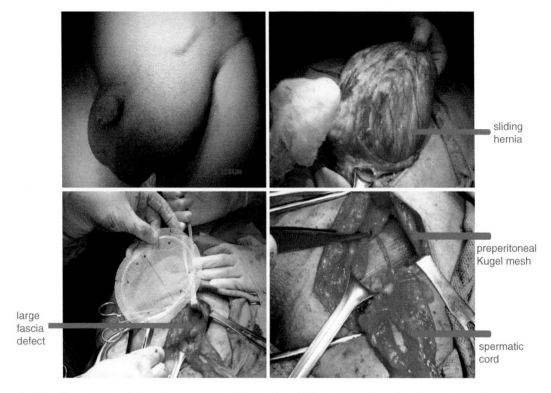

Fig. 8.7 Total posterior failure (huge rec type IV), use 11 × 14 Kugel preperitoneal sublay mesh repair, treated as ventral-incisional hernia

Table 8.2 Database of tension-free repair (2001–2015, prospective data collection)

	Period	P'ts/sides	For recurrent P'ts/sides
Lichtenstein (Progrip/Surgisis/Marlex)	2001–2015	103/124	N/A
PerFix Plug and Patch	2001–2015	964/1105	131/158
PHS/UHS	2001–2015	1494/1727	158/173
Kugel and Modified Kugel	2004–2015	738/894	149/168
Total	2001–2015	3299/3850	438/499

Table 8.3 Long-term results

Complications and recurrences	No	Percents
Seroma		2%
Scrotal hematoma/bleeding		1.8%
Superficial wound infection		0.5%
Testicular atrophy (in rec hernia)	1	
Chronic groin pain		6.9%
Chronic severe groin pain		0.8%
Recurrence (re-recurrences)		0.43% (∗2%)
Mesh extraction	2	
Impotence?	3	

∗2% re-recurrence for recurrent hernia pts (86% follow-up rate at 2 year, 73% at 5 year)

8.6 Conclusions

Tailored open tension-free repair of groin hernia is simple and effective, while over-treatment (pain/discomfort) and under-treatment (recurrence) can be avoided, the complications and long-term results of tailored approach are satisfactory. Key points for successful TFR are: proper dissection of the anterior and/or preperitoneal space with adequate selection of mesh and mesh position according to the MPO pathology.

References

1. Lomanto D, Cheah W-K, Faylona JM, et al. Inguinal hernia repair: toward Asian guidelines. Asian J Endosc Surg. 2015;8:16–23.
2. Awad SS, Fagan SP. Current approaches to inguinal hernia repair. Am J Surg. 2004;188:9S–16S.
3. Jacobs DO. Mesh repair of inguinal hernias—redux. N Engl J Med. 2004;350:1895–7.
4. Simons MP, Aufernacker T, Bay-Nielsen M, Bouillot JL, et al. European Hernia Society guidelines on the treatment of inguinal hernia in adult patients. Hernia. 2009;13:343–403.
5. Miserez M, Peeters E, Aufenacker T, et al. Update with level 1 studies of the European Hernia Society guidelines on the treatment of inguinal hernia in adult patients. Hernia. 2014;18:151–63.
6. Lichtenstein II, Shulman AG, Amid PK. The tension-free hernioplasty. Am J Surg. 1989;157:188–93.
7. Chastan P. Tension-free open hernia repair using an innovative self-gripping semi-resorbable mesh. Hernia. 2009;13:137–42.
8. Rutkow IM. "Tension-free" inguinal herniorrhaphy: a preliminary report on the "mesh plug" technique. Surgery. 1993;114:3–8.
9. Millikan KW, Doolas A. A long-term evaluation of the modified mesh-plug hernioplasty in over 2000 patients. Hernia. 2008;12:257–60.
10. Kugel RD. Minimally invasive, nonlaparoscopic, pre-peritoneal, and sutureless, inguinal herniorrhaphy. Am J Surg. 1999;178:298–302.
11. Li J, Zhang Y, Hu H, et al. Early experience of performing a modified Kugel hernia repair with local anesthesia. Surg Today. 2008;38:603–8.
12. Huang CS. Macroporous partially absorbable light-weight mesh materials reduce postoperative pain for patients with groin hernia repair. Chin J Hernia Abdom Wall Surg. 2013;7(2):115–8.
13. Huang CS, Huang CC, Lien HH. Prolene hernia system compared with mesh plug technique: a prospective study of short- to mid-term outcomes in primary groin hernia repair. Hernia. 2005;9:167–71.
14. Awad SS, Yallalampalli S, Srour AM, et al. Improved outcomes with the Prolene Hernia System mesh compared with the time-honored Lichtenstein onlay mesh repair for inguinal hernia repair. Am J Surg. 2007;193:697–701.
15. Gilbert AL. Combined anterior and posterior inguinal hernia repair: intermediate recurrence rates with three groups of surgeons. Hernia. 2004;8(3):203–7.
16. Wong JU, Leung TH, Huang CC, Huang CS. Comparing chronic pain between fibrin sealant and suture fixation for bilayer polypropylene mesh inguinal hernioplasty: a randomized clinical trial. Am J Surg. 2011;202(1):34–8.

Total Extraperitoneal Repair of Groin Hernias

Pradeep Chowbey

Surgery for inguinal hernia repair is a routinely performed procedure across the globe [1], which makes it a traditional training ground for surgeons to build on their existing technical skills.

Broadly, surgical procedures are classified into: open repair without the use of a mesh implant (i.e. sutured), open repair with a mesh, and laparoscopic repair with a mesh [also known as (1) transabdominal preperitoneal (TAPP) repair when done through the peritoneal cavity and (2) total extraperitoneal (TEP) repair when done without entering the peritoneal cavity].

TEP is a minimally invasive procedure that requires an expertise in performing the procedure. With this technique hernias are repaired using a mesh which is placed behind the muscle of the abdominal wall. Minimal invasive inguinal hernia surgery has gained popularity with gratifying results in terms of early return to work, reduced post-operative pain, decline in mesh infection and minimal recurrence.

9.1 Introduction

Inguinal hernia is a benign disease following a static course but their consequent complications may be drastic and frequent. Surgical repairs done under emergency conditions are invariably morbid in nature. Hence, an elective and planned surgery is always a preferred choice for a surgeon.

Open hernia repairs have been standard methods of treatment. With current trends in surgery, the majority of surgical techniques, open or laparoscopic, are performed with mesh for tension-free repair. In the past two decades laparoscopic techniques have been introduced for the treatment of hernias, which includes transabdominal preperitoneal (TAPP) method and totally extraperitoneal (TEP) approach [2, 3].

Surgery is not generally advised in most cases if the hernia is asymptomatic; watchful waiting is the recommended option. Surgery is usually recommended with symptomatic hernia. However, with higher frequency of femoral hernias in women, even asymptomatic patients who are medically fit should be offered surgical repair as the procedures provide coverage of the femoral space (e.g. laparoscopic repair) at the time of initial operation, which is advisable for women.

The laparoscopic inguinal hernia repair involves a 'tension-free' repair by the placement of a prosthetic mesh to cover the entire groin area, including the sites of direct, indirect and femoral hernias, thus completely reinforcing the myopectineal orifice. The effectiveness of this type of repair has been well established by the open operation of Stoppa [4, 5]. It mimics the conventional open technique; the difference lies in the reduced extent of surgical invasion.

P. Chowbey (✉)
Institute of Minimal Access, Metabolic and Bariatric Surgery, Max Super-Speciality Hospital, New Delhi, India

© Springer Nature India Private Limited 2020
P. Chowbey, D. Lomanto (eds.), *Techniques of Abdominal Wall Hernia Repair*,
https://doi.org/10.1007/978-81-322-3944-4_9

9.1.1 Indications of TEP

The indications for performing a laparoscopic hernia repair are essentially the same as repairing the hernia conventionally. However, the endoscopic approach may offer definite benefit over its open counterpart to the patients suffering from bilateral inguinal hernias and recurrent inguinal hernias.

Surgeons during their early experience should preferably operate on the following patients:

- Small, direct, uncomplicated hernias.
- Incomplete, indirect reducible hernia.
- Thin patients.
- Fit for general anaesthesia.
- Patients who can safely withstand a longer duration of surgery.

9.1.2 Contraindications of TEP

- Strangulated hernia
- Massive scrotal hernia
- Previous history of pelvic lymph node resection
- Non-reducible, incarcerated inguinal hernia
- Previous history of laparoscopic herniorrhaphy
- Patients unfit for general anaesthesia

9.1.3 Pre-operative Preparation

- Patient should be explained the basic mechanism of herniation, exact disease process, and its treatment.
- Patient should be briefed about the post-operative sequelae of post-operative pain, possible temporary discoloration of the groin and scrotum, and seroma formation within the first few post-operative days.
- Patient has to be explained the various available modalities of treatment with their potential benefits and material risks.
- A written consent is mandatory after explaining to the patient and relatives the possibility

of conversion to open surgery if technical difficulties are envisaged, or in the interest of the patient's safety and well-being.

- A thorough medical history of the patient must be taken. Special measures must be taken if the patient is on drugs such as anticoagulants (due to hypertension and coronary artery disease); if the patient is on acetyl salicylic acid and related drugs (these must be discontinued at least a week before surgery); and if the patient is on oral warfarin (should be placed on heparin or its long-acting derivatives).
- Apart from the routine blood and urine investigations, a coagulation profile must always be performed, as an intractable coagulopathy is an absolute contraindication for endoscopic surgery.
- A pre-anaesthetic check-up must be done to get clearance for surgery.
- The patient is given a light dinner and kept fasting overnight.
- In male patients with an inguinal hernia, the operative area from the umbilicus to the pubic bone and laterally to the anterior superior iliac spine is shaved and prepared (Fig. 9.1).
- A catheter may be introduced when the surgery is expected to be of longer duration.
- An antibiotic prophylaxis is administered before anaesthesia.

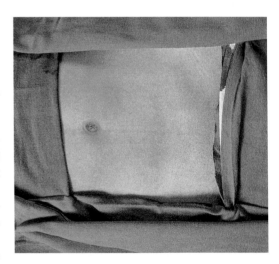

Fig. 9.1 The prepared abdomen

- After induction, complete reduction of the contents of the hernial sac is done by manual manipulation, if possible.
- Patients need to be explained about the occurrence of seromas post-operatively and their resemblance to recurrent hernia.

9.1.4 Operation Theatre Layout

1. The patient is placed in the Trendelenburg position with both the arms secured by the sides.
2. The monitor is positioned at the foot end of the patient. The surgeon stands on the side opposite the hernia with the assistant (camera-person) on the same side as the hernia (Fig. 9.2a, b).
3. In bilateral repairs, the positions are switched between the surgeon and assistant to repair the contralateral side.

9.1.5 Surgical Technique

- *Extraperitoneal access*
  An infraumblical, transverse 12 mm incision is made to expose the anterior rectus sheath. (Fig. 9.3a).
  To avoid inadvertent opening of the peritoneum, a transverse incision is made on anterior rectus sheath to one side of midline

Fig. 9.2 (**a**) OT layout for the repair of right-sided inguinal hernia; and (**b**) a patient in the OT

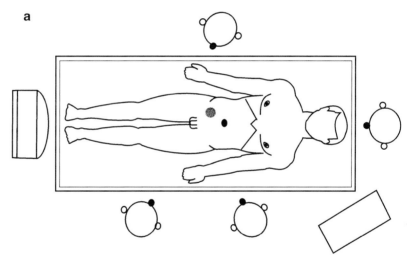

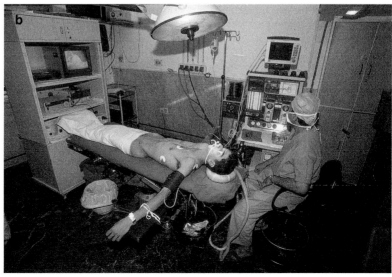

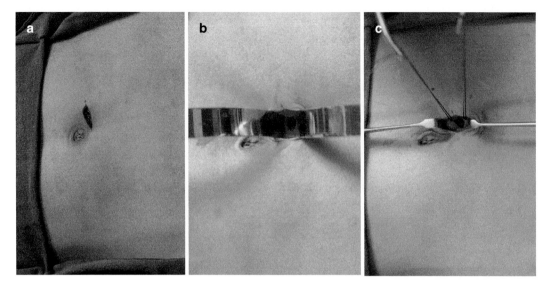

Fig. 9.3 (**a**) Subumbilical skin incision; (**b**) transverse incision on the rectus sheath; and (**c**) stay sutures

(Fig. 9.3b). The margins of incised sheath are held with stay sutures using vicryl 1-0 (Fig. 9.3c).

- *Balloon dissection of the extraperitoneal space*

  Balloon dissection has been recommended for creating the extraperitoneal space. Although various balloon trocars are available, we prefer to use our indigenous balloon for preperitoneal dissection because it is cheap and as effective as the commercial ones. We take two finger-stalls of a size 8 latex surgical glove (Fig. 9.4a) and tie one on top of the other on the tip of a 5 mm laparoscopic suction cannula (Fig. 9.4b). This is then introduced into the preperitoneal space and inflated with 100–150 mL of saline (Fig. 9.4c–f). It not only creates an initial working space but also brings about haemostasis by balloon tamponade. The balloon is deflated after 3–5 min and the cannula removed.

- *Trocar placement*

  A 10 mm Hasson cannula (blunt tip) is introduced into the preperitoneal tunnel through the infraumbilical incision and is secured with stay sutures. Insufflation is begun with the pressure setting at 12 mmHg. A pressure of >12 mmHg should be avoided as it may lead to subcutaneous emphysema.

A 10 mm 30° telescope mounted on the camera head is introduced through the subumbilical port. Next, two working ports are placed in the preperitoneal space. First, a 5 mm port is placed ~2 cm above the pubis in the midline, after which a 5 mm port is placed midway between the two placed ports (subumbilical and suprapubic) in the midline (Fig. 9.5a, b). Along with the three midline ports, additional ports, if required, can be placed lateral to the rectus muscle below the linea semicircularis. Use of ribbed trocars is preferred as the ribbing prevents repeated slippage during change of instruments.

- *Dissection of hernial sac*

  Dissection of the extraperitoneal space begins in the midline with the surgeon standing on the side opposite to the side of the hernia. Beginners are advised to use a curved dissector in place of scissors during the learning curve. Dissection of the loose areolar tissue is performed using a combination of sharp and blunt dissection supplemented by short bursts of cautery (Fig. 9.6a, b). The aim is to identify the first anatomical landmark, i.e. the pubic bone (Fig. 9.6c), which appears as a white glistening structure in the midline, marking the distal limit of dissection.

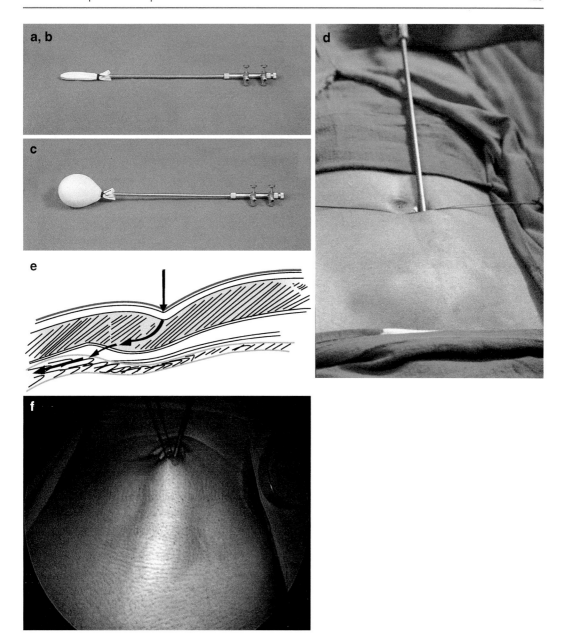

Fig. 9.4 (**a**) Suction cannula with fingerstalls; (**b**) prepared ballon; (**c**) inflated balloon; (**d**) inflated balloon in the extraperitoneal space; (**e**) Sketch of the path to the extraperitoneal space; and (**f**) creation of the preperitoneal space using an inflated balloon; the direction of the balloon cannula is towards the pubic bone

The space below the pubic bone (retropubic space/space of Retzius) is exposed for 2–3 cm to accommodate the lower margin of the mesh (Fig. 9.7a, b). Extreme caution should be exercised during this dissection as the urinary bladder and venous plexus around the prostate could be traumatized easily.

The pubic bone is traced laterally towards the side of the hernia. The next anatomical structure to be identified at this stage is the Cooper ligament (Fig. 9.7a, b).

In case of a direct hernia, it may become difficult to identify the Cooper ligament as

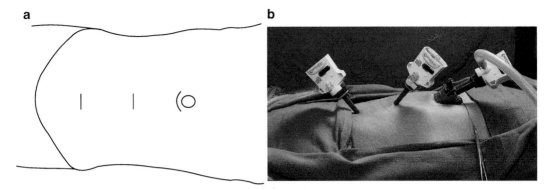

Fig. 9.5 (**a** and **b**) Port sites

this area may be occluded by the hernial sac (Fig. 9.8a, b).

An attempt is made to reduce this direct sac by traction on the peritoneal extrusion and counter-traction on the fascia transversalis. Once the complete sac is reduced, a definitive defect would be seen in the anterior abdominal wall (Fig. 9.9a, b). The anatomical landmarks that would now become visible are the Cooper ligament, the iliopubic tract, femoral ring, and inferior epigastric vessels (Fig. 9.10a, b).

It is suggested that the direct sac should be inverted and anchored to the Cooper ligament to decrease the risk of seroma formation.

The lateral extension of the pubic bone is seen in the form of a Y-shaped fork. The superior limb of the fork is formed by the ileopubic tract whereas the Cooper ligament forms the inferior limb. The femoral ring lies at the junction of the two limbs. Superior to the iliopubic tract on the anterior abdominal wall lies the direct hernial defect, which is bounded laterally by the inferior epigastric vessels and medially by the lateral border of the ipsilateral rectus muscle.

In case of a small direct hernia, ligation is not needed once the sac has been reduced. Complete reduction of the sac is ensured by identifying the margins of the defect. The spermatic cord lies immediately inferior and lateral to the inferior epigastric vessels. The lateral plane of dissection is created between the cord structures below and anterior abdominal wall above, just lateral to the inferior epigastric vessels. Flimsy adhesions

around the cord are lysed with extreme caution as the external iliac vessels lie just below the cord structures.

An indirect hernial sac is identified as a white, glistening structure lying anterolateral to the cord (Fig. 9.11a, b). An incomplete sac is dissected off the cord and completely reduced. No attempt should be made to reduce a complete sac, as extensive dissection may result in severe post-operative testicular oedema and pain. Such a sac should be separated from the cord and ligated using 2-0 vicryl (Fig. 9.12a, b). The sac is then divided distal to the ligature, leaving the distal end of the sac open. Complete reduction is ensured by identifying the reflection of the peritoneum on the spermatic cord (Fig. 9.13). The cord should be completely parietalized to the extent where the vas deferens is seen turning medially. This manoeuvre exposes the triangle of doom.

The triangle of doom is bound medially by the vas deferens and laterally by the testicular vessels. The peritoneum forms the base of the triangle and the deep inguinal ring forms the apex (Fig. 9.14a, b). Dissection should be best avoided within this triangle as the external iliac vessels are contained within it. A lipoma of the cord, if present, should be completely reduced. A large indirect sac may be ligated proximally and divided distally. In case of indirect hernia, lateral to the inferior epigastric vessels, the peritoneal sac is dissected away from the cord structures, both medially and laterally until it is completely separated and then dealt with appropriately.

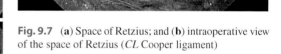

Fig. 9.7 (a) Space of Retzius; and (b) intraoperative view of the space of Retzius (*CL* Cooper ligament)

extent of dissection in this space is the psoas muscle (Fig. 9.15a, b), whereas the lateral limit is the anterior superior iliac spine, as seen from outside. Cranially, the peritoneum would be seen to be densely adherent to the abdominal wall at the level of the arcuate line. This needs sharp dissection to further expand the extraperitoneal space in a cranial direction. The extraperitoneal space is now fully prepared for mesh insertion and fixation (Fig. 9.16a, b).

In the case of bilateral hernias, the surgeon and camera assistant change sides and a similar dissection is performed on the opposite side.

- *Mesh preparation and placement*
  The minimum size of the polypropylene mesh to be used on each side should not be less than 15 cm × 13 cm (Fig. 9.17a). The mesh should be taken out of its packaging under absolutely

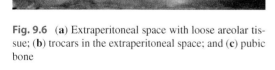

Fig. 9.6 (a) Extraperitoneal space with loose areolar tissue; (b) trocars in the extraperitoneal space; and (c) pubic bone

Adequate space has to be created lateral to the cord structures as the lateral part of the mesh would lie in this space. This space contains only loose areolar tissue, which is completely divided using sharp and blunt dissection. The inferior

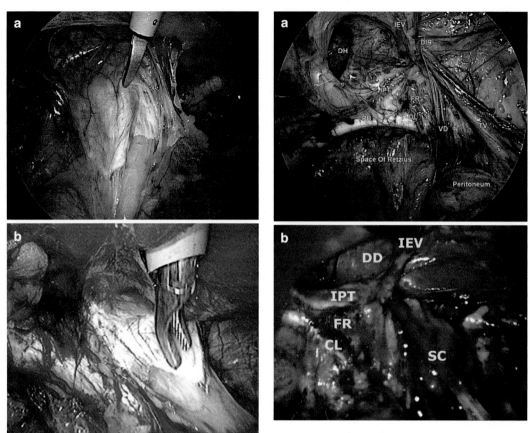

Fig. 9.8 (**a**) Direct sac; and (**b**) intraoperative view of a direct hernia

Fig. 9.10 (**a**) Anatomical landmarks seen after reduction of a direct sac; and (**b**) Intraoperative view of the structures seen after reduction of a direct sac (*CL* Cooper ligament; *DD* direct defect; *FR* femoral ring; *IPT* iliopubic tract; *IEV* inferior epigastric vessels; *SC* spermatic cord)

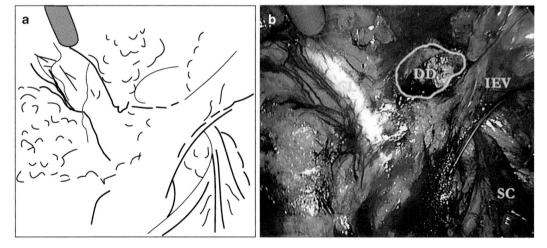

Fig. 9.9 (**a**) Appearance after reduction of a direct sac; and (**b**) operative view after reduction of a direct sac (*CL* Cooper ligament; *DD* direct defect; *IEV* inferior epigastric vessels; *SC* spermatic cord)

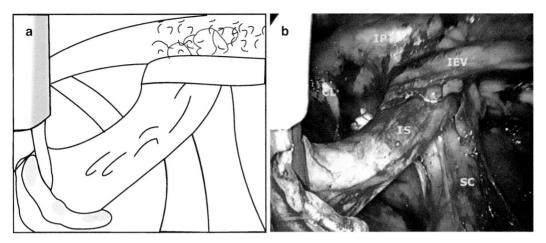

Fig. 9.11 (**a**) Indirect sac dissected; and (**b**) Laparoscopic view of the dissected indirect sac (*CL* Cooper ligament; *IPT* iliopubic tract; *IEV* inferior epigastric vessels; *SC* spermatic cord; *IS* Indirect sac)

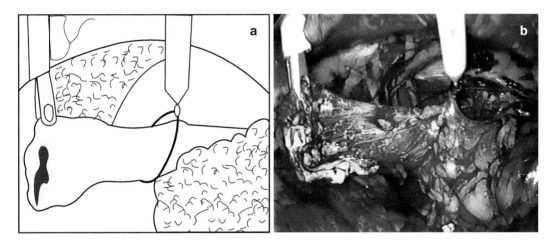

Fig. 9.12 (**a**) Transected and ligated indirect sac; and (**b**) Endoscopic view of the transected and ligated indirect sac

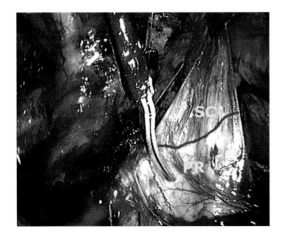

Fig. 9.13 Peritoneal reflection on the spermatic cord (*SC* spermatic cord; *PR* peritoneal reflection)

sterile conditions just before introduction into the site. To handle a mesh of this size in the restricted preperitoneal space is not easy. We have developed a technique of introducing a rolled mesh in this space for easy handling and accurate fixation.

The mesh is rolled like a carpet to two-thirds of its length, leaving 5 cm free. Two stay sutures are tied on the roll using an absorbable suture (Vicryl 2-0) 3 cm away from the margins to keep the rolled mesh in position (Fig. 9.17b, c).

The rolled mesh is then held with a 5 mm grasper and introduced into the preperitoneal space through the 10 mm subumbilical port.

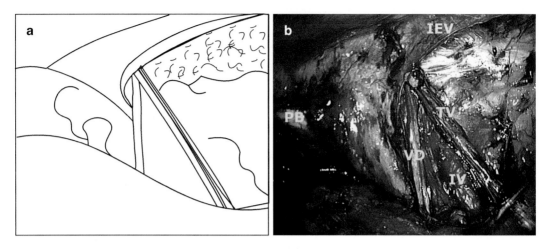

Fig. 9.14 (**a**) Triangle of doom; and (**b**) Laparoscopic view of the triangle of doom (*PB* pubic bone; *IEV* inferior epigastric vessels; *TV* testicular vessels; *VD* vas deferens; *IV* iliac vessels)

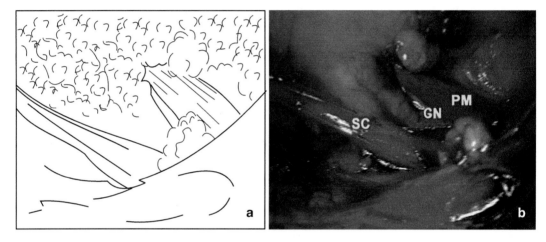

Fig. 9.15 (**a**) Psoas muscle with femoral branch of genitofemoral nerve; and (**b**) endoscopic view of the psoas muscle with femoral branch of genitofemoral nerve (*SC* spermatic cord; *GN* genitofemoral nerve; *PM* psoas muscle)

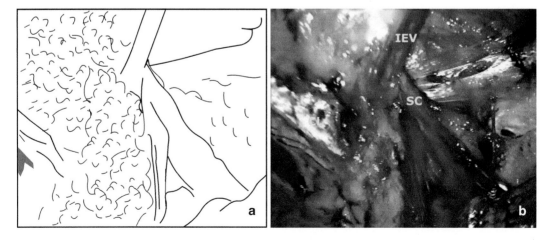

Fig. 9.16 (**a**) Completely dissected right extraperitoneal space; and (**b**) intraoperative view of the completely dissected right extraperitoneal space (*SC* spermatic cord; *CL* Cooper ligament; *IEV* inferior epigastric vessels)

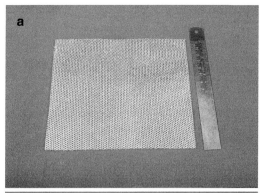

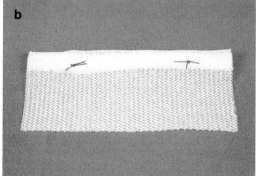

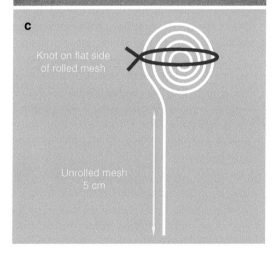

Fig. 9.17 (**a**) 15 × 15 cm polypropylene mesh; (**b**) rolled mesh; and (**c**) sheath of roll

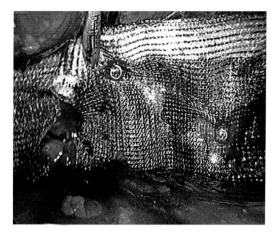

Fig. 9.18 Two-point fixation of the mesh

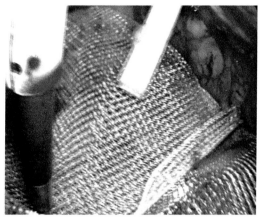

Fig. 9.19 Unrolled mesh after cutting the stay sutures

- *Mesh fixation*

  The mesh is placed such that the medial margin extends for 2–3 cm beyond the midline and 2–3 cm below the pubic bone inferomedially. Laterally, the inferior margin of the mesh should lie over the psoas muscle. It should be ensured that no extraperitoneal fat lies beneath the lower margin of the mesh. The fold of the peritoneum should lie below the inferior margin of the mesh.

  The mesh is fixed at two places on the Cooper ligament using a 5 mm fixation device—ProTack™ (Autosuture, Tyco Healthcare, US Surgicals, Norwalk, CT, USA; Fig. 9.18). No fixation should be done laterally for fear of cutaneous nerve entrapment. In the case of bilateral hernias, a similar fixation of the mesh is done on the opposite side with a 2–3 cm overlap in the midline.

  After removing the stay sutures, the mesh is unrolled to lie within the extraperitoneal space (Fig. 9.19). After keeping the unrolled mesh in position, CO_2 is exsufflated and the trocars are removed. As the extraperitoneal space is an artificial space, it gets obliterated after exsufflation of CO_2. It should be ensured that the mesh lies flat at the time of exsufflation.

- *Wound closure*
  After removal of the Hasson trocar from the subumbilical port, the two stay sutures on the anterior rectus sheath are tied to each other, ensuring complete sheath closure. The skin of all three ports is closed using skin clips/sutures, depending on the surgeon's choice. Complete exsufflation of CO_2 from the extraperitoneal space must be ensured before wound closure.

9.1.6 Post-operative Care

- Patients are ambulated once fully conscious.
- Patients are encouraged to get up and walk around on the same day.
- Clear fluids are given immediately on recovery from anaesthesia. The quantity of oral liquids is gradually increased.
- Patients are discharged the next morning on a normal diet.
- Oral analgesics are administered for 3 days post-operatively. Injectable diclofenac is administered only on demand.
- All port sites are covered with waterproof dressings and patients are permitted to have a shower.
- No restriction on normal physical activity is advised as it is a 'tension-free' repair.
- Wound stitches/clips are removed on the first post-operative visit, i.e. at 1 week post-surgery.

9.1.7 Post-operative Complications

The complication of laparoscopic hernia repair can be summarized as follows:

1. Seroma/haematoma—This is the most common complication of TEP repair. The incidence varies from 5 to 25% [2]. Seroma usually occurs in a large hernia, and more often in an indirect than a direct hernia. Division of the sac of an indirect hernia without excessive dissection of the sac from the cord structures decreases the incidence of cord haematoma and seroma formation. In direct hernia, the transversalis fascia can be pulled into the extraperitoneal space and fixed over the pubic bone to decrease the incidence of seroma formation. If a seroma develops, it usually subsides automatically in 2–6 weeks. Aspiration is best avoided and the patient should be reassured. In rare cases in which aspiration is required, it should be performed under aseptic conditions as it may lead to contamination and chances of mesh infection. An ultrasound should be performed to confirm the diagnosis before performing aspiration.

2. Neuralgia—This is usually transient. Neuralgic pain over the lateral aspect of the thigh is the commonest. Pain may also be referred to the knee joint. Neuralgia is caused by irritation of the genitofemoral nerve and/or lateral cutaneous nerve of the thigh, and the intermediate cutaneous branch of the femoral nerve. The irritation can be due to the mesh placed in that region or entrapment of the nerve in the fixation device (tacks used for staples). To minimize the incidence of neuralgia, the fascia over the psoas muscle should not be dissected and the mesh should only be fixed medially. No staples should be applied lateral to the cord structures. If the mesh has to be fixed laterally (in the case of a large, indirect hernia) it should be fixed on the anterior abdominal wall above the iliopubic tract.

3. Testicular swelling and pain—This is usually present in the immediate post-operative period and is caused by excessive dissection of the sac of an indirect hernia from the cord structures. This should be avoided. Scrotal support for a few days is of help, although the condition usually subsides spontaneously.

4. Wound infection—The incidence of infection is usually low in the case of TEP repair. Occasionally, there may be slight discharge from the subumbilical port because of a small haematoma in the area. It usually subsides by drainage of the haematoma and use of antiseptic dressings.

5. Mesh infection—Mesh infection is a rare but serious complication of TEP repair [3]. The iso-

lated microflora in mesh-related infections is usually associated with the following bacteria: *Staphylococcus* species, especially *S. aureus*; *Streptococcus* species, including group B streptococci; and Gram-negative (mainly enterobacteriaceae) and anaerobic bacteria [6]. In addition to these organisms, mesh infections with pathogenic, waterborne atypical mycobacteria are being recognized in recent years (Ref). These organisms include three major pathogenic species: *Mycobacterium fortuitum*, *Mycobacterium chelonae* and *Mycobacterium abscessus*. *M. chelonae* is known to cause nosocomial skin and soft-tissue infections following contaminated injections, surgical procedures and laparoscopic surgery. The source of infection is contamination of the wound directly or indirectly with colonized tap water. Most cases of mesh infections after laparoscopic surgery can be attributed to deficiencies in the sterilization technique.

In early cases of infection, patients present with fever, chills or rigor, focal tenderness, erythema and swelling. Late infections are more indolent and presentations are varied. Symptoms can be chronic, recurrent or totally absent until the progression of sepsis. Sinus formation, swelling, pain or fever of unknown etiology may be encountered. The treatment of mesh infections initially involves administration of antibiotics, local wound care, and drainage. In deep-seated mesh infections, prolonged antibiotic treatment in combination with percutaneous or open drainage has been reported to be effective in restraining the infectious process [2]. However, in the presence of an extensive infection, caused by biofilm formation and limited penetration of the drug in the area, mesh removal and surgical cleaning of the wound provide the best possible treatment to eradicate infection. It should be emphasized that early surgical intervention is desirable in the presence of extensive infection and abscess formation.

6. Osteitis pubis—It is a rare but reported complication after TEP repair. It can be an extremely disabling condition with severe pain and persistent symptoms after surgery. The use of penetrating fixation devices and excessive cautery on the pubic bone should be avoided. Osteitis pubis presents as persistent pain over the pubic bone, which generally settles with anti-inflammatory drugs.

7. Recurrence—Recurrence after endoscopic hernia repair is low [7]. Factors causing recurrence in the early post-operative period are as follows:
   (a) Use of a small-sized mesh
   (b) Migration or folding of the mesh into the defect
   (c) Displacement of the mesh by a haematoma
   (d) Folding of the mesh
   (e) Missed indirect sac in the case of a direct hernia
   (f) Inadequate dissection of the extraperitoneal space.

8. The incidence of recurrence can be reduced by taking the following precautions:
   (a) Using a mesh that is 15 cm × 13 cm on both sides
   (b) Fixing the mesh medially to the Cooper ligament
   (c) Ensuring complete proximal dissection of the peritoneum from the spermatic cord
   (d) Maintaining proper haemostasis to prevent haematoma formation
   (e) Adequate training of surgeons.

9.2 Summary

- Laparoscopic surgery for inguinal hernia is an advanced laparoscopic procedure. A surgeon should first have adequate experience of basic laparoscopic procedures before attempting a laparoscopic hernia repair.
- A complete knowledge of the laparoscopic anatomy of the preperitoneal space is an important prerequisite for performing a TEP repair.
- For beginners, proper selection of a case is important. A small, direct, right inguinal hernia is ideal.
- Creation of the preperitoneal space is the most important step and all necessary precautions should be taken.

- Accessing and enlarging the preperitoneal space helps in creating adequate space and ensuring proper haemostasis.
- The urinary bladder should be voided before surgery.
- In the case of a direct inguinal hernia, an indirect sac should always be looked for along the cord structures and treated accordingly.
- In the case of an indirect hernia, minimum dissection should be performed while separating the sac from the cord structures.
- The peritoneum should be well reflected proximally from the cord structures and laterally from the psoas muscle so that the mesh can be placed accurately.
- A mesh of at least 15 cm × 13 cm should be used.
- The mesh should be fixed medially over the Cooper ligament. This prevents migration and rolling of the mesh, which can cause recurrence of a hernia after surgery.
- Lateral fixation below the iliopubic tract should be avoided, as it may cause neuralgia.

Key Points
- The proper access between fascia transversalis and peritoneum is important.
- Pubic bone is the first landmark in the midline, which needs to be identified at the start of dissection.
- As the dissection proceeds laterally to pubic bone, one should be aware of the presence of 'corona mortis'.

- Inferior epigastric vessels should be identified on roof when creating lateral space.
- Dissect laterally till the lateral border of psoas muscle to create adequate space.
- While parietalization, caution should be exercised while dissecting the triangle of Doom and Bendavid circle.

References

1. Garren MJ. Laparoscopic inguinal hernia repair total extraperitoneal (TEP) approach. In: Illustrative handbook of general surgery. Berlin: Springer International; 2016. p. 539–45.
2. Chowbey P. Endoscopic repair of abdominal wall hernias. Delhi: Byword Books Private Limited; 2012.
3. Konik RD, Narh-Martey P, Bogen G. Recurrence of an inguinal hernia containing the dome of the bladder following laparoscopic repair with mesh: a case report. Int J Surg Case Rep. 2016;25:218–20.
4. Shah T, Shah S, Joshi BR, Karkee RJ, Gupta RK. Total extraperitoneal approach in large inguino-scrotal hernias: an institutional approach. J Soc Surg Nepal. 2016;18(3):51.
5. Utiyama EM, Damous SH, Tanaka EY, Yoo JH, de Miranda JS, Ushinohama AZ, Faro MP, Birolini CA. Early assessment of bilateral inguinal hernia repair: a comparison between the laparoscopic total extraperitoneal and Stoppa approaches. J Minim Access Surg. 2016;12(3):271.
6. Chowbey PK, Khullar R, Sharma A, Soni V, Baijal M, Garg N, Najma K. Laparoscopic management of infected mesh after laparoscopic inguinal hernia repair. Surg Laparosc Endosc Percutan Tech. 2015;25(2):125–8. https://doi.org/10.1097/SLE.0000000000000056.
7. Gutlic N, Rogmark P, Nordin P, Petersson U, Montgomery A. Impact of mesh fixation on chronic pain in total extraperitoneal inguinal hernia repair (TEP): a nationwide register-based study. Ann Surg. 2016;263(6):1199–206.

Transabdominal Pre-peritoneal (TAPP) Repair for Groin Hernias

10

George Pei Cheung Yang

10.1 Transabdominal Pre-peritoneal Groin Hernia Repair

Transabdominal pre-peritoneal (TAPP) groin hernia repair is one of the two mature techniques of laparoscopic groin hernia repair. Compared to TEP, TAPP provides an easier correlation between the pre-peritoneal and peritoneal anatomy for the surgeon. It involves intraperitoneal diagnostic laparoscopy, incision of the peritoneum to gain access to the pre-peritoneal space, creation of the peritoneal flap, reduction of the groin hernia and its sac, placement of the synthetic mesh, and closure of the peritoneal flap. The mesh should not come into contact with the bowel. Therefore any defect in the peritoneal flap should be closed properly to avoid bowel adhesion and fistulation to the mesh. (Fig. 10.1).

10.2 Operative Set-Up, Positioning, and Ports Placement

The patient is placed in supine position. In majority of cases, pre-operative voiding is all that is necessary to prevent the bladder from obstructing

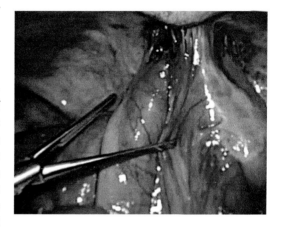

Fig. 10.1 Bowel adhesion to mesh leading to bowel obstruction after previous laparoscopic groin hernia repair

the operative field. For those patients with history of cystitis, outflow obstruction like prostatic hypertrophy, or those with previous pelvic irradiation, foley catheter should be considered to better empty the bladder to improve operative field vision. Also with these patients the surgeon should keep in mind that there might be bladder adhesion to the anterior abdominal wall such that caution should be taken during dissection to avoid bladder injury.

The monitor screen should be place at the patient's foot end, with the surgeon standing on the contralateral side of the hernia. The assistant to hold the laparoscope can either stand behind the surgeon or on the opposite side. The anesthetist should be reminded to position the external tubing of the laryngeal mask on the angle of the

G. P. C. Yang (✉)
Hong Kong Adventist Hospital,
Happy Valley, Hong Kong
e-mail: george.yang@hkah.org.hk

© Springer Nature India Private Limited 2020
P. Chowbey, D. Lomanto (eds.), *Techniques of Abdominal Wall Hernia Repair*,
https://doi.org/10.1007/978-81-322-3944-4_10

patient's mouth to avoid collusion between the tubbing and the cable of the laparoscope.

Under general anesthesia, with the patient supine and in Trendelenburg position 30° or so, the first port is inserted at subumbilicus for diagnostic laparoscopy. Pneumoperitoneum is created with carbon dioxide generally at 12–15 mmHg pressure.

The operation can be performed with the three ports approach or single port approach depending on the surgeon's preference. The benefit of single port trans-umbilical approach is only for postoperative cosmetic result. The operative steps and attentions are exactly the same.

With the three ports approach, one can consider the two different methods (Fig. 10.2). On the right side, the laparoscope is placed through the mid-clavicular line port allowing the surgeon to have a better vision on the retropubic space of retzius. On the left side, the laparoscope is placed through the subumbilical port with two working trocars on either side. This allows the surgeon to

perform repair on both sides with these three ports, but the vision at the retropubic space of retzius may be obscured by the peritoneum and the median umbilical ligament. With a 30° laparoscope one may rotate the scope to obtain a better vision.

10.3 TAPP Consist of the Following Operative Steps

Diagnostic peritoneal laparoscopy is one of the main advantages of laparoscopic hernia repair. It allows the surgeon to correctly identify the site and number of any hernia in the groin region. It is not uncommon for a patient especially female to have additional ipsilateral and/or bilateral groin hernia apart from the clinically obvious one. Therefore laparoscopic repair should be offered for female patients [1]. Figure 10.3 shows an elderly lady presented with left femoral hernia,

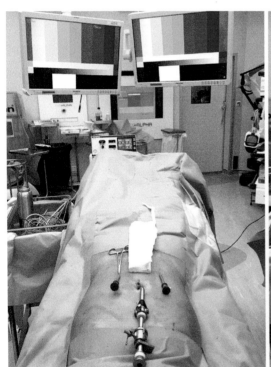
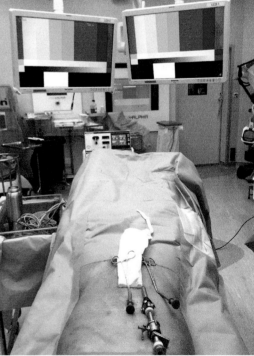

Fig. 10.2 Ports placement for TAPP: Left—camera port at subumbilical wound with two working ports one on each side; Right—camera port at mid-clavicular line, one working port at subumbilical wound and another one lateral to the camera port

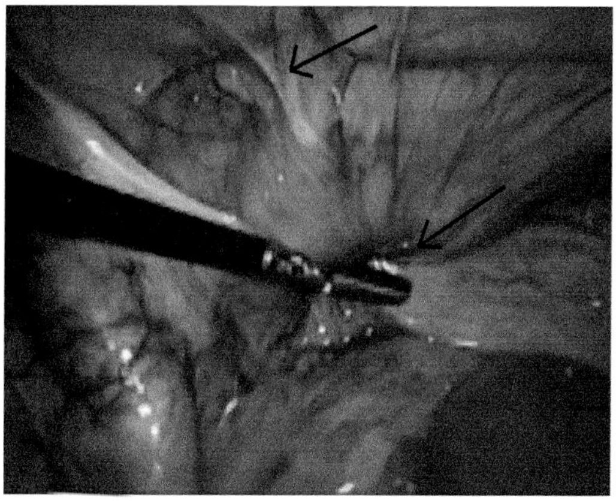

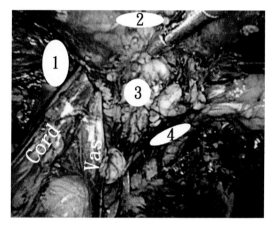

Fig. 10.3 Left femoral and obturator hernia

Fig. 10.4 1 indirect inguinal; 2 direct inguinal; 3 femoral; 4 obturator hernias

with an additional left obturator hernia. Laparoscopic preperitoneal mesh placement not only allows intra-abdominal pressure to spread out evenly over the mesh, it also allows the mesh to cover all myopectineal orifices where potential hernia might occur (Fig. 10.4). Currently in both EHS and Asian hernia guidelines [1, 2], laparoscopic repair is recommended for bilateral inguinal hernia, recurrent inguinal hernia from previous open anterior repair, and female patients.

The incision of the peritoneum and creation of the peritoneal flap is the next step. Whether to start medial or lateral to the medial umbilical ligament depends on the surgeon's preference. With this step, it is vital to first identify the inferior epigastric vessels (the lateral umbilical fold) to avoid injury to this vessel, which can result with unnecessary bleeding. Some surgeons will create a high flap and some prefer a low flap. Nonetheless, the peritoneal flap should be large enough not only to allow proper placement of the synthetic mesh but also to allow 1–2 cm gap caudally to avoid exposing the edge of the mesh after closure of the peritoneal flap. If the flap is too low with limited pre-peritoneal space, the surgeon will be forced to shift the mesh down or crumble up the mesh in order to accommodate it. This leads to suboptimal mesh positioning and placement. For high flap the incision should start about 5 cm below the level of umbilicus.

During dissection the surgeon should have clear understanding of the pre-peritoneal anatomy in order to avoid injury to vessels and nerves, especially the structures that lie in the triangle of doom and the triangle of pain. Structures including the inferior epigastric vessels and its origin from the external iliac artery and vein, transverse vessels over the pubic arch the "corona mortis," the genitofemoral nerve and its medial genital branch, and the lateral femoral cutaneous nerve. The handling of the spermatic cord and vas deferens require caution to avoid direct trauma to these structures and their blood supply, in order to prevent postoperative cord structures related complications like testicular ptosis, testicular atrophy, dysejaculation, and infertility.

Mesh placement is one of the vital elements in determining the success of repair in the long term. While the debate on mesh fixation or not is forever running, most surgeons agreed that for high-risk hernia it will be better to fix the mesh [3–7]. These include M1-3 hernia (EHS Classification) [8], inguinoscrotal hernia, and sliding hernia. Generally the goals of mesh fixation are first to avoid migration of the mesh, and secondly to avoid folding up of the mesh. Not uncommonly we found recurrence after previous laparoscopic repair caused by folding up of the mesh, either of its inferior medial (Fig. 10.5) or inferior lateral (Fig. 10.6) part, which allow the hernia to recur underneath the mesh. These areas covered by the mesh also contain vital

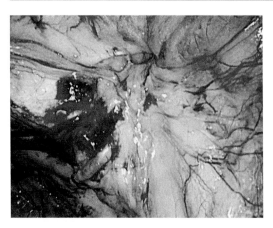

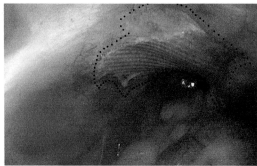

Fig. 10.7 Dotted line outlines the old mesh

Fig. 10.5 Vascular triangle

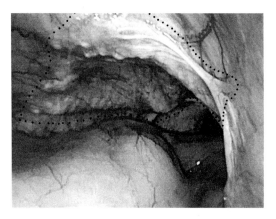

Fig. 10.6 Dotted line outlines the old mesh

structure like the iliac vessels and major nerves (triangle of pain and triangle of doom). Nonpenetrating type of fixation like biocompatible glue or self-gripping mesh may be superior in these areas to avoid injury to the great vessels and nerve. Fixing the mesh to the rectus muscle probably offers no advantages unless in M3 hernia. For bilateral M1-3 hernia, the left and right meshes should overlap each other in the midline. In male the spermatic cord may also cause problem by slinging up the medial inferior part of the mesh, which may allow hernia to slip through in the future. It is therefore important to properly lay the mesh down against the psoas muscle and external iliac vessels. Alternatively there are meshes available in the market designed to have a slit open lateral end with

proper overlapping laterally. This allows the surgeon to place the inferior lateral slip of the mesh posterior to the spermatic cord to avoid the mesh being sling up by the cord (Fig. 10.7).

After proper placement of the mesh, the peritoneal flap is then closed. It can be closed with tacker/ staple devise like absorbable tackers or running suture. It is again important to note the position of the inferior epigastric vessel in order to avoid injury. Injuring this vessel at this stage without being noticed by the surgeon may lead to significant bleeding, because the large perperitoneal space can accommodate large volume of blood. If using tacker/staple to close the peritoneum, it is important to have less than 1 cm gap between each tacker/staple in order to reduce the chance of bowel herniating into the peritoneal flap. Running suture may be a better alternative [9].

Towards the end of the operation, it is strongly advised to check the peritoneal flap for proper closure and for any defect which may expose the mesh. These defects in the peritoneal flap should all be closed by suture under direct vision rather than tackers to avoid injury to the vessel and nerve behind the flap. There is no study to show how small a size of peritoneal defect will not cause problem such as bowel adhesion or fistulation. In my opinion, if you can see the mesh through the defect it should be closed. Mesh-related bowel adhesion and fistulation are major morbidities which are difficult to manage and treat (Fig. 10.1).

10.4   Indication for TAPP

As with TEP, TAPP should only be consider when expertise including surgeon and supporting nursing staffs are available, as well as equipment and mesh. For bilateral groin hernia, pelvic floor hernia (Fig. 10.8), recurrent hernia after previous open anterior repair, female patients with groin hernia, TAPP can be considered as an alternative to TEP repair. Laparoscopic repair (TEP/TAPP) should be seriously considered for patients with pelvic floor hernia because of the risk of bilateral occurrence and better coverage and positioning of the mesh.

For complex groin hernia like sliding inguinal hernia (Fig. 10.9), incompletely reduced groin hernia, groin hernia with adhesion around the ori-

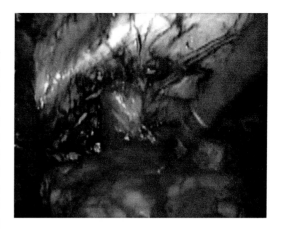

Fig. 10.10 Obturator hernia

fice, or when difficulty arises during TEP repair, TAPP should be the technique of choice. It is because TAPP allows the surgeon to have better correlation between the pre-peritoneal and peritoneal condition, such that inadvertent injury can be avoided to the herniate content (Fig. 10.10).

10.5   Postoperative Complications

10.5.1 Recurrence

Proper placement of mesh especially its inferior flap is important to prevent folding up of the mesh and recurrence. Inadequate lateral coverage of the hernia orifice increases the risk of recurrence because the mesh will shrink by 20–50% over time which may re-expose the hernia orifice. Diagnostic laparoscopy is vital to identify concurrent ipsilateral hernia to prevent recurrence (Figs. 10.11 and 10.12).

10.5.2 Bleeding

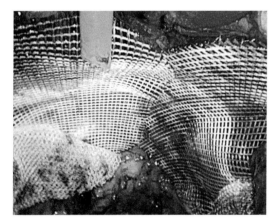

Fig. 10.8 Overlapping mesh

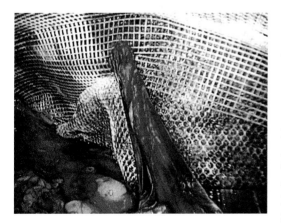

Fig. 10.9 Cord through mesh

Major bleeding usually comes from inferior epigastric vessel or pubic branches veins injury. Caution during dissection and early identification of these vessels is the key to prevent injury. Patients who are on anticoagulation should be identified pre-operatively and the anticoagulation medication adequately stopped before the

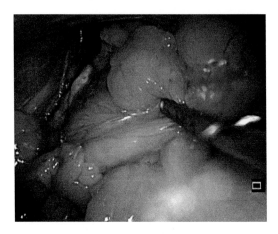

Fig. 10.11 Sliding right indirect inguinal hernia

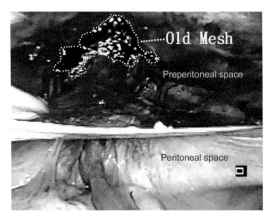

Fig. 10.12 TAPP view allows correlation reference between pre-peritoneal structures with peritoneal condition

operation. They should be warned of possible bruising that may track down into the scrotum after the operation.

10.5.3 Seroma

Most surgeons will agree that seroma is present in all patients after laparoscopic groin hernia repair; the size determines its clinical presentation. It is considered as a normal physiological body response to a dead space which was previously occupied by the hernia. Almost all seromas will resolve over several months' time. It is recommended not to aspirate asymptomatic seroma which may increase the risk of infection [2, 10].

10.5.4 Mesh Infection

Wound infection in laparoscopic repair is extremely rare, so is mesh infection. Prophylactic intravenous antibiotic is not required from evidence base [1, 2, 11], but nonetheless it is still commonly given by many surgeons. What is more important is the handling of the mesh during surgery. The surgeon's gloves should be changed when it comes to the placement of the mesh. The surgeon should employ a non-touch technique, keeping the mesh in the factory sterile packing if possible, using forceps to grasp it, removing from the packing, and placing it through the 10 mm trocar.

10.5.5 Postoperative Pain

Postoperative pain should be minimal and mostly subside completely within 1–2 weeks. Most patients complain of swollen sensation of the lower abdominal wall and scrotum, this also should subside completely over 1–2 weeks postoperatively.

To minimize the risk of chronic pain, tacker should be avoided especially inferior to the pectineal line (Triangle of pain). Alternatively anatomical mesh, self-adhesive mesh, or non-traumatic fixation with glue can be an alternative.

10.6 Special Considerations

10.6.1 Contraindication for TAPP

TAPP requires the patient to undergo general anesthesia and pneumoperitoneum, so for those who are not suitable for general anesthesia and pneumoperitoneum open groin hernia repair should be considered.

Age itself should not be a contraindication [2], since even for 90-year-olds, as long as their cardiac function is optimal, laparoscopic groin hernia repair can be performed safely.

Previous abdominal surgery no longer is an absolute contraindication, because of the advancement in laparoscopic surgical technique and improvement in endoscopic vision technology. More and more laparoscopic surgeries are being performed for patients who had previous open abdominal surgery, such as laparoscopic repair of incisional hernia.

Previous pelvic irradiation may cause problem because of the induced fibrosis and adhesion in the pelvis. One should consider open repair if there is dense adhesion around the iliac vessel and myopectineal orifices in the pre-peritoneal space.

10.7 Strangulated and Incarcerated Groin Hernia

This is no longer a contraindication for laparoscopic repair. However for these conditions the surgeon should be experienced. Diagnostic laparoscopy should be performed first to clearly identify the site of strangulation and whether there is any other concurrent hernia present in the ipsilateral or contralateral side. Having the strangulated hernia reduced, the surgeon can proceed to laparoscopic repair. Reduction of the strangulated herniated content should be done very carefully; our experience showed that external compression under laparoscopic guidance may be safer than to rely only on laparoscopic pulling by grasping instrument, which may cause bowel injury. The stretching and distension of the abdominal wall by pneumoperitoneum, together with the external compression of the herniated content to decrease its oedema, will allow most of the strangulated hernia to be reduced. Some author suggested incising the posterior fascia to release the strangulated content [12]; this should be done by an expert in this field with extreme caution. Compared to open repair for strangulated hernia, laparoscopic repair results in lower wound infection rate, relatively lower laparotomy, and lower bowel resection rate. The use of mesh in these conditions did not show any increase in mesh infection rate. In open repair for strangulated hernia many surgeons will also choose Lichtenstein repair [13].

Another frequently asked question for laparoscopic repair in strangulated or incarcerated groin hernia is shall we perform TAPP or TEP after reduction of the strangulated content? I would suggest TEP, because in TAPP, having the dissecting instruments especially endoscopic scissor goes through the port in and out of peritoneum many times with distended bowel imposes a higher risk of injury to the bowel. Incising and closing the peritoneum in TAPP with the presence of distended bowel also creates additional risk. So after reduction of the strangulated herniate content, if the surgeon proceeds to TEP repair, it seems to be safer.

10.8 Conclusion

Laparoscopic groin hernia repair is a technically demanding operation; it requires a thorough understanding of the pre-peritoneal anatomy. The attitude to the operation, together with the handling and placement of mesh, plays a vital role in determining the success of the surgery. It has great benefits in managing recurrent, bilateral, and pelvic floor hernias. Especially for pelvic floor hernia like femoral and obturator hernias, the undoubtable superiority of diagnostic laparoscopy plus the accurate placement of mesh in the pre-peritoneal space to cover all potential hernia orifices in the groin make it the technique of choice. A surgeon should not only acquire one technique, both TAPP and TEP should be acquired and under certain situations one should adjust their approach accordingly.

References

1. Simons MP, Aufenacker, Bay-Nielsen M, Bouillot JL, Campanelli G, Conze J, Lange D, Fortelny R, Heikkinen T, Kingsnorth A, Kukleta J, Morales-Conde S, Nordin P, Schumpelick V, Smedberg S, Smietanski M, Weber G, Miserez M. European Hernia Society guidelines on the treatment of inguinal hernia in adult patients. Hernia. 2009;13:343–403.
2. Lomanto D, Cheah WK, Faylona JM, Huang CS, Lohsiriwat D, Maleachi A, Yang GPC, Li MKW, Tumtavitikul S, Sharma A, Hartung RU, Choi YB, Sutedja B. Inguinal hernia repair: toward asian guidelines. Asian J Endosc Surg. 2015;8:16–23.

3. Khajanchee YS, Urbach DR, Swanstrom LL, et al. Outcomes of laparoscopic herniorrhaphy without fixation of mesh to the abdominal wall. Surg Endosc. 2001;15:1102–7.

4. Kathouda N, Mavor E, Friedlander MH, et al. Use of fibrin sealant for prosthetic mesh fixation laparoscopic extraperitoneal inguinal hernia repair. Ann Surg. 2001;233(1):18–25.

5. Lau H. Fibrin sealant versus mechanical stapling for mesh fixation during endoscopic extraperitoneal inguinal hernioplasty: a randomized prospective trial. Ann Surg. 2005;242(5):670–5.

6. Lovisetto F, Zonta S, Rota E, et al. Use of human fibrin glue (Tissucol) versus staples for mesh fixation in laparoscopic transabdominal perperitoneal hernioplasty: a prospective randomized study. Ann Surg. 2007;245(2):222–31.

7. Olmi S, Scaini A, Erba L, et al. Quantification of pain in laparoscopic transabdominal preperitoneal (TAPP) inguinal hernioplasty identifies marked difference between prosthesis fixation system. Surgery. 2007;142(1):40–6.

8. Miserez M, Alexandre JH, Campanelli G, Corcione F, Cuccurullo D, Hidalgo Pascual M, Hoeferlin A, Kingsnorth AN, Mandala V, Palot JP, Schumpelick V, Simmermacher HK, Stoppa R, Falment JB. The European hernia society groin hernia classification: simple and easy to remember. Hernia. 2007;11:113–6.

9. Kapiris SA, Brough WA, Royston CMS, et al. Laparoscopic transabdominal preperiotneal TAPP hernia repair. A 7-year two-center experience in 3017 patients. Surg Endosc. 2001;15:972–5.

10. Peiper C, Conze J, Ponschek N, et al. Value of subcutaneous drainage in repair of primary inguinal hernia. A prospective randomized study of 100 cases. Chirurg. 1997;68:63–7.

11. McCormack K, Wake B, et al. Transabdominal preperitoneal (TAPP) versus totally extraperitoneal (TEP) laparoscopic techniques for inguinal hernia repair: a systematic review. Cochrane Database Syst Rev. 2005;25(1):CD004703.

12. Ferzli G, Shapiro K, Chaudry F, et al. Laparoscopic extraperitoneal approach to acutely incarcerated inguinal hernia. Surg Endosc. 2004;18:228–31.

13. Yang GPC, Chan CTY, Lai ECH, et al. Laparoscopic versus open repair for strangulated groin hernias: 188 cases over 4 years. Asian J Endosc Surg. 2012;5(3):131–7. ISSN 1758-5902.

Open and Laparoscopic Repair of Femoral Hernia

11

Deepraj S. Bhandarkar

11.1 Introduction

A femoral hernia is the protrusion of the preperitoneal fat, bladder or a peritoneal sac through the femoral ring, which is bounded superiorly by the iliopubic tract, inferiorly by Cooper ligament, laterally by the femoral vein, and medially by the junction of the iliopubic tract and the lacunar ligament (Fig. 11.1). A femoral hernia is commonly seen in patients between ages of 40 and 70 years, and is 2–5 times more common in women than in men. Typically, it produces a bulge below the inguinal ligament but in some cases the sac may ascend in a cephalad direction resulting in a swelling above the inguinal ligament. Alternately it presents with incarceration and produces a painful groin swelling in conjunction with signs of intestinal obstruction. Though physical examination remains the mainstay of diagnosis of femoral hernias, the sensitivity and positive predictive value of physical examination has been shown to be 50% and 37.5%, respectively [1].

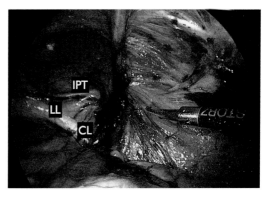

Fig. 11.1 Laparoscopic view showing area of the femoral ring. *IPT* iliopubic tract, *CL* Cooper's ligament and *LL* lacunar ligament

11.2 Indications for Surgery

All patients with diagnosed femoral hernias should be advised elective repair. The reason for this is twofold. Firstly, femoral hernias are associated with a higher risk of developing complications than inguinal hernias. In one study, the rates of strangulation were 22% and 45% at 3 and 21 months after diagnosis for femoral hernias, compared with 2.8% and 4.5% for inguinal hernias [1]. Secondly, strangulation of a femoral hernia necessitates a bowel resection in 23% [2] (as compared to 5% of inguinal hernias) and the mortality of the emergency surgery is 6–23% [3].

D. S. Bhandarkar (✉)
Department of Minimal Access Surgery, Hinduja Hospital, Mumbai, Maharashtra, India

11.3 Contraindications

There are no contraindications to the performance of surgical repair of femoral hernia as even in those with significant co-morbidity the surgery can be undertaken safely under local anaesthesia. Elective repair of femoral hernia during pregnancy is generally contraindicated and this is best carried out 4–6 weeks postpartum after the abdominal wall regains its normal tone. In patients with active groin infection or systemic sepsis requiring surgery, a non-mesh repair can be safely undertaken.

11.4 Approaches to Repair of Femoral Hernia

The three approaches to repair of a femoral hernia are (a) femoral, (b) inguinal and (c) preperitoneal. A laparoscopic repair via a trans-abdominal pre-peritoneal (TAPP) or a totally extraperitoneal (TEP) route constitutes a variant of the preperitoneal approach. Each technique has its distinct advantages and disadvantages and the factors determining the choice include familiarity of the surgeon with a particular technique, patient's general condition, co-morbidities, elective versus emergent situation and presence/suspicion of strangulation.

11.4.1 Femoral Approach

This is the simplest of the three approaches requiring minimum of dissection and can be performed under local anesthetic. However, in presence of incarceration or strangulation this approach is difficult to employ, as the visualization of the femoral ring may be suboptimal.

11.4.1.1 Technique

The patient is in supine position with the bladder having been emptied or catheterized. Under local or regional anaesthesia an inguinal or subinguinal incision is made and carried down to the external oblique aponeurosis. The hernial sac located infe-rior to the aponeurosis is identified, dissected and opened. The contents of the sac are examined and reduced. Following this the femoral ring is closed with non-absorbable sutures or a polypropylene plug sutured to the inguinal ligament, fascia lata and pectineal fascia. If the hernia is incarcerated, better exposure may be obtained by dividing the lacunar ligament medially.

11.4.1.2 Results

Glassow et al., reported on suture repair of 1138 femoral hernias with 1.9% recurrence [4]. Swarnkar et al., repaired 43 femoral hernias with a polypropylene mesh plug without any recurrence at a median follow up of 2 years [5].

11.4.2 Inguinal Approach

This approach provides excellent exposure of the femoral ring, release of incarcerated contents and resection of bowel when necessary. Thus, this is the preferred approach for incarcerated hernia.

11.4.2.1 Technique

Via an inguinal incision the external oblique aponeurosis is exposed and opened. The cord structures are mobilized and presence of an inguinal hernia is ruled out. The floor of the inguinal canal (transversalis fascia) is opened to expose the femoral hernial sac. The sac is opened and contents are examined carefully to exclude compromise of vascularity. The exposure can be improved by dividing fibres of lacunar ligament and iliopubic tract medially. Division of the inguinal ligament to gain exposure should be avoided as far as possible as this increases the likelihood of recurrence. After confirming the viability of bowel it is returned to the peritoneal cavity and the sac is closed. A repair is performed by approximating the Cooper's ligament to the iliopubic tract. In an elective setting a polypropylene mesh is chosen to obliterate the femoral canal. Though plugs of various shapes were popular in the past, a flat sheet of polypropylene covering the femoral canal as well as the floor of the inguinal canal is preferred.

11.4.2.2 Results

Bendavid have reported a recurrence of 1.8% in 329 patients with femoral hernia repaired with an umbrella-shaped mesh placed via an inguinal approach [3].

11.4.3 Open Preperitoneal Approach

This approach can be used both in the elective and emergent settings and offers excellent exposure, ability to identify and when necessary resect non-viable bowel and also place a large mesh that can cover all the three potential defects in the myopectineal orifice of Fruchaud.

11.4.3.1 Technique

A transverse lower abdominal incision is made 2.5–3 cm above the inguinal ligament to expose the external oblique aponeurosis and the anterior rectus sheath. The anterior rectus sheath is incised and the rectus is retracted medially to gain access to the extraperitoneal space. The sac is opened, contents are examined and dealt with appropriately and the sac is closed. The repair is in the form of 3–5 interrupted sutures of a non-absorbable material between Cooper's ligament and iliopubic tract. Alternately, a mesh covering the femoral, direct and indirect defects is placed and fixed in place.

11.4.3.2 Results

Chen et al reported a randomized trial comparing a preperitoneal mesh repair ($n = 45$) and mesh plug repair ($n = 40$) in patients with primary femoral hernias [6]. No patient in preperitoneal group experienced a recurrence, whereas there were 10% recurrences in the mesh plug group. Moreover, 15% patients who had a mesh plug put in complained of a foreign body sensation.

11.4.4 Laparoscopic Preperitoneal Approach

With the increasing interest and experience in application of laparoscopic techniques to the repair of groin hernias, femoral hernias are commonly repaired by this approach today. The laparoscopic operation offers the advantage of excellent exposure (as well as mesh coverage) of the entire myopectineal orifice, ability to pick up occult hernias, reduced postoperative pain and faster recovery. The two laparoscopic approaches are (a) trans-abdominal pre-peritoneal (TAPP) and (b) totally extra-peritoneal (TEP). In a patient with an incarcerated/strangulated femoral hernia the TAPP approach is preferred.

11.4.4.1 Technique of TAPP

The technique of TAPP, including position of the patient, port positions and steps, is described in detail in Chap. 11. Figure 11.2 shows view of the right groin with direct inguinal and femoral hernial orifices. In brief, a peritoneal incision is made from the anterior superior iliac spine (ASIS) to the medial umbilical ligament 2.5–3 cm above the internal ring. The peritoneum is dissected downward to expose the medial (Retzius) and lateral (Bogros) spaces. The femoral hernial sac is identified carefully dissected taking care not to injure the external iliac vein. Concomitant direct or indirect hernial sacs are also dealt with. The peritoneum is dissected downwards from the cord structures so as to parietalize them (Fig. 11.3). In females the round ligament may be coagulated and divided. A wide mesh (minimum 15 cm × 12 cm) is placed to cover all the three hernial defects (Fig. 11.4). This is then secured in place with the help of fixation devices or sutures. The peritoneal incision is carefully closed with a

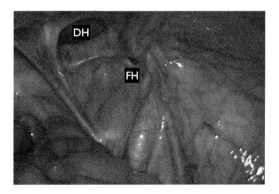

Fig. 11.2 Laparoscopic view of the right groin showing direct inguinal (DH) and femoral hernial (FH) orifices

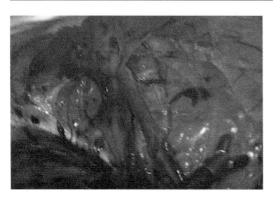

Fig. 11.3 Laparoscopic dissection to expose the myopectineal orifice

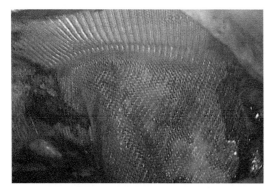

Fig. 11.4 A mesh is placed to cover the indirect, direct and femoral hernial orifices and fixed

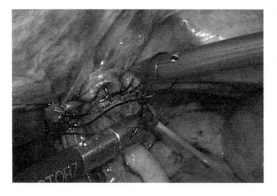

Fig. 11.5 Peritoneal incision is closed with a running suture

running suture (preferably) or with tacks (Fig. 11.5). The fascia at the 10 mm port site and skin incisions are closed.

11.4.4.2 Technique of TEP
The technique of TEP, including position of the patient, port positions and steps is described in

detail in Chap. 10. In brief, the extraperitoneal space is entered with an infra-umbilical incision and dissected either with the help of a balloon dissector or the laparoscope. Further dissection is undertaken either with instruments introduced via two midline ports or one midline port and another placed near the ASIS on the side of the hernia. Wide dissection of the extra-peritoneal space, placement and fixation of the mesh as described above follows.

11.4.4.3 Results
Hernandez-Richter et al., [7] performed TAPP in 1097 patients including 51 with femoral hernia. There were no recurrences at 1-year follow-up. Felix et al., used both TAPP and TEP in 1173 patients with groin hernias, 16 out of which were femoral hernias and 69 had a femoral component along with inguinal hernias [8]. There were no recurrences at 2 years in the 85 patients with femoral hernias.

11.5 Postoperative Care

Patients undergoing elective open or laparoscopic repair of femoral hernia under general anaesthetic are commenced on liquids within 4–6 h and rapidly progressed to solids. Commencement of orals may be delayed in patients undergoing emergency surgery for obstruction or in whom bowel has been resected. Intravenous analgesics and one to three doses of antibiotics are administered. Most patients should be able to get discharged within 24–36 h after surgery on oral analgesics. A follow-up is scheduled 7–10 days after surgery, at which time the incisions are checked, sutures, if any, are removed and in case of a laparoscopic repair a seroma is excluded.

Key Points
- Femoral hernia may present as a bulge in the groin or with signs of intestinal obstruction.
- All patients are advised repair upon diagnosis due to high risk of complications.
- The various approaches to repair of femoral hernia are (a) femoral, (b) inguinal, (c) open preperitoneal and (d) laparoscopic (TAPP or TEP).

- Factors such as associated medical co-morbidities, elective versus emergent presentation and surgeon comfort with a particular approach dictate the choice of technique.
- In elective settings a laparoscopic repair is superior to an open operation.

References

1. Hair A, Paterson C, O'Dwyer PJ. Diagnosis of a femoral hernia in the elective setting. J R Coll Surg Edinb. 2001;46:117–8.
2. Dahlstrand U, Wollert S, Nordin P, Sandblom G, Gunnarsson U. Emergency femoral hernia repair. A study based on a national register. Ann Surg. 2009;249:672–6.
3. Bendavid R. Femoral hernia (part III): an "umbrella" for femoral hernia repair. In: Bendavid R, editor. Prostheses and abdominal wall hernias. Boca Raton: CRC; 1994. p. 413.
4. Glassow F. Femoral hernia: review of 2105 repairs in a 17-year period. Am J Surg. 1985;150:353–6.
5. Swarnkar K, Hopper N, Nelson M, Feroz A, Stephenson BM. Sutureless mesh-plug hernioplasty. Am J Surg. 2003;186:201–2.
6. Chen J, Lv Y, Shen Y, Liu S, Wang M. A prospective comparison of preperitoneal tension-free open herniorrhaphy with mesh plug herniorrhaphy for the treatment of femoral hernias. Surgery. 2010;148:976–81.
7. Hernandez-Richter T, Schardey HM, Rau HG, Schildberg FW, Meyer G. The femoral hernia: an ideal approach for the transabdominal preperitoneal technique (TAPP). Surg Endosc. 2000;14:736–40.
8. Felix EL, Michas CA, McKnight RL. Laparoscopic repair of recurrent hernias. Surg Endosc. 1995; 9:135–8.

Groin Hernia in the Elderly

12

K. G. Mathew

12.1 Introduction

Groin hernias are amongst the most commonly performed surgical operations, with over 71,000 groin hernia repairs carried out in the UK in 2014/2015 [1]. About 600,000 groin hernia surgeries are performed in the United States yearly. Inguinal hernia classically presents maximally in early childhood, and then in the elderly, whereas femoral hernia does not exhibit this bimodal type of prevalence [2] (Fig. 12.2). Men have a 27–43% lifetime risk of groin hernia, whereas in women it is 3–6%. The only cure for inguinal hernia is surgery. The asymptomatic patients with groin hernias are a minority and even with watchful waiting 70% convert to surgery within 5 years. Though most groin hernias in adults are operated in the older age groups the various guidelines do not clearly address the issues of operating in this age group.

12.2 Defining the Elderly

Sixty years is generally considered the onset of old age and people more than 60 years are categorized as elderly. However, this cut off age is usually based on the pensionable age of various

governments, and does not have any basis of the time when physiological ageing is significant. Senior citizens over 60 years of age today differ vastly from what their parents were at that age, and in fact they bear no similarities to their grandparents at that age. Thus calculating old age from a fixed time point could be biased.

Ryder's concept in 1975 that the age of a human being is to be calculated based on the number of years the person is expected to live is indeed interesting. He takes a step further to emphasize that a person is deemed 'old' when he/she is expected to live a maximum of 10 years from their present age [4] (Fig. 12.1).

On the other hand, Shoven in 2010 was of the opinion that beginning of old age could be ascertained by comparing the morbidity rate at every age at a specified period. A combination of both these theories can guide physicians to plan treatment. As an example, in the US the cutoff age for elderly in 1933 was 48.7 and rose to 56.6 in 2005—a 16.22% increase. In other words, in 1933 a 55-year-old would be termed 'elderly' and be part of the senior most category. However in 2005 this 55 year old is younger than in 1933 based on life expectancy of a 55-year-old being 19.2 years in 1933 and 26.7 years in 2005. Hence for therapeutic purposes it may be useful to classify the elderly based on their life expectancies and offer treatment accordingly. One example is knee joint replacement surgery which is now often performed in people above age 70. It would

K. G. Mathew (✉)
Department of Surgery, NMC Specialty Hospital, Dubai, UAE

© Springer Nature India Private Limited 2020
P. Chowbey, D. Lomanto (eds.), *Techniques of Abdominal Wall Hernia Repair*,
https://doi.org/10.1007/978-81-322-3944-4_12

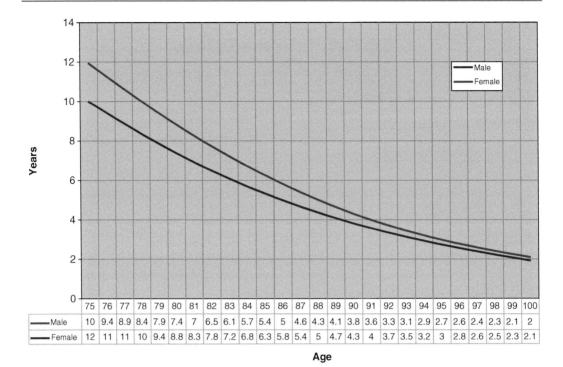

	75	76	77	78	79	80	81	82	83	84	85	86	87	88	89	90	91	92	93	94	95	96	97	98	99	100
Male	10	9.4	8.9	8.4	7.9	7.4	7	6.5	6.1	5.7	5.4	5	4.6	4.3	4.1	3.8	3.6	3.3	3.1	2.9	2.7	2.6	2.4	2.3	2.1	2
Female	12	11	11	10	9.4	8.8	8.3	7.8	7.2	6.8	6.3	5.8	5.4	5	4.7	4.3	4	3.7	3.5	3.2	3	2.8	2.6	2.5	2.3	2.1

Age

Fig. 12.1 Life expectancy by age 2003–2005. Office for the National Statistics: interim life tables 2003–2005. Newport:ONS:2005

not make much sense to do this is if he/she has not got sufficient active life expectancy irrespective of the age at which surgery is done.

In short, we could term life expectancy as the total number of years a person is expected to live considering the mortality rates to remain constant in the future. In Japan, the normal life expectancy of a person is 83.7 years while all over the world it is 71.0 years (2010–2013 UN World Population Report). Hence in Japan old age can be said to start at 70 years.

While emergency surgery is inevitable at any age, elective surgery for asymptomatic or minimally symptomatic conditions needs to consider not only the life expectancy in that country but also the quality of life enjoyed by the person at that point of time. A surgeon has the duty to maintain the person's quality of life and irrespective of age if surgery can improve or prevent deterioration of that person's quality of life, the same should not be withheld only based on age.

So, for treatment purposes, what is important is the life expectancy and physiological age rather than the chronological age. For studies/research we could classify the elderly into three segments namely elderly (65–70 years), elderly elderly (70–75 years), and late elderly (more than 75 years).

The studies do not define what segment of the elderly is studied. In today's changing definition of what defines an elderly and with improved surgical techniques and peri operative care, it is prudent to consider a different therapeutic approach in the above 80s, who in most parts of the world are the true physiological elderly. People in their 60s and 70s can be operated using the same guidelines as younger people.

12.3 Pathophysiology Wound Healing in Elderly

For a holistic appreciation of hernia surgery in the elderly an understanding of wound healing and bio-material incorporation is useful in planning the optimum treatment. Optimizing hernia surgery in the elderly will avoid complications of poor wound healing and recurrence.

Wound healing is age dependent. Foetuses up to the 24th week heal without scarring (Dang et al. [5]). As one grows older, the healing is impaired, but there is no definitive transition age. At present, healing of wounds in the healthy elderly is quite normal despite alterations to individual processes, as long as associated morbidity factors are controlled [6].

12.4 Wound Healing Phases [7]

Phase 1: Various cytokines such as tumor growth factor (TGF-B), platelet-derived growth factor (PDGF), fibroblast growth factor (FGF) and epidermal growth factor (EGF) are released to provide the first phase of the inflammatory response.

Phase 2: Inflammatory phase: The inflammatory cells neutrophils, macrophages and lymphocytes migrate to the area of injury.

Phase 3: Proliferative phase: Largely under the influence of the macrophages. There occurs angiogenesis and proliferative fibroblast. T-lymphocytes migrate to the wound.

Phase 4: Fibroblasts produce collagen: In hernia surgery the key area is the phase 4 of wound healing. Proliferating fibroblasts produce and secrete procollagen, which converts extracellularly to tropocollagen. The collagen produced by the fibroblasts is rich in amino acids, Lysine and Prolene. These amino acids in the presence of oxygen, vitamin C and iron undergo hydroxylation to hydroxylysine and hydroxyprolene, which are in turn responsible for cross linking of the collagen. Reorientation of collagens occurs and this increases the tensile strength from the fifth day and the strength continues to increase up to 1 year. In wound healing, type I and III are important collagens. Type III dominates in the early phases of wound healing, while type I is most abundant in later scar tissue.

High levels of type III collagen compared to type I may affect strength of wound as type III collagen is soluble and not strong.

12.5 Alteration of the Connective Tissue in the Hernia Patient

Sir Arthur Keith 1924 [8]: "We are so apt to look on tendons, facial structures and connective tissue as dead passive structures (which they are to anatomists dissecting cadavers). They are certainly alive, and the fact that hernias are so often multiple in middle age and old people leads me to suspect that a pathological change in the connective tissue of the belly wall may render certain individuals particularly liable to hernia."

12.6 Wound Healing in the Elderly

Though healing of wounds are generally delayed in the elder category, of significance in hernia surgery is effective collagen production. This depends on a fine balance between production of appropriate collagen by fibroblasts and degradation by metalloproteinase enzymes (MMP). It has been reported that synthesis becomes lower while rate of degradation of collagen gets higher with increasing age [9].

In the transversus abdominis fascia, significantly higher levels of MMP-2 (metalloproteinase) have been found in patients with direct inguinal hernia. MMP-2 is an enzyme that degrades collagens types 4, 5, 7, 10, 11, elastin, gelatin, fibronectin and other matrix proteins and hence may reflect proteolysis of connective tissue as a possible mechanism of recurrence in direct inguinal hernia. In wound healing MMP-2 is important during the prolonged phase of matrix remodeling, whereas MMP-9 derived primarily from neutrophils is important in the early phases of the repair. A recent study of hernia wound healing assessed wound fluid collagenases in an implanted ePTFE mesh. High levels of MMP-9 were found 24 h after surgery with decline 48 h after surgery reflecting the inflammatory activity of PMN leukocytes and Monocyte macrophages. The concentration of MMP-9 after the first postoperative day was negatively associated with the amount of collagen deposited in the implanted ePTFE mesh after 10 days, indicating that the concentration of MMP-9 may be a predictor of healing in this type of wound [10, 11].

It has been reported that with increase in age collagen synthesis reduces but degradation of collagen increases. This has been attributed to the decreased motility of the fibroblasts, decreased proliferative capacity and chemotactic response. Ashcroft et al. have shown an up-regulation of the activity of MMP-9, which means less collagen is deposited.

Goodson and Hunt [12] concluded based on their animal experiments that in the older mice wounds that had been incised gain strength, whereas in the case of open wounds they contracted slowly. Slower tissue remodeling ultimately leads to a fine scar but with less tensile strength.

Some other aspects of wound healing in the elderly that may have a practical significance are:

1. Decreased vascularity of the dermis and loss of subcutaneous fat
2. Decreased oxygenation of tissues which leads to more inflammatory response and less collagen
3. Increased tendency for bacterial adhesion
4. Capillary fragility and easy bruising leading to a tendency for ecchymosis or even hematomas at surgical sites.

However, wound healing and mesh incorporation in the elderly can proceed normally if associated co-morbidities are controlled and potential deterrents to wound healing are overcome with appropriate perioperative care.

12.7   Is Watchful Waiting an Option in the Elderly?

A review of mortality after hernia surgery, especially in the elderly is an useful exercise for planning treatment. Hernia surgery should in principle have no mortality/avoidable mortality, considering that the procedure is very common at all ages.

Nielssen and his group have made a study of the rate of mortality after hernia surgery keeping in mind various factors of age, sex, emergency/ elective and hernia anatomy. Their findings were based on patients who were 15 years and above who had undergone groin hernia surgery during the period 1 Jan. 1992–31 Dec 2004. This analysis was based on cases from hernia surgery centres which were part of the Swedish Hernia Registry. The post-operative risks of mortality were termed as SMR; Standardized Mortality Ratio. This was the ratio between the expected deaths and the unexpected deaths which occurred within a span of 30 days post surgery. The mortality increase was significant for both genders after emergency femoral hernia surgery. Elective inguinal hernia operations have no mortality SMR 0.63 (0.52–0.76), whereas for emergency inguinal operations the mortality spikes to SMR 5.94 (4.99–7.01) Groin hernia surgeries are more often done in the older population in Sweden, and this holds true more for the femoral hernias. In fact it was noted that both men and women who required emergency hernia surgery were older than patients who were admitted for elective surgery. Inguinal hernia patients were generally found to be younger than femoral hernia patients.

The mortality is related to emergency surgery (inguinal/femoral) and if bowel resection is done, mortality is increased two fold. So mortality is not to be considered when there is every indication for surgery in a person who shows a clear case of hernia as elective hernia repair does not carry an increased risk even at higher age groups.

Emergency groin hernia repair carries increased morbidity and mortality at any age. Add to this the risk of other co-morbid factors that the elderly may be burdened with. Hence emergency surgery has significantly increased morbidity and mortality in the very elderly and dictates that we prevent such a situation and electively repair groin hernias in the elderly. The same conclusion is derived from a retrospective study from UK [13]. All residents who died from abdominal hernia between January 1989 and 31 March 1995 were identified (65 cases). Those who died from inguinal hernia were mostly elderly men, and over half of these had been diagnosed by their GPs, but surgery was deferred due to age and minimal symptoms. They ultimately presented as emergency

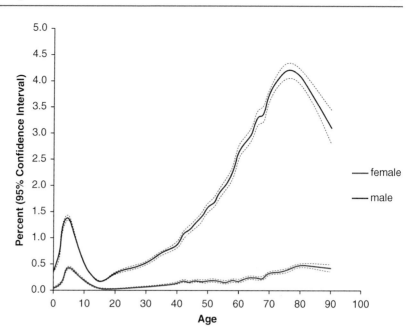

Fig. 12.2 Prevalence of groin hernia repair, (inguinal and femoral combined), stratified by age and gender. The results indicate the percentage of persons at a given age in the population who were operated for a groin hernia during the study period. Example: 4.19% CI (4.04–4.34% of all males aged 75–80 years in Denmark were operated for a groin hernia at least once during the study period (Ref: [3])

and with a final fatal outcome that could have been prevented by early surgery. This suggests that in the elderly with an inguinal hernia, the option of elective surgery should be considered even in the absence of symptoms. In patients with a femoral hernia age is no bar to proceed with surgery due to the high risk of complications.

The prevalence of groin hernia in the elderly is not known, but it is seen that most groin hernia surgeries are in the above 60 age group (Fig. 12.2). The elderly usually have associated co-morbid factors that increase the risk of surgery and hence a limitation to offering surgery electively. One limitation of offering elective surgery in the elderly is the high incidence of associated co morbidities in this group.

In 2013 a study conducted by Amato et al. [4] showed that high risk (ASA III-IV) elderly could undergo inguinal hernia surgery in the non-emergent setting and have no increased mortality. Two hundred and ninety-two patients were included and in ages of (a) under 75 (b) between 75 and 85 (c) over 85 but with no unstable medical condition and BMI less than 32. ASA grades ranged from 1 to 4 and surgery was by open mesh repair with local anaesthesia plus or minus deep sedation. There were no deaths or major complications. Shows that age alone is no bar for cor-

recting asymptomatic or minimally symptomatic groin hernias even with associated co morbidities as long as the morbidities are controlled.

While on this topic it is worthwhile to have a look at the INCAS trialists collaboration published in 2010 [14] (Table 12.1). This is an extensive review on the topic of elective compared with watchful waiting in the elderly male patients with an inguinal hernia. Mean mortality associated with elective hernia repair was 0.2% (0–1.8%) while emergency repair had a mortality of 4.0% (0–22.2%). Four retrospective cohort studies investigated rate of incarceration and/or strangulation as primary outcomes. The data after computation yielded a 0.4% incidence of yearly rate of irreducibility associated with a non-operative approach. Two randomized trials reported the crossover rate and combining these figures from the two 13% (8.0–19.5%) of mildly symptomatic and asymptomatic inguinal hernia patients assigned to watchful waiting management will cross over to surgery.

Sensitivity analysis showed the optimal decision to be related to the procedural mortality rates and annual risk of incarceration/strangulation. Hence, since mortality associated with emergency repair is lower than its threshold value of 4.2% (average mortality is 4.0%) the optimal

Table 12.1 Mortalities associated with elective and emergency inguinal hernia repair and risk at incarceration and/or strangulation in case of nonsurgical inguinal hernia treatment

First author	Mortality elective repair			Mortality emergency repair			Risk of incarceration and/or strangulation of non-surgically treated hernia		
	n	Death	Mortality rate %	n	Death	Mortality rate %	n	Annual risk of incarceration/ strangulation, %	Type of event: incarceration and/or strangulation
Williams [3]	222	4	1.8	48	6	12.5	NA	NA	NA
Neuhauser [15]	71,651	NR	0.5	7495	NR	4.7	8633	0.4	Strangulation or incarceration
Tingwald [7]	44	0	0	15	1	22.2	NA	NA	NA
Nehme [16]	1044	14	1.3	235	18	7.7	NA	NA	NA
Allen [17]	49	0	0	15	1	22.2	NA	NA	NA
Gallegos [18]	417	0	0	22	0	0	439	1.5	Strangulation
Oishi [19]	1758	0	0	67	2	3.0	NA	NA	NA
Primatesta [20]	27,937	28	0.1	2738	47	1.7	NA	NA	NA
MRC Group [21]	915	0	0	NA	NA	NA	NA	NA	NA
Bay-Nielsen [22]	23,695	55	0.2	1156	81	7.0	NA	NA	NA
Ohana [23]	200	0	0	67	4	6.0	NA	NA	NA
Neumayer [24]	1983	4	0.2	NA	NA	NA	NA	NA	NA
Fitzibbons [25]	294	0	0	NA	NA	NA	256	0.2	Acute hernia incarceration without strangulation
O'Dwyer [26]	75	1	1.3	NA	NA	NA	75	0.9	Acute hernia
Nilsson [27]	66,897	95	0.1	4167	134	3.2	NA	NA	NA
Alvarez [28]	NA	NA	NA	70	2	2.9	NA	NA	NA
Neurra [29]	NA	NA	NA	31	NA	12.0	46,608	0.4[a]	Incarceration and strangulation
Rai [30]	NA	NA	NA	181	11	6.3	NA	NA	NA
Kulah [31]	NA	NA	NA113	4	3.5	6.1	NA	NA	NA
Hair [32]	NA	NA	NA	10	0	0	61	27	Irreducibility requiring operation
NMR, Prismant [33]	45,026	34	0.1	1631	49	3.0	NA	NA	NA
Total average	242,207	596	0.2	18,092	715	4.0	56,072	0.4	

NA not applicable, *NMR* National Medical Registration, *NR* not reported
(Ref: INCA trialists collaboration: Table 2: P255)

choice is observation. Also, if elective repair has a mortality that is more than 0.2% (average is 0.2%) or risk of incarceration and/or strangulation lower than its threshold value of 0.5% (average 0.4%), the optimal choice is observation. The conclusion is that the life expectancy for elderly male inguinal patients associated with watchful waiting or operation does not differ, and so

watchful waiting is a choice for elderly males with asymptomatic or minimally symptomatic inguinal hernias.

However this detailed mathematical analysis has to be weighed against other studies which show that emergency repairs have an increased mortality and advocating elective repair even in the very elderly.

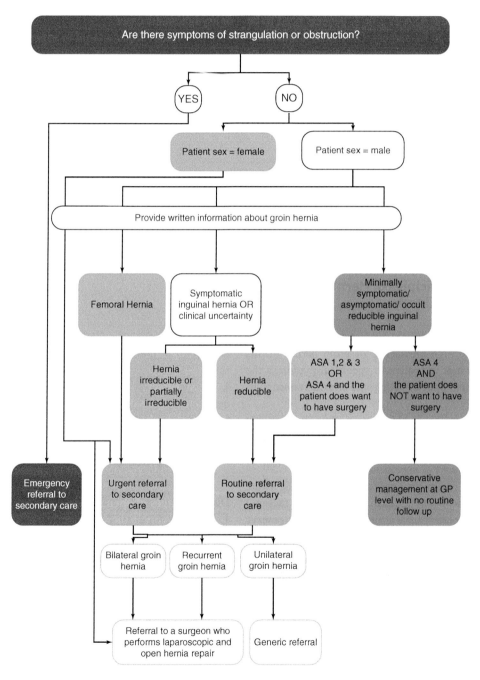

Fig. 12.3 British Hernia Society Commissioning Guide 2016. Ref [1]

26. O'Dwyer PJ, et al. Observation or operation for patients with an asymptomatic inguinal hernia: a randomized clinical trial. Ann Surg. 2006;244:167–73.
27. Nilsson H, et al. Mortality after groin hernia surgery. Ann Surg. 2007;245:656–60.
28. Alvarez JA, et al. Incarcerated groin hernias in adults presentation and outcome. Hernia. 2004;8:121–6.
29. Neutra R, et al. Risk of incarceration of inguinal hernia in cell Colombia. J Chronic Dis. 1981; 34:561–4.
30. Rai S, et al. A study of the risk of strangulation and obstruction in groin hernias. Aust N Z J Surg. 1998;68:650–4.
31. Kulah B, et al. Emergency hernia repairs in the elderly patients. Am J Surg. 2001;182:455–9.
32. Hair A. What effect does the duration of an inguinal hernia have on patient symptoms? J Am Coll Surg. 2001;193:125–9.
33. National Medical Registration (LMR). Dutch Hospital Statistics–procedures. http://www.prismant.nl.
34. Malik AM, et al. Factor influencing morbidity and mortality in elderly population undergoing inguinal hernia surgery. J Pak Med Assoc. 2010;60(1):45–7.
35. Ageing and its influence on wound healing. Clin Rev Wounds UK. 2007;3(1).
36. Ashcroft GS, et al. Age related differences in the temporal and spatial regulation of matrix metalloproteinases (MMPs) in normal skin and acute cutaneous wounds of healthy humans. Cell Tissue Res. 1997;290(3):581–91.
37. Ashcroft GS, et al. Age related changes in the temporal and spatial distribution of fibrillin and elastin mRNAs and proteins in acute cutaneous wounds in healthy humans. J Pathol. 1997;183(1):80–9.
38. Kulah B. Emergency hernia repairs in elderly patients. Am J Surg. 2001;182:45–459.
39. Amato B, Compagna R, et al. Day-surgery inguinal hernia repair in the elderly: single centre experience. BMC Surg. 2013;13(suppl 2):528.
40. Cerimele D, et al. Physiological changes in aging skin. Br J Dermatol. 1990;122(S35):13–20.
41. de Goed B, et al. Watchful waiting versus surgery of mildly symptomatic or asymptomatic inguinal hernia in men aged 50 years and older: a randomized controlled trial. Ann Surg. 2018;267(1):42–9.
42. Desai H. Aging and wounds part 1: fetal and post natal healing. J Wound Care. 2003;6(4):192–6.
43. Desai H. Aging and wounds part 2 healing in old age. J Wound Care. 1997;6(4):192–6.
44. Garavello A, et al. Inguinal hernia in elderly. Indications, techniques, results. Minerva Chir. 2004;59(3):271–6.
45. Nilson H, et al. Mortality after groin hernia surgery. Ann Surg. 2007;245(4):656–60.
46. Howes EL, et al. The age factor in the velocity of the growth of fibroblasts in the healing wound. J Exp Med. 1932;55(4):577–84.
47. INCA Trialist Collaboration. Operation compared with watchful waiting in elderly male inguinal hernia patients: a review and data analysis. Chicago: American College of Surgeons; 2011.
48. Kondo H, et al. Effects of serum from human subjects of different ages on migration in vitro human fibroblasts. Mech Aging Dev. 1989;47(1):25–37.
49. Kaltic MR. Chapter 6. Principles of geriatric surgery. 2011. p. 93. Table 6.1.
50. Palumbo LT, et al. Primary inguinal hernioplasty in the elderly patients. Geriatrics. 1954;9:8–14.
51. Compogna R, Rossi R, et al. Emergency groin hernia repair: implications in elderly. From 26th National Congress of the Italian Society of Geriatric Surgery Naples, Italy, 19–22 June 2013. BMC Surg. 2013;13(Suppl 2):S21.
52. Sgnoc R, Gruber J. Age related aspects of cutaneous wound healing: a mini review. Gerontology. 2013;59:159–64.
53. Lars NJ, Finn G. The role of collagen in hernia genesis. In: Bendavid R, Abrahmson J, et al., editors. Abdominal wall hernia: Principles and management; 2001. p. 19.
54. Simons MP, et al. Europena Hernia Society guidelines on the treatment of inguinal hernia in adult patients. Hernia. 2009;13:343–403.
55. Schumpelick V, et al. Inguinal hernia repair in adults. Lancet. 1994;344:375–9.
56. Guo S, DiPietro LA. Factors affecting wound healing: critical reviews in oral biology and medicine. J Dent Res. 2010;89(3):219–29.
57. Van De Kerkhof PCM, et al. Age related changes in wound healing. Clin Exp Dermatol. 1994;19:369–74.
58. Anderson WC, Scherbov S. A new perspective on population aging. Demogr Res. 2007;16(Article 2):27–58.

Sportsman Hernia

13

Yen Ping Tan and Jaideepraj Rao

13.1 Introduction

Chronic groin pain is a fairly common presenting complaint among athletes, which can also happen in general population. This condition is known to most as sportsman hernia. But in fact, it is a misnomer as usually, there is no real hernia involved. No general consensus has yet been reached concerning the actual existence of sportsman hernia, the relevant pathology, diagnosis, management or even the name that should apply to this condition [1]. Other terms that have been used include athletic pubalgia, Gilmore's groin, footballer's groin injury complex and pubic inguinal pain syndrome. In the latest consensus meeting, this condition is better defined and accepted as inguinal disruption [2]. This condition involved almost males exclusively. More than 90% of affected individuals are males. Although more prevalent among professional athletes, it can also affect amateur athletes and general populations [3]. Symptoms, ranging from mild to severe, are usually recurrent and chronic and it can potentially endanger an athlete's career [1, 3–6]. Types of sports that are more prevalent to be affected by this condition usually involved repetitive kicking, twisting, turning or cutting movements such as in football, ice hockey and rugby [7]. This chapter will further discuss the clinical presentations, role of imaging and further management and controversy of sportsman hernia.

13.2 Main Contents

13.2.1 Clinical Presentations and Pathophysiology

The presenting complaint is frequently exercise-related groin pain. Typically, pain localized over the lower lateral edge of the rectus abdominis, and may radiate towards testis, suprapubic area or adductor longus origin [8, 9]. Onset of pain is usually insidious, but some known cases came with initial sudden tearing sensation. The pain is usually aggravated by sudden accelerations, twisting and turning, repetitive kicking, [7] even coughing or sneezing. Pain will generally persist for 1–2 days after sports. Despite adequate rest in between, pain will usually reassert upon resumption of sports. Sportsman hernia also presented with vague clinical sign on examination. Usually, all one can find is localized tenderness just above the pubic crest. Palpable or visible cough impulse for hernia is usually absent.

Y. P. Tan · J. Rao (✉)
Department of General Surgery, Tan Tock Seng
Hospital, Singapore, Singapore

© Springer Nature India Private Limited 2020
P. Chowbey, D. Lomanto (eds.), *Techniques of Abdominal Wall Hernia Repair*,
https://doi.org/10.1007/978-81-322-3944-4_13

The pathophysiology of sportsman hernia is still a topic of controversy, varies to different beliefs. General belief is that there is disequilibrium between upward and oblique pull of abdominal muscles on the pubis against the downward and lateral pull of the adductors. General consensus on the pathophysiology includes [2]:

1. Weakened posterior wall of the inguinal canal
2. Disruption of external oblique aponeurosis, may appear as tears or scarring
3. Dilatation of external ring, conjoint tendon tears and inguinal ligament dehiscence

Also, it is important to exclude other causes of chronic groin pain during history and physical examination such as pubic rami occult fractures, bursitis, osteitis pubis, acetabular injury femoroacetabular impingement and even early osteoarthritis changes. Pathology of the hip and hamstring should also be excluded [7, 10].

13.2.2 Diagnosis

Diagnosis of sportsman hernia can be difficult as chronic groin pain is a common complaint which may be caused by various differential diagnoses across different specialties. It remains a diagnosis of exclusion. Thus, before we can diagnose a sportsman hernia, we first have to exclude other causes i.e.: genitourinary, intraabdominal, gynaecological, hip/lumbar spine or muscular in origin [8, 9].

According to the recently published British consensus on sportsman hernia [2], the diagnosis of sportsman hernia can be made if at least three out of the five clinical features are detectable:

1. Pinpoint tenderness over the pubic tubercle at the point of insertion of the conjoint tendon;
2. Palpable tenderness over the deep inguinal ring;
3. Pain and/or dilation of the external ring with no obvious hernia evident;
4. Pain at the origin of the adductor longus tendon; and
5. Dull, diffused pain in the groin, often radiating to the perineum and inner thigh or across the midline.

13.2.3 Role of Imaging

Sportsman hernia is a clinical diagnosis. Role of imaging is more importantly to exclude or diagnose associated injuries or pathology. Modalities of imaging include:

1. Ultrasound of the groin
   - This is a relatively cheap and widely available modality. However, its downside will be that it is operator dependent.
   - Ultrasound is useful to detect a real hernia, and also posterior wall weakness. It is especially sensitive when the ultrasound is performed real time. It can be done upon patient standing up or exerting cough or abdominal pressure in order to diagnose occult hernia [11, 12].
2. MRI of the groin
   - This is a useful modality in the case of suspected sportsman hernia. MRI can visualize the inguinal canal and its surrounding muscle and aponeurosis clearly thus detecting any abnormality. As what being said, its role still more importantly to diagnose other underlying muscular or bony pathology. Diagnoses such as osteitis pubis, adductor compartment injury, rectus abdominis tendon injury or pathology involving pubic symphysis can be detected via MRI [13–15]
   - Decision for operative intervention for sportsman hernia remains a clinical decision. However at present climate it is accepted that while approaching athletes with chronic groin pain, MRI is inevitably one of the modality for assessment especially for professional athlete before planning for any surgical intervention [2]

13.2.4 Management Strategy

The aim of treatment for those who presented with sportsman hernia is to resolve their symptoms and to minimize the time they are away from their sporting activities. This is especially true for professional athletes. The decision to conserve or to offer surgery remains difficult and controversial till date. There is still no conclusive evidence to guide us on indication for surgery and whether surgery is superior to conservative therapy in terms of treatment outcome.

Treatment options include:

1. Physiotherapy and sports rehabilitation
   - Currently, general belief is for trial of physiotherapy and sports rehabilitation initially for athletes who present with sportsman hernia. As sportsman hernia invariably is associated with some muscular strain and injury, up to 2 months of physiotherapy and sports rehabilitation is generally recommended to wait for resolution of symptoms. It is recommended that physiotherapy and rehab program is sports/occupation centered as much as possible to improve treatment outcome [16–18]
2. Screening and prevention
   - As we make advancements in sports medicine and understand human body more and more, screening and prevention of high-risk athletes are imperative to reduce incidences of sportsman hernia. Posture, muscles, gait, movement and flexibility of athletes should be analysed and high-risk athletes should be identified [2]. Athletes with previous history of groin complaints should be identified. Training regime should be more individualized especially to the high-risk group to reduce risk of developing sportsman hernia.
   - As surgeons we may not have adequate expertise in physiotherapy, rehab or screening, thus it is recommended to involve physiotherapy, rehab physician as well as the athletes' team physio, coaches and doctors in order to have a multidisciplinary approach and multimodality treatment for the involved athlete [18]
3. Local injection and image-guided intervention
   - Local injection of anaesthetic agents, sclerosants, cortisone [19], platelet-enriched plasma etc., can be given based on the clinician's individual decision. However, there is yet to be any strong evidence to

suggest it will improve the eventual treatment outcome.
   - If imaging studies picked up a specific abnormality or injury, image-guided injection can be targeted to the involved muscle/joints to alleviate symptoms. Example such as symphysis pubic articular injection [20], adductor longus soft tissue injections are treatment options to alleviate symptom but more study are required to prove its worth and safety profile.
   - A recent randomized trial in Australia hypothesized that inflammation around ilioinguinal nerve is the main culprit of chronic groin pain in athletes. Thus, they did a randomized study on radiological-guided radiofrequency denervation (RFD) of inguinal nerve compared to local injection of anaesthetic and found that pain is much improved in the RFD group [21]
4. Surgery
   - In general, discussion for surgical intervention should be carried out only after an appropriate period of physiotherapy and sports rehab failed to alleviate the problem and involved athlete is unable to return to normal sports activities [22]
   - Role of surgery is to identify the pathology involved, release tension on the inguinal canal and mesh repair of the posterior wall weakness.
   - The recommended surgical approach is open or laparoscopic (TEP or TAPP) hernia repair with mesh [8, 10]. No other surgical technique so far has shown to be superior to conventional open or laparoscopic hernia mesh repair.
   - To date, there are still very limited randomized controlled trials done on surgical intervention for sportsman hernia. A recent RCT published compared 60 patients with sportsman hernia underwent laparoscopic mesh hernia repair versus 2 months of conservative physiotherapy [10]. It concluded that more surgical arm patients have less chronic groin pain after 1 month and returned to sports within 3 months compared to the conservative managed arm.

- So far, there is no evidence to show any difference in outcome between open or laparoscopic approach. However, we generally believe that minimally invasive technique will shorten duration of recovery, hospital stay and athletes can return to their sports activities faster. However, there are differing opinions on that as the pathology of sportsman hernia will require an open anterior approach to examine closely the rectus abdominis muscle, conjoint tendon and ilioinguinal nerve. As there is still no hard evidence to decide on that, surgery of choice (open vs. laparoscopic) should be based more on individual surgeon's preference and available expertise.
- Pre- and post-operatively it is important to have a multimodal collaboration with the physiotherapist and rehab physicians to individualise a rehab program for the athletes in order to return to their sports activities as soon as possible [18].

13.3 Summary

Sportsman hernia is a complex exercise-related chronic groin pain that happens almost exclusively in males and more commonly among athletes. Diagnosis of sportsman hernia remains a challenge but a careful history and physical examinations are imperative to approach this problem. The key to diagnosis of sportsman hernia is to exclude other underlying pathologies first that can also cause chronic groin pain. Imaging modalities can be helpful but the diagnosis and decision for surgical intervention for sportsman hernia remains a clinical one. Recommended approach for treatment will be for physiotherapy and sports rehabilitation initially before consideration of surgery if symptoms do not improve. The role of surgery is to identify pathology, release abnormal tension on inguinal canal and to repair the posterior wall weakness. Selection of surgical candidate is important and more indicated when patient involved has failed conservative treatment after an appropriate

period. Recommended surgery is either open or laparoscopic (TEP or TAPP) hernia mesh repair approach. Multidisciplinary approach involving surgeons, physiotherapists, rehab physicians as well as athlete's team coaches and physio are important to manage this complex problem holistically and to improve patient's outcome. There is still very limited evidence and randomized trial on sportsman hernia. Thus, more studies are needed in the future in order for us to come out with a guideline or protocol to optimize treatment for sportsman hernia.

Key Points

- Key to rule out other differential diagnoses for chronic groin pain before diagnosing and treating as sportsman hernia
- Physiotherapy with sports/occupation-centered rehabilitation has shown to alleviate symptom and return athletes to their sports activities earlier
- Laparoscopic or open approach for hernia mesh repair is the recommended surgery depending on surgeon's preference and expertise
- A multidisciplinary approach for sportsman hernia is recommended to optimize treatment plan and improve outcome for sportsman hernia

References

1. Moeller JL. Sportsman's hernia. Curr Sports Med Rep. 2007;6(2):111–4.
2. Sheen AJ, Stephenson BM. Treatment of the sportsman's groin: British Hernia Society's 2014 position statement based on the Manchester Consensus Conference. Br J Sports Med. 2014;48:1079–87.
3. Farber AJ, Wilckens JH. Sports hernia: diagnosis and therapeutic approach. J Am Acad Orthop Surg. 2007;15:507–14.
4. Swan KG Jr, Wolcott M. The athletic hernia: a systematic review. Clin Orthop Relat Res. 2007;455:78–87.
5. Joesting DR. Diagnosis and treatment of sportsman's hernia. Curr Sports Med Rep. 2002;1(2):121–4.
6. Diesen DL, Pappas TN. Sports hernias. Adv Surg. 2007;41:177–87.
7. Falvey EC, Franklyn-Miller A, McCrory PR. The groin triangle: a patho-anatomical approach to the diagnosis of chronic groin pain in athletes. Br J Sports Med. 2009;43:213–20.

8. Edelman DS, Selesnick H. "Sports" hernia: treatment with biologic mesh (surgisis): a preliminary study. Surg Endosc. 2006;20(6):971–3.
9. Deysine M, Deysine GR, Reed WP Jr. Groin pain in the absence of hernia: a new syndrome. Hernia. 2002;6(2):64–7.
10. Paajanen H, Brinck T, Hermunen H, et al. Laparoscopic surgery for chronic groin pain in athletes is more effective than nonoperative treatment: a randomised clinical trial with magnetic resonance imaging of 60 patients with sportsman's hernia (athletic pubalgia). Surgery. 2011;150:99–107.
11. Lilly MC, Arregui ME. Ultrasound of the inguinal Xoor for evaluation of hernias. Surg Endosc. 2002;16(4):659–62.
12. Lorenzini C, SoWa L, Pergolizzi FP, Trovato M. The value of diagnostic ultrasound for detecting occult inguinal hernia in patients with groin pain. Chir Ital. 2008;60(6):813–7.
13. Barile A, Erriquez D, Cacchio A, De Paulis F, Di Cesare E, Masciocchi C. Groin pain in athletes: role of magnetic resonance. Radiol Med (Torino). 2000;100(4):216–22.
14. Verrall GM, Henry L, Fazzalari NL, Slavotinek JP, Oakeshott RD. Bone biopsy of the parasymphyseal pubic bone region in athletes with chronic groin injury demonstrates new woven bone formation consistent with a diagnosis of pubic bone stress injury. Am J Sports Med. 2008;36(12):2425–31.
15. Paajanen H, Hermunen H, Karonen J. Pubic magnetic resonance imaging findings in surgically and conservatively treated athletes with osteitis pubis compared to asymptomatic athletes during heavy training. Am J Sports Med. 2008;36(1):117–21.
16. Hölmich P, Uhrskou P, Ulnits L, et al. Effectiveness of active physical training as treatment for long-standing adductor-related groin pain in athletes: randomized trial. Lancet. 1999;353:439–43.
17. Hölmich P, Larsen K, Krogsgaard K, et al. Exercise program for prevention of groin pain in football players: a cluster-randomised trial. Scand J Med Sci Sports. 2010;20:814–21.
18. Weir A, Jansen JA, van de Port IG, et al. Manual or exercise therapy for long-standing adductor-related groin pain: a randomised controlled clinical trial. Man Ther. 2011;16:148–54.
19. Lynch SA, Renström PA. Groin injuries in sport: treatment strategies. Sports Med. 1999;28(2):137–44.
20. Schilders E, Bismil Q, Robinson P, O'Connor PJ, Gibbon WW, Talbot JC. Adductor-related groin pain in competitive athletes. Role of adductor enthesis, magnetic resonance imaging, and entheseal pubic cleft injections. J Bone Joint Surg Am. 2007;89(10):2173–8.
21. Comin J, Obaid H, Lammers G, et al. Radiofrequency denervation of the inguinal ligament for the treatment of 'sportsman's hernia': a pilot study. Br J Sports Med. 2013;47:380–6.
22. Kaplan O, Arbel R. Sportsman's hernia—a plea for conservative therapeutical approach. Harefuah. 2005;144(5):351–6, 381.

Complications Inguinal Hernias: Strangulated Incarcerated and Obstructed Hernias

14

Pradeep Chowbey

14.1 Introduction

Inguinal hernia is the commonest of all groin hernias. An inguinal hernia is an abnormal protrusion of intra-abdominal tissue through a fascial defect in the groin. Inguinal hernia is a benign disease following a static course but their consequent complications may be drastic and frequent. Inguinal hernias are repaired mainly to relieve symptoms like pain and reduce the risk of acute incarceration/strangulation. Surgical repairs done under emergency conditions are invariably morbid in nature. Hence, an elective and planned surgery is always a preferred choice for a surgeon.

Strangulated hernias are described in which the blood supply to the contained part has been impeded, or cut off usually by a constriction, or band intrinsic to the hernia itself. Incarcerated hernia is an irreducible hernia but the blood supply to the contained part is intact [1]. The cause of hernia undergoing strangulation is unknown [1]. Large series [2, 3] of study on strangulated hernia have concluded that pathology intrinsic to the hernia itself or its content is not only the cause of strangulation. Indeed, less than 1% of hernias have a band or other abnormality that can clearly be implicated as causing strangulation.

Condon [4] noted "the essential substrate" that permits the development of a strangulating hernia is the presence of a small opening in the abdominal wall with rigid margins. Strangulated groin hernia is a life-threatening condition and requires immediate surgical intervention. The incidence of strangulated inguinal hernia ranges between 0.29 and 2.9% [1]. The prevalence worldwide of strangulated inguinal hernia is 0.3–2.9% of all the inguinal hernias in the adults [5, 6]. All groin hernias have a potential for strangulation. For inguinal hernia, the neck of the sac is responsible for 80% of obstruction and external ring for 20% [1]. Factors that initiate strangulation in a hernia that has been present chronically for many years is poorly understood. Perhaps it is through intestinal odema, or a large bolus passing into the contained intestine, that the rigid confines of the hernia itself can now act as a true obstructing mechanism.

A delay in diagnosis for more than 6–12 h increases the chance of intestinal necrosis with the need for bowel resection in 15% of cases [6, 7]. The diagnostic delay increases morbidity and mortality [8]. Literature shows a mortality rate varying from 2.6 to 9% during management of strangulated hernia. The prompt recognition and surgical management is imperative for this condition.

The surgical basics consist of obtaining a good exposure and an easy access if resection is necessary; the hernial sac and its contents are to

P. Chowbey (✉)
Metabolic and Bariatric Surgery, Max Super
Specialty Hospital, New Delhi, India

© Springer Nature India Private Limited 2020
P. Chowbey, D. Lomanto (eds.), *Techniques of Abdominal Wall Hernia Repair*,
https://doi.org/10.1007/978-81-322-3944-4_14

be reduced without causing any damage or inducing a bowel perforation, and the hernia should be repaired adequately through the same incision. Laparoscopy is feasible and allows an easy diagnosis of bowel suffering with a 4% morbidity rate [9, 10].

14.2 Presentation and Diagnosis

Early diagnosis of strangulated hernia is essential to prevent the complications and reduce the morbidity. There are various conventional and newer diagnostic modalities which have been used by laparoscopic surgeons. The foremost diagnostic tools are thorough history and the physical examination of the patient. The common clinical presentation in the emergency department is an irreducible mass in the abdominal wall and localized pain. Mechanical bowel obstruction, constipation, diarrhea, vomiting are also some of the signs and symptoms of patients presenting with strangulated bowel. Strangulate hernias which are neglected may lead to bowel perforation and haemodynamic instability.

Systemic and haemodynamic imbalance also indicate strangulation. In these situations, haemoconcentrations, leucocytosis and lactic acidosis, which are not resolved with volume rescuscitation, can indicate obstruction and strangulation. Viewing the data from strangulated bowel obstructions, it is difficult to differentiate the incarceration from strangulation based on clinical findings alone. Majority of the patients are obese, where a small part of the intestine is strangulated and hernia is occulted. In these cases, radiological imaging is an aid for diagnosis. Plain abdominal radiographs may be useful to show the evidence of bowel obstruction. Computed tomography clearly delineates the incarcerated organ and helps in establishing the diagnosis. Pneumatosis intestinalis, fat stranding, or even free air within the hernia sac suggest the vascular compromise of hernia contents.

A definitive diagnosis of strangulated hernia is through surgical exploration; when intestinal ischaemia is suspected. There are very limited studies to proclaim exploratory laparotomy or laparoscopy as the only means of surgical diagnostics. Midline laparotomies have showed increased incidence of morbidity, due to possible intestinal resections. Laparoscopy is the choice of procedure for bowel ischaemia diagnosis especially in geriatric patients with comorbidities; thus decreasing both the negative and non-therapeutic laparatomy rates. Romain et al. [11] have studied and demonstrated prognostic factors affecting postoperative morbidity after incarcerated groin hernia repair. Midline laparotomy has been established to be an independent prognostic factor for medical and surgical complications. The advanced techniques help in safe assessment of hernia contents during incarcerated and strangulated hernia repair and avoiding midline laparotomy. It raises the difficulty index for surgeons to evaluate the viability of previously incarcerated hernia contents.

The major concern for strangulated hernia has been bowel ischaemia. ICG (indocyanine green) fluorescence technique has been a newer modality to evaluate the intestinal blood flow and limiting the number of bowel resections. With this technique, blood flow can be observed on injecting the ICG dye. It allows wide area of observation and is convenient for the surgeon for assessment of strangulated hernia [12].

14.3 Management of Strangulated and Obstructed Inguinal Hernias

The goals for the management of strangulated and obstructed inguinal hernias

- To ensure complete reduction of hernia contents
- To assess the viability of contents
- To resect the gangrenous bowel
- To repair the defect

Traditional techniques like Bassini and Shouldice repairs have been preferred choice from contemporary tension free techniques. Hernandez-Irrizary et al. [13] found that 60% of emergency inguinal hernia repairs used open and non-mesh technique. Literature shows majority of clinicians have preferred open non-mesh technique to decrease the incidence of mesh infection in cases of emergency obstructed, strangulated and inguinal hernias. The standard method of open repair is done via anterior groin incision and repair. The fascia of the external oblique muscle is divided and hernia sac is assessed for contents and inspected for viability. Resection of gangrenous bowel is performed through the same incision if encountered. Occasionally, it is difficult to reduce the contents through anterior approach. Once the hernia sac is opened, the defect is expanded for reduction of incarcerated contents. In indirect inguinal hernias, the deep inguinal ring is incised medially to avoid injury to the vas deferens. It is important to ensure the inferior epigastric vessels are properly ligated to avoid haemorrhagic complication. For direct hernias, transversalis fascia needs division either medially or laterally. Extensive lateral division demands vigilance of inferior epigastric arteries.

The high recurrence rate post open repair has been recognized; the utility of laparoscopic techniques for acute inguinal hernia repair has gradually altered traditional thinking. Several drawbacks with traditional open approach include difficulty in avoiding tension in the swollen and edematous tissues leading to higher recurrence rate, possible contamination of mesh and need for proper evaluation to rule out ischemic bowel for any further bowel resection [14]. Laparoscopic surgeries are technically more demanding and require surgical expertise. Laparoscopic inguinal hernia repair has gradually gained acceptance due to its potential advantages of fast recovery, better cosmesis, reduced postoperative pain and lower rate recurrence [15].

In incarcerated inguinal hernias, it is important to assess the hernia content viability. Mesh repair in situations of incarcerated hernia has always been a subject of debate due to increased risk of mesh infection rates [16–20]. Tension-free repairs have gained popularity worldwide for elective as well as complicated inguinal hernia repairs. Inguinal hernia is mostly encountered as an emergency condition in surgical clinics. The

first case of laparoscopic repair of acutely incarcerated groin hernia was reported in 1993 [21]. There has been a debate ever since the case was reported regarding the laparoscopic approach for incarcerated hernia repair. Transabdominal preperitoneal (TAPP) approach has been commonly used for reduction and repair of incarcerated inguinal hernias. Elective TAPP repair and total extraperitoneal (TEP) approach used for incarcerated hernia have been compared in various studies. Mortality rate comparison with that of elective TAPP repairs and emergency hernia repairs found no significant differences in a prospective study of 194 TAPP repairs [22]. Felix et al. [23] also concluded TAPP was the choice for incarcerated inguinal hernias. Easy examination of incarcerated bowel for signs of necrosis and relative simplicity for bowel resection have led surgeons to be in favour of this approach. An added advantage of TAPP is having a sufficient time to observe the return of color and peristalsis of bowels if the viability is initially doubtful [24–26]. In contrast open technique where surgeons have few minutes to make a decision on bowel resection, TAPP allows the reassessment of the viability of bowels at the end of procedure and circumvent the need for unnecessary bowel resection. Moreover, TAPP approach facilitates the inspection of contralateral hernia orifices and unsuspected hernia which are not possible in TEP approach [26]. A study by Siow et al. [27], retrospectively reviewed their experience with TAPP and limited open technique in treatment of 20 incarcerated scrotal hernias. Study concluded that laparoscopic with its modified technique is safe and effective in patients with incarcerated scrotal hernias.

However, Ferzli et al. [28] have described their experience with totally extraperitoneal repair for acutely incarcerated hernias. Number of patients were limited to 11, 3 of which converted into open. Follow up period was from 9 to 69 months and no recurrence was reported. The advantage of limited mobility of hernia contents for reduction, easy placement of additional trocar and creation of medial tissue release for incarcerated direct hernias, TEP has also been preferred by few authors. Although, there are limited studies for using TEP approach than TAPP approach for incarcerated inguinal hernias.

The combination approach TAPP for initial view, reduction of hernia contents and proceeding with standard TEP approach has become convenient approach. The combined laparoscopic approach for incarcerated inguinal hernia takes an advantage of each separate approach. The combined approach was described by Lavonius [29], open anterior approach was used for repair and exploratory laparoscopy was used for reduction and evaluation of bowel viability.

Ferzli et al. [30] reviewed 1890 hernia TEP repairs. Ninety-four cases of large scrotal hernias were identified of which, nine cases required conversion into open and six underwent combined approach with no recurrence. Authors advocated that a combined laparoscopic and open approach assist in visualization and dissection of the periperitoneal space. Yang et al. [31] conducted a retrospective study on 188 patients who underwent emergency surgical repair of strangulated groin hernias. Fifty-seven patients underwent laparoscopic repairs and 131 received open repairs. The incidence of laparotomies were higher in open group 19 vs. 0 in case of laparoscopic repairs. The postoperative recovery was better with shorter hospital stay (4.39 vs. 7.34) in the laparoscopic group. According to the latest European hernia guidelines [32], TEP approach for the large, difficult scrotal hernia may serve as an adjunct to dissection and definition of preperitoneal space allowing for easier hernia and mesh placement once the case is "converted" to open repair.

The common difficulties faced by the surgeons during repair of incarcerated and strangulated hernias without mesh are high incidence of recurrence rates (5–21%) and high wound infection rates (6–14%) [16, 19]. There are numerous studies which have compared the use of mesh and primary repairs in patients with incarcerated and strangulated hernias [33, 34]. The common prosthetic materials in tension free hernia mesh repairs are polymers, polypropylene, and polyster. Propylene is prosthesis of choice as it provides the best prosthesis leading to fibroblast activation [35]. The pore size of mesh also con-

tributes to the association and incidence of mesh infection. The pore size greater than 75 μm is favourable due to easier penetration of macrophages into the tissue, minimizing the risk of mesh infection [36]. Current meta-analysis on risk factors associated with mesh infection after hernia surgery is reported to be 5% [37].

Various situations and recommendations during emergency hernia repair are as follows [38].

1. Clean surgical field
2. Potentially contaminated surgical field
3. Contaminated-dirty surgical field

Clean surgical field: The preferred technique depends on amount of contamination, size of hernia and surgical expertise. Prosthetic mesh repair is recommended with intestinal incarceration and no signs of strangulation or concurrent bowel resection.

Potentially contaminated surgical field: With intestinal strangulation and bowel resection, primary direct suture is advised and synthetic repair can be performed with utmost caution. Biological meshes may be considered for managing hernia in contaminated surgical field.

Contaminated-dirty surgical field: Patients with strangulation, obstruction and peritoneal spillage by bowel perforation, direct tissue suture or anatomic repair is done when the defect is small. Biological mesh is suggested depending on degree of contamination and defect size. In patients experiencing sepsis, open management with delayed repair is the mainstay to prevent abdominal compartment syndrome. Early definitive closure of abdomen is vital once patient stabilizes.

14.4 Conclusion

Strangulated inguinal hernia is an incidence of acute abdomen which requires emergency surgery. The emerging acceptance for elective hernia repair has reduced the incidence of strangulation but has not eradicated completely. Prompt recognition and treatment is crucial. The immediate objectives of operation are reduction of hernia contents, resection of gangrenous tissue and repair of hernia defect. The use of prosthetic mesh repair is not an absolute contraindication in emergency hernia repairs. The parameters are dependent on surgeon acumen and expertise to handle the challenging situation. However, multiple studies are in favour of both using meshes and laparoscopic techniques in acute abdomen with perforated bowel but in the absence of frank peritonitis.

References

1. Pollack R. Strangulated external hernias. In: Nyhus LM, Condon RE, editors. Hernia. 3rd ed. Philadelphia: Lippincott Company Ltd.; 1989. p. 273–84.
2. Frankau C. Strangulating hernias: a review of 1987 cases. Br J Surg. 1932;19:176–99.
3. Denis C, Enguist IF. Strangulating external hernia. In: Nyhus LM, Condon RE, editors. Hernia. 3rd ed. Philadelphia: Lippincott Company Ltd.; 1978. p. 279–29.
4. Condon RE. Strangulating hernias. In: Nyhus LM, Condon RE, editors. Hernia. 3rd ed. Philadelphia: Lippincott Company Ltd.; 1989. p. 284.
5. Gallegos NC, Dawson J, Jarvis M, Hobsley M. Risk of strangulation in groin hernias. Br J Surg. 1991;78:1171–3.
6. Tanaka N, Uchida N, Ogihara H, Sasamoto H, Kato H, Kuwano H. Clinical study of inguinal and femoral incarcerated hernias. Surg Today. 2010;40:1144–7.
7. Bekoe S. Prospective analysis of the management of incarcerated and strangulated inguinal hernias. Am J Surg. 1973;126:665–8.
8. Nilsson H, Stylianidis G, Haapamäki M, Nilsson E, Nordin P. Mortality after groin hernia surgery. Ann Surg. 2007;245:656–60.
9. Deeba S, Purkayastha S, Paraskevas P, Athanasiou T, Darzi A, Zacharakis E. Laparoscopic approach to incarcerated and strangulated inguinal hernias. JSLS. 2009;13:327–31.
10. Rebuffat C, Galli A, Scalambra MS, Balsamo F. Laparoscopic repair of strangulated hernia. Surg Endosc. 2006;20:131–4.
11. Romain B, Chemaly R, Meyer N, Brigand C, Steinmetz JP, Rohr S. Prognostic factors of postoperative morbidity and mortality in strangulated groin hernia. Hernia. 2012;16:405–10.
12. Jafari MD, Wexner SD, Martz JE, McLemore EC, Margolin DA, Sherwinter DA. Perfusion assessment in laparoscopic left sided/anterior resection (PILLAR) II: a multi-institutional study. J Am Coll Surg. 2015;220:82–92.
13. Hernandez-Irizarry R, Zendejas B, Ramirez T, et al. Trends in emergent inguinal hernia surgery in Olmsted County, MN: population-based study. Hernia. 2012;16(4):397–403.
14. Hoffman A, Leshem E, Zmora O, Nachtomi O, Shabtai M, et al. The combined laparoscopic approach for the treatment of incarcerated inguinal hernia. Surg Endosc. 2010;24(8):1815–8.
15. Mahon D, Decadt B, Rhodes M. Prospective randomized trial of laparoscopic (transabdominal preperitoneal) vs. open (mesh) repair for bilateral and recurrent inguinal hernia. Surg Endosc. 2003;17:1386–90.
16. Papaziogas B, Lazaridis C, Makris J, et al. Tension-free repair versus modified Bassini technique (Andrews technique) for strangulated inguinal hernia: a comparative study. Hernia. 2005;9:156–9.
17. Simons MP, Aufenacker T, Bay-Nilsen M, et al. European hernia society guidelines on the treatment of inguinal hernia in adult patients. Hernia. 2009;13:343–403.
18. Nieuwenhuizen J, Van Ramshorst GH, Ten Brinke JG, et al. The use of mesh in acute hernia: frequency and outcome in 99 cases. Hernia. 2011;15:297–300.
19. Derici H, Unalp H, Nazli O, et al. Prosthetic repair of incarcerated inguinal hernias: is it a reliable method? Langenbecks Arch Surg. 2010;395:575–9.
20. Atila K, Guler S, Inal A. Prosthetic repair of acute lyincarcerated groin hernias: a prospective clinical observational cohort study. Langenbecks Arch Surg. 2010;395:563–8.
21. Watson SD, Saye W, Hollier PA. Combined laparoscopic incarcerated herniorrhaphy and small bowel resection. Surg Laparosc Endosc. 1993;3:106–8.
22. Leibl BJ, Schmedt CG, Kraft K, Kraft B, Bittner R. Laparoscopic transperitoneal hernia repair of incarcerated hernias: is it feasible? Surg Endosc. 2001;15:1179–83.
23. Felix EL, Michas CA, Gonzales MH. Laparoscopic hernioplasty: TAPP vs TEP. Surg Endosc. 1995;9:984–9.
24. Ishihara T, Kubota K, Eda N, Ishibashi S, Haraguchi Y. Laparoscopic approach to incarcerated inguinal hernia. Surg Endosc. 1996;10:1111–3.
25. Legnani GL, Rasini M, Pastori S, Sarli D. Laparoscopic transperitoneal hernioplasty (TAPP) for the acute management of strangulated inguino-crural hernias: a report of nine cases. Hernia. 2008;12:185e188.
26. Jagad RB, Shah J, Patel GR. The laparoscopic transperitoneal approach for irreducible inguinal hernias: perioperative outcome in four patients. J Minim Access Surg. 2009;5:31–4.
27. Siow SL, Mahendran HA, Hardin M, Chea CH, Nik Azim NA. Laparoscopic transabdominal approach and its modified technique for incarcerated scrotal hernias. Asian J Surg. 2013;36(2):64–8.
28. Ferzli G, Shapiro K, Chaudry G, et al. Laparoscopic extra-peritoneal approach to acutely incarcerated inguinal hernia. Surg Endosc. 2004;18:228–31.
29. Lavonius MI, Ovaska J. Laparoscopy in the evaluation of the incarcerated mass in groin hernia. Surg Endosc. 2000;14:488–9.
30. Ferzli GS, Rim S, Edwards ED. Combined laparoscopic and open extraperitoneal approach to scrotal hernias. Hernia. 2013;17(2):223–8.
31. Yang GP, Chan CT, Lai EC, Chan OC, Tang CN, Li MK. Laparoscopic versus open repair for strangulated

groin hernias: 188 cases over 4 years. Asian J Endosc Surg. 2012;5(3):131–7.

32. Bittner R, Montgomery MA, Arregui E, Bansal V, Bingener J, Bisgaard T, Buhck H. Update of guidelines on laparoscopic (TAPP) and endoscopic (TEP) treatment of inguinal hernia (International Endohernia Society). Surg Endosc. 2015;29(2):289–321.

33. Abdel-Baki NA, Bessa SS, Abdel-Razek AH. Comparison of prosthetic mesh repair and tissue repair in the emergency management of incarcerated para-umblical hernia: a prospective randomized study. Hernia. 2007;11:163–7.

34. Wysocki A, Kulawik J, Pozniczek M, Strzalka M. Is the Lichtenstein operation of strangulated groin hernia a safe procedure? World J Surg. 2006;30:2065–70.

35. Tatar C, Tüzün İS, Karşıdağ T, Kızılkaya MC, Yılmaz E, et al. Prosthetic mesh repair for incarcerated inguinal hernia. Balkan Med J. 2016;33:434–40.

36. Amid PK. Classification of biomaterials and their related complications in abdominal wall hernia surgery. Hernia. 1997;1:15–21.

37. Mavros MN, Athanasiou S, Alexiou AG, Pantelis K, Mitsikostas PK, Peppas G, Falagas ME. Risk factors for mesh-related infections after hernia repair surgery: a meta-analysis of cohort studies. World J Surg. 2011;35:2389–98.

38. Sartelli M, Coccolini F, van Ramshorst GH, Campanelli G, Mandalà V, Ansaloni L, Moore EE. WSES guidelines for emergency repair of complicated abdominal wall hernias. World J Emerg Surg. 2013;8(1):50. https://doi.org/10.1186/1749-7922-8-50.

Recurrent Inguinal Hernia

15

Rajesh Khullar

15.1 Introduction

Groin hernias are defined as protrusion of a viscus or part of a viscus or any abdominal content through an opening in the groin region. They constitute the majority of all abdominal wall hernias. Treatment of groin hernias is surgical repair of the defect, unless the condition of the patient precludes any surgical intervention. The success of a procedure is therefore determined by the permanence of the repair; a corollary, recurrence, defines a repair's failure.

The journey of groin hernia repair is one of the finest examples of evolution of surgical science in the understanding of human anatomy, physiology and histopathology, to minimize or eliminate the chance of a recurrence. Along a spectrum of continuing evolutionary debates, the current accepted principle of groin hernia repair is a tensionless, prosthetic reinforcement of the hernial defect. Surgical repairs based on these principles are anterior repairs like Lichtenstein, anterior preperitoneal repairs like Stoppa's and posterior endoscopic repairs like total extraperitoneal repair (TEP) and transabdominal preperitoneal repair (TAPP).

Laparoscopic/endoscopic inguinal hernia repair entails placement of the mesh in the posterior most potential space of the anterior abdominal wall between the peritoneum and the fascia transversalis. The space is created specifically for the repair and allowed to collapse at the end of the procedure. In principle the collapse should grip the mesh and keep it in position thus decreasing chances for a recurrence. The success of a surgical procedure for groin hernia is judged by the incidence of recurrence following the repair. Accepted recurrence rates of ~10% for primary repair and 25% for recurrent hernia repair in the pre-prosthetic era have shown a significant decrease to <5% following tensionless mesh repairs [1]. The risk of recurrence doubles following repair for recurrent groin hernia versus primary hernia. The recurrence rates reported for laparoscopic repairs are:

- Trans-abdominal Pre-peritoneal (TAPP)— 1.0–4.3% [2]
- Totally Extra Peritoneal (TEP)—0–0.4% [3].

Although comprising only a small fraction, the actual number of these procedures performed worldwide makes this fraction figure of recurrence a sizable health hazard and socioeconomic problem. An understanding of the potential risk factors and mechanisms of recurrence enables efficient negation of their effect, along with standardization of the procedure.

R. Khullar (✉)
Institute of Minimal Access, Metabolic and Bariatric Surgery, Max Super-Specialty Hospital, New Delhi, India

© Springer Nature India Private Limited 2020
P. Chowbey, D. Lomanto (eds.), *Techniques of Abdominal Wall Hernia Repair*,
https://doi.org/10.1007/978-81-322-3944-4_15

15.2 Risk Factors and Mechanism of Recurrence

The identified risk factors for recurrence following an endoscopic repair are primarily technical. Non-controllable patient- or pathology-related risk factors play a small role in recurrences following endoscopic repairs.

Technical factors may be related to surgeon's expertise and surgical technique or the prosthesis being used.

1. **Surgeon's Expertise:** Laparoscopic groin hernia repair is labelled as a technically advanced laparoscopic procedure with a steep learning curve. The learning curve being adjudged by the improvement in the number of conversions, operative time, complications and recurrences during the surgeon's learning phase before reaching a comfortable level of competency. Competency being defined by values of the surgical outcomes being comparable to acceptable outcomes of a standard procedure. Numerous studies quote varying number of cases, 40–250, mandated for acquiring sufficient technical expertise [4–7]. The incidence of recurrence is seen to stabilize over the first 100 cases; however, operative time, conversions and complications have been seen to improve even after 250 cases [7], implying that factors other than surgical expertise and surgeon's competence operate in the causation of recurrences. Most studies report on experience of single surgeons' or single institutions' attaining of adequate competence levels; however, the common observation shows majority of recurrences and complications to occur in the initial 50–100 cases [8, 9]. In the 2012 EAES consensus development conference a recurrence rate of 0–5%, 5 years down the practice was voted as a target to be achieved by the practicing endoscopic surgeon to be considered competent [10].

2. **Technical factors**
   (a) **Incomplete dissection**: Inadequate space—Laparoscopic repair requires a complete exposure of the myopectineal orifice, so that all potential hernial sites are adequately overlapped by the mesh. An inadequate space results in limited exposure of the operative field, precluding the placement of an adequately sized mesh. Insufficient space may result in use of either a small mesh made to fit the available space or folding/rolling of a larger mesh [11]. Both situations can cause recurrence. This occurs because a small mesh is prone to migration into the hernial defect by the same forces that caused the hernia and a larger but rolled/folded mesh can slide away from the defect due to intra-abdominal shearing forces. A large-sized mesh placed in a small space can also balloon out through the defect resembling a recurrence.

   (b) Missed hernias and cord lipomas—Missing a cord lipoma or a hernia and ineffectual mesh fixation are other accepted reasons of recurrences [12]. A cord lipoma originates from the pre-peritoneal fat and therefore forms an unnatural constituent of the cord. Often a tongue of peritoneum may get pulled up along with the lipoma resulting in a true hernial sac. Failure to properly parietalize the cord structure by stripping away the peritoneum and defining the triangle of Doom is the cause for missed hernias and recurrences. The cord should be parietalized till the vas deferens is seen to curve medially towards the pelvis and the testicular vessels seen laterally to retreat proximally up the retroperitoneum.

   (c) Hematoma's—A pre-peritoneal hematoma or urinary retention in the post-operative period may also lift the mesh from its position predisposing to hernia recurrence.

   The space needed for laying down a 15×12 cm^2 mesh stretches from the pubic symphysis in the midline and 2–3 cm behind the pubic bone inferomedially to the psoas major muscle infero-laterally and transversus abdominis muscle superolaterally, the lateral limit being determined by finger indentation at the anterior superior iliac spine (ASIS).

(d) **Inappropriate fixation**: After a prosthetic hernia repair, tissue-mesh interface is the weakest link and is commonly the site where the repair gives way. This may occur due to poor grip provided by the already weakened tissue or avulsion of the fixation device due to pressures and strain acting on the mesh. Mesh implantation involves three important components for ensuring a secure attachment, which are

- Length of mesh beyond edge of defect,
- Site of fixation and
- Strength of fixation.

On principle the mesh should be fixed using devices with adequate tissue penetration to counter the intra-abdominal forces, to tissues with strong inherent strength, well away from the hernia site. Tissues in and around the hernial defect are weak and likely to give way under stress. Although there are several studies and meta-analysis that have found no difference in recurrence following fixation or non-fixation of mesh [13–16], there is also sufficient evidence suggesting non-fixation to be one of the causes of recurrences [11, 17, 18]. Majority of surgeons recommend mesh fixation in large hernias to prevent early displacement, mesh migration and recurrence. Also by their own admission the authors conducting the meta-analysis have hinted at the need for better quality of trials before saying a final word on this subject [16].

One of the earlier studies on causes for recurrence following laparoscopic hernia repair by Phillips EH et al., note the causes of recurrence as a smaller mesh in 60% cases, insufficient fixation in 30% cases, a non-repair in 20% cases and the hernia recurring due to clips pulling out of tissues in 8% cases [19]. The study involved a large number of patients across high volume centres with sufficient surgical experience. What is notable is that none of the patients undergoing TEP reported a recurrence.

(e) **Mesh material**: There are several trials and meta-analyses comparing heavy weight and light weight meshes both in open and in laparoscopic inguinal hernioplasties [20, 21]. The type of mesh used does not affect the incidence of recurrence. The decision of which mesh to use will therefore lie with whatever the operating surgeon is comfortable using. As the position of the mesh is extraperitoneal, the non-coated mesh suffices for covering the defect. What remains as a choice is therefore low weight or heavy weight. Theoretically, however, a heavy weight mesh, known to contract more may predispose to delayed recurrences. Similarly a light weight mesh is more prone to folding and may get lifted up from the lower edge during desufflation resulting in a recurrence.

(f) **Mesh size**—Small meshes provide inadequate coverage of myopectineal orifice and increase recurrence. Also meshes contract and shrink with time, which should be taken into consideration before deciding on the mesh size.

(g) **Mesh slitting**: Slitting a mesh results in a defect in the mesh with the potential to allow a recurrence to occur. A retrospective assessment of causes for recurrences by Leibl et al. in 2000 addressed the issue of mesh-slitting as one of the causes for recurrence [22]. It was concluded that a non-slit mesh was safer to avoid a recurrence. A large mesh with no slit, smoothly covering a well-dissected myopectineal orifice fixed medially to the pubic periosteum and Cooper's ligament and laterally to the transversus abdominis sheath provided the best defense against a recurrence.

Laparoscopic groin hernia repair requires advanced laparoscopic skills for mastering a new approach and a new technique with a steep learning curve. The surgical approach is posterior, making necessary a reorientation of the groin anatomy. The anatomical region contains vital structures like the external iliac vessels, periprostatic venous plexus and the cutaneous nerves, which require good technical knowledge and skill for safe dissection and handling. The complexity of the approach therefore lies in creating an adequate space safely and exposing the entire myopectineal orifice for a smooth prosthetic reinforcement of the region. All these factors add to procedural difficulties and are contributory to the development of recurrences. In fact the technical factors listed above are responsible for nearly all recurrences [22–24]. Yet the incidence of recurrence following posterior mesh repairs whether anterior or endoscopic is very low and superior to all anterior repairs. A longitudinal study from the Swedish hernia registry has shown the pre-peritoneal repair, both endoscopic and open, to have the best outcomes for recurrent hernias, irrespective of what the primary repair was [25].

3. **Patient factors**

Recurrences may still develop, even after all technical factors have been appropriately addressed. This small yet persistent incidence reflects the effect of non-technical factors such as the ones related to the disease or the patient, which contribute to the occurrence of recurrences. These include:

Modifiable risk factors

1. Smoking is associated with increased recurrence
2. Obesity—moderate evidence to link obesity with increased recurrence
3. Malnutrition, anemia
4. Diabetes
5. Chronic lung disease
6. Steroids

Non-controllable patient-related risk factors

7. Collagen disease—decreased type I/III ratio has higher recurrence rates
8. Gender—females have higher recurrence
9. Hernia anatomy

10. Hernia type—direct hernias and sliding hernias are more likely to recur
11. Age

These factors are common to all types of repairs and affect the risk of recurrence. What is perhaps common to them all is a common pathway through which their effect on recurrence is expressed. The effect of smoking, malnutrition, diabetes, steroids, collagen disorders or size and type of hernia (direct/indirect) is expressed in the composition of the scar and quality of collagen tissue in the healing wound, which determines its strength and contractility. There is a strong lobby of herniologists who have been arguing for hernia to be labelled as a systemic disease with local manifestations. There is now sufficient evidence in literature supporting this theory. It is possible that the underlying pathophysiology of the different inguinal hernia types could affect the overall recurrence risk as well as the risk of developing a specific type of recurrent inguinal hernia [26–29].

15.3 Evaluation

A detailed evaluation begins with a detailed history of hernia, past surgical, past medical history. Previous operative records with findings should be carefully examined. Detailed local and systemic examination should be performed on all patients. In most cases a recurrence can be diagnosed after clinical examination. In case of doubt, ultrasound of the groin should be performed; if suspicion of recurrence still exists despite a normal sonogram, dynamic CT or MRI should be considered. Repair of a recurrent hernia is always difficult and should be undertaken only by experienced surgeons in a specialised center.

15.4 Management

There is no evidence to support that conservative management in recurrent groin hernia and surgery should be offered to all patients. Patient should be explained by the surgeon in detail the advantages and disadvantages of each procedure after which the patient can take an informed decision.

Patients with history of previous tissue repairs are candidates for both open(anterior) and laparoscopic (posterior) repair. However, laparoscopic approach avoids a previously scarred area and is the preferred technique.

In cases where open (anterior) mesh repair has been performed, laparoscopic approach is the procedure of choice as it involves entering virgin tissue planes and carries less risk of nerve entrapment and injury to vas. However, laparoscopic approach in recurrent hernias has longer operative times than primary procedure and increased incidence of peritoneal injury.

In cases of recurrence after a previous laparoscopic repair, anatomy is completely distorted and an anterior (open) approach is the surgery of choice. Few centres do report the feasibility of TAPP in recurrent hernias after TEP/TAPP, but it should be undertaken only by an experienced surgeon.

Management of cases where both anterior and posterior approaches have failed is a difficult task. In such cases a TAPP or a laparoscopic IPOM can be undertaken by the experienced surgeon.

Principles of repair
1. The approach to hernia should be through undisturbed tissue planes to avoid scarred area with distorted anatomy.
2. Dissection should be slow and meticulous. One must always try to restore the normal anatomy.
3. Recurrent inguinal hernia repair must include exploration of the entire groin region so femoral hernias are not missed and subsequent recurrence is prevented.
4. Previous mesh need not be removed. No evidence to support increased risk of chronic pain. Removal of mesh may increase the risk of bleeding, injury to urinary bladder.
5. Mesh should be of adequate size and placed over the previous mesh so as to cover the previous displaced mesh.

15.5 Summary

Recurrence of inguinal hernia remains a challenging situation for an operating surgeon. Standardization of surgical technique helps to decrease the recurrence rates. Guidelines are available to aid the process of decision-making regarding which procedure to perform after a recurrence. When operating on a recurrent inguinal hernia, a meticulous surgical technique should be employed to ensure optimal outcomes.

Recurrence is the prime factor for determining the success of any surgical repair of a hernia be it groin or ventral. Endoscopic groin hernia repair fairs favorably amongst different approaches to groin hernia repairs with low recurrence rates and a rapid recovery. Recurrences following endoscopic groin hernia repair are mainly technical errors, some of which like extent of dissection and mesh size have already been standardized. Developing standard training protocols for teaching and training in this approach will benefit young aspiring herniologists keen to learn this approach.

References

1. Gopal SV, Warrier A. Recurrence after groin hernia repair-revisited. Int J Surg. 2013;11:374–7.
2. Burcharth J. The epidemiology and risk factors for recurrence after inguinal hernia surgery. Dan Med J. 2014;61(5):B4846.
3. Bendavid R. Expectations of hernia surgery (inguinal and femoral). In: Paterson-Brown S, editor. Principles and practice of surgical laparoscopy. Philadelphia: Saunders; 1994. p. 387–414.
4. Bansal VK, Krishna A, Misra MC, Kumar S. Learning curve in laparoscopic inguinal hernia repair: experience at a tertiary care centre. Indian J Surg. 2016;78(3):197–202.
5. Lim JW, Lee JY, Lee SE, Moon JI, Ra YM, Choi IS, Choi WJ, Yoon DS, Min HS. The learning curve for laparoscopic totally extraperitoneal herniorrhaphy by moving average. J Korean Surg Soc. 2012;83(2):92–6.
6. Choi YY, Kim Z, Hur KY. Learning curve for laparoscopic totally extraperitoneal repair of inguinal hernia. Can J Surg. 2012;55(1):33–6.
7. Schouten N, Simmermacher RK, van Dalen T, Smakman N, Clevers GJ, Davids PH, Verleisdonk EJ, Burgmans JP. Is there an end of the "learning curve" of endoscopic totally extraperitoneal (TEP) hernia repair? Surg Endosc. 2013;27(3):789–94.

8. Feliu-Palà X, Martín-Gómez M, Morales-Conde S, Fernández-Sallent E. The impact of the surgeon's experience on the results of laparoscopic hernia repair. Surg Endosc. 2001;15(12):1467–70.

9. Aikoye A, Harilingam M, Khushal A. The impact of high surgical volume on outcomes from laparoscopic (totally extra peritoneal) inguinal hernia repair. J Clin Diagn Res. 2015;9(6):PC15–6.

10. Poelman MM, Van den Huevel B, et al. EAES consensus development conference on endoscopic repair of groin hernias. Surg Endosc. 2013;27(10):3505–19.

11. Lowham AS, Filipi CJ, Fitzgibbons RJ, Stoppa R, Wantz GE, Felix EL. Mechanisms of hernia recurrence after preperitoneal mesh repair: traditional and laparoscopic. Ann Surg. 1997;225:422–31.

12. Felix E, Scott S, Crafton B, Geis P, Duncan T, Sewell R, et al. Causes of recurrence after laparoscopic hernioplasty. A multicenter study. Surg Endosc. 1998;12:226–31.

13. Claus CM, Rocha GM, Campos AC, Bonin EA, Dimbarre D, Loureiro MP, Coelho JC. Prospective, randomized and controlled study of mesh displacement after laparoscopic inguinal repair: fixation versus no fixation of mesh. Surg Endosc. 2016;30(3):1134–40.

14. Garg P, Nair S, Shereef M, Thakur JD, Nain N, Menon GR, Ismail M. Mesh fixation compared to nonfixation in total extraperitoneal inguinal hernia repair: a randomized controlled trial in a rural center in India. Surg Endosc. 2011;25(10):3300–6.

15. Teng YJ, Pan SM, Liu YL, Yang KH, Zhang YC, Tian JH, Han JX. A meta-analysis of randomized controlled trials of fixation versus nonfixation of mesh in laparoscopic total extraperitoneal inguinal hernia repair. Surg Endosc. 2011;25(9):2849–58.

16. Sajid MS, Ladwa N, Kalra L, Hutson K, Sains P, Baig MK. A meta-analysis examining the use of tacker fixation vs. no-fixation of mesh in laparoscopic inguinal hernia repair. Int J Surg. 2012;10(5):224–31.

17. Knook MT, Weidema WF, Stassen LP, van Steensel CJ. Endoscopic total extraperitoneal repair of primary and recurrent inguinal hernias. Surg Endosc. 1999;13:507–11.

18. Jago R. Stapled and nonstapled laparoscopic transabdominalpreperitoneal inguinal hernia repair. Surg Endosc. 1999;13:766.

19. Philips EH, Rosenthal R, Fallas M, Caroll B, Arregui M, Corbott J, et al. Reasons for early recurrence following laparoscopic hernioplasty. Surg Endosc. 1995;9:140–5.

20. Sajid MS, Kalra L, Parampalli U, Sains PS, Baig MK. A systematic review and meta-analysis evaluating the effectiveness of lightweight mesh against heavy weight mesh in influencing the incidence of chronic groin pain following laparoscopic inguinal hernia repair. Am J Surg. 2013;205(6):726–36.

21. Currie A, Andrew H, Tonsi A, Hurley PR, Taribagil S. Lightweight versus heavyweight mesh in laparoscopic inguinal hernia repair: a meta-analysis. Surg Endosc. 2012;26(8):2126–33.

22. Leibl BJ, Schmedt CG, Kraft K, Ulrich M, Bittner R. Recurrence after endoscopic transperitoneal hernia repair (TAPP): causes, reparative techniques and results of the reoperation. J Am Coll Surg. 2000;190:651–5.

23. Kukleta JF. Causes of recurrence in laparoscopic inguinal hernia repair. J Minim Access Surg. 2006;2:187–91.

24. Dehal A, Woodward B, Johna S, Yamanishi F. Bilateral laparoscopic totally extraperitoneal repair without mesh fixation. JSLS. 2014;18(3).

25. Sevonius D, Gunnrsson U, et al. Recurrent groin hernia surgery. Br J Surg. 2011;98(10):1489–94.

26. Henriksen NA, Yadete DH, Sorensen LT, Agren MS, Jorgensen LN. Connective tissue alteration in abdominal wall hernia. Br J Surg. 2011;98(2):210–9.

27. Henriksen NA, Mortensen JH, Lorentzen L, Agren MS, Bay-Jensen AC, Jorgensen LN, Karsdal MA. Abdominal wall hernias-A local manifestation of systemically impaired quality of the extracellular matrix. Surgery. 2016;160(1):220–7. https://doi.org/10.1016/j.surg.2016.02.011.

28. Klinge U, Binnebosel M, Mertens PR. Are collagens the culprits in the development of incisional and inguinal hernia disease? Hernia. 2006;10:472–7.

29. Antoniou SA, Antoniou GA, Granderath FA, Simopoulos C. The role of matrix metalloproteinases in the pathogenesis of abdominal wall hernias. Eur J Clin Invest. 2009;39(11):953–9.

Part III

Abdominal Wall Hernia

Biomaterials for Abdominal Wall Hernia Repair

16

Asim Shabbir and Sujith Wijerathne

16.1 Introduction

The evolution of hernia surgery is greatly influenced by the discovery of new biomaterials. These biomaterials have helped surgeons to overcome limitations in surgical techniques to achieve greater heights in better quality of care for their patients. Their advent has helped surgeons to overcome the most significant technical challenge faced in the past that is tension. With tension-free repair the incidence of recurrence has dropped significantly and synthetic meshes have made the possibility of achieving a tension-free repair easier.

Biomaterials in abdominal wall hernia repair can be broadly divided in to absorbable and the more popular non-absorbable synthetic meshes. Additionally there are biologic meshes which can be allograft or even xenograft. The properties of these biomaterials are different when comparing to each other, this makes them unique and reserved for different types of hernia repairs.

This article highlights the properties of meshes used in inguinal and ventral hernia repairs, their specific indications with available data on safety and feasibility and the current guidelines available on the choice of biomaterials for abdominal wall hernia repairs.

The three most common prostheses used for abdominal wall hernia repair today are polypropylene, polyester and polytetrafluoroethylene (PTFE). These materials differ from each other in material composition, weight, burst strength and the inflammatory response. When choosing a specific mesh for abdominal wall hernia repair, the above properties are taken into consideration in conjunction with the available evidence.

16.2 Meshes for Inguinal Hernia Repair

There are countless amounts of inguinal hernia repaired around the world annually in the present era and still most of these hernias are repaired with open technique using various prosthetic materials. These prosthetics can range from polyester to polypropylene and in some parts of the developing world where access is limited to these new biomaterials, even sterilized mosquito nets are used as prosthetics [1, 2]. With the evolvement of minimal access surgery concept, laparoscopic hernia repair is increasingly gaining popularity and utilize similar biomaterials that are used in the open technique with proven benefits of low recurrence rates and complications [1]. The technique of tension-free repair using a prosthetic mesh have become the gold standard

A. Shabbir · S. Wijerathne (✉)
Department of Surgery, Minimally Invasive Surgical
Centre, National University Health System,
Singapore
e-mail: sujith_wijerathne@nuhs.edu.sg

© Springer Nature India Private Limited 2020
P. Chowbey, D. Lomanto (eds.), *Techniques of Abdominal Wall Hernia Repair*,
https://doi.org/10.1007/978-81-322-3944-4_16

for inguinal hernia repairs [3]. In the earlier stages of development of this technique there were concerns about placing a mesh in an acute or incarcerated hernia, but later on evidence supporting mesh placement appeared to be safe [4], even in the setting of bowel necrosis [5]. There are numerous types and commercial brands of meshes marketed for inguinal hernia repair. Mesh materials are processed in numerous ways and are available as simple flat mesh types in various sizes, with or without precut segments, and also available as three-dimensional forms which closely conform to the contours of inguinal anatomy reducing the need for fixation. Some meshes have additional components incorporated to them to reduce adhesions, to facilitate fixation and to prevent infection [1].

Historically inguinal hernia repairs were done without any prosthesis. Surgeons gradually started using variety of wires and sutures to reinforce the repair, which lead to the development of early forms of meshes which were initially made from stainless steel and these meshes were too stiff. Subsequently nylon meshes were used, but they disintegrated too rapidly, and later on meshes made out of polypropylene were found to be more durable and became popular in inguinal hernia repair [6–8].

Initially meshes were used to just buttress or reinforce suture repairs. In 1980 Irving Lichtenstein performed a tension-free hernia repair with a mesh placed anterior to the transversalis fascia, and soon the "Lichtenstein repair" became the gold standard for inguinal hernia repair. This technique is simple and can be safely performed even under local anesthesia, and has an acceptable recovery period and a complication rate [9–11].

There are three basic polymers currently available for production of meshes and namely these are polyester, polypropylene and polytetrafluoro-ethylene (PTFE). Polyester polymers were discovered in 1946. Polyester was first used for an inguinal hernia repair by Wolstenholme in 1956 [12]. Polypropylene was introduced by Usher in 1958 as a prosthetic material and soon it became the most commonly used prosthetic for inguinal hernia repairs [13]. Polypropylene has much better tensile strength, it was less prone to infection and there was evidence of connective tissue infiltration when implanted to animal models compared to the other meshes available in the market during the time it was introduced. Though PTFE was discovered by DuPont in 1938 and it was only used in hernia repair in 1950s. Modifications were made to expand PTFE in 1960s to produce a uniform structure with enhanced mechanical strength (ePTFE) [1, 13].

The development of laparoscopic inguinal hernia repair positively affected the evolution of these three basic polymers making multiple alterations in them to produce more lighter, durable and user-friendly meshes. Alterations that were made to the texture and porosity of these meshes resulted in different tissue reactions and subsequently better mesh incorporation in to the host tissues [1].

Polyester is commonly used in the clothing industry and it is also used as a biomaterial for abdominal wall hernia repair but less commonly now compared to polypropylene. Polyester polymers are made of an ester in the main chain (Fig. 16.1). In studies comparing these two meshes, there were no differences in recurrence rates [14, 15]. One study showed slightly higher incidence of chronic inguinal pain and "feeling of the mesh" in patients where polypropylene mesh was used [14]. The main concern regarding the polyester mesh has been the degradation overtime with loss of tensile strength.

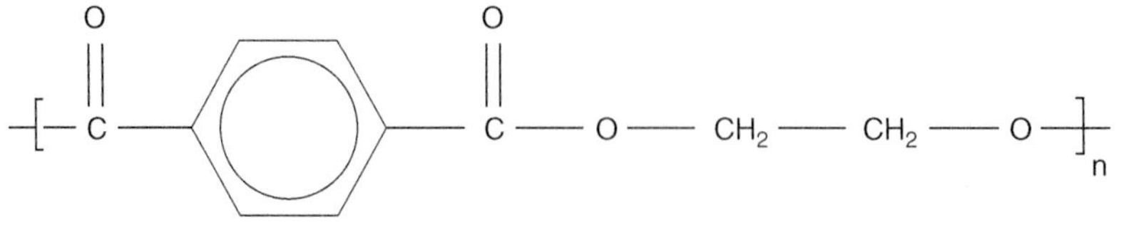

Fig. 16.1 Biochemical arrangement of polyester

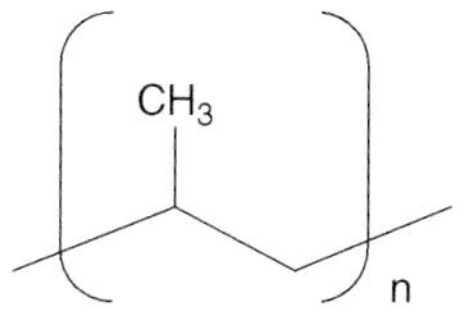

Fig. 16.2 Biochemical arrangement of polypropylene

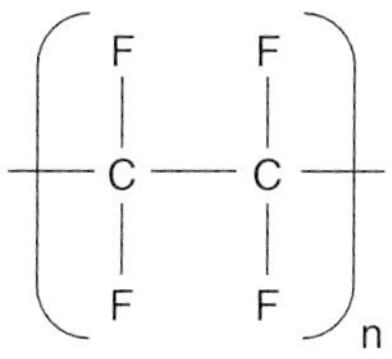

Fig. 16.3 Biochemical arrangement of PTFE

Polypropylene was discovered in 1954 by Giulio Natta and Karl Ziegler. It is a thermoplastic polymer which consists of an ethylene with a methyl group attached to it (Fig. 16.2). This material is hydrophobic, resistant to biological degradation and electrostatically neutral. In these polypropylene meshes the weight, filament size, pore size and architecture affect its biologic reactivity, in addition to the individual host response [1]. Polypropylene meshes can be monofilament, multifilament or compound. Langenbach et al., compared these three types of meshes in laparoscopic inguinal hernia repair and found that patients who had hernia repaired with monofilament polypropylene had superior outcomes compared to those with multifilament polypropylene. The monofilament group took significantly longer time to return to work, had higher pain scores and demonstrated more impairment in everyday activities compared to patients with a multifilament polypropylene [14]. The flexibility of these meshes can be altered by either using knitted or woven materials [15]. It was initially thought that the pore size should be at least 0.75–1 mm to prevent infection, but this varied between different manufacturers [16].

An ideal prosthetic material should be able to provide maximum strength with minimal amount of foreign body implanted to a patient, and this depends on the size of the fibers and pores. Lightweight polypropylene meshes are designed to achieve these goals. Some studies show an improvement of post-operative pain when lightweight polypropylene meshes are used compared to heavyweight meshes [17–20]. Initially there were concerns about increased recurrence rates with lightweight meshes but subsequent studies failed to demonstrate this especially when it is used in laparoscopic inguinal hernia repair [1].

Coda et al., have categorized these meshes based on their weight and composition [21]. Based on the weight they have categorized polypropylene monofilament knitted/woven prosthetics as Ultra-light <35 g/m^2, Light $\geq 35 < 70$ g/m^2, Standard $\geq 70 < 140$ g/m^2 and Heavy ≥ 140 g/m^2. According to the biomaterial composition they have classified the meshes as simple, composite, combined and biologic. Prosthetics made of one pure biomaterial are considered simple and those made of two or more different layers and called composite meshes. Prosthetics made of two or more materials knitted or woven together are called combined [21].

PTFE is a synthetic fluoropolymer of tetrafluoroethylene that has numerous applications (Fig. 16.3). It has been used in inguinal hernia repair mainly with intra-peritoneal on-lay mesh technique, but due to higher recurrence and infection rates PTFE did not become popular [22, 23]. PTFE also has a small pore size which results in insufficient molecular permeability leading to poor clearance of fibrinous and proteinaceous materials which eventually results in formation of post-operative seroma [1].

To overcome some of the disadvantages faced with the use of pure synthetic biomaterials, manufacturers started combining them with various other materials. Beta-glucan-coated polypropylene prosthetics is an example for this [1]. Beta-glucan is a product of plant origin that is used to promote healing and also has an immune-modulatory effect. The meshes coated with this have shown a decrease in the incidence of chronic pain and recurrence compared to pure polypropylene meshes [24, 25]. Some meshes combine non-absorbable material with a barrier layer on the side facing bowel to prevent adhesions. If the peritoneal coverage is being violated, then these meshes are useful to separate the synthetic prosthesis from intra-abdominal contents [1].

Some of the prosthetic meshes are made by combining non-absorbable material with absorbable materials and with time this technique reduces the foreign material in the body. Combination of polypropylene and polyglactine is an example for a composite prosthetic. Polyglactine fibers are resorbed in approximately 60 days leaving the polypropylene fibers behind [1]. But studies show no difference between this composite mesh and standard polypropylene mesh with regards to perioperative complications, post-operative pain and recurrence [26, 27].

Prosthetics have also been modified to reduce the need for fixation. Polypropylene mesh with a nitinol frame and titanium-coated monofilament polypropylene meshes like TiMESH® (GfE, Medizintechnik GmbH, Germany) are examples for those meshes that have been modified to reduce the need for fixation. Figure 16.4 shows a TiMESH® placed in the pre-peritoneal space during a laparoscopic inguinal hernia repair performed at our institution. It is believed that the reduced need for fixation may reduce the risk of post-operative pain. Three-dimensional meshes which conform to the contours of the pelvic and inguinal anatomy also reduces the need for fixation. Studies have shown that these anatomically contoured prosthetics have minimal risk of post-operative and chronic pain, low recurrence rates and may not even require fixation [28, 29].

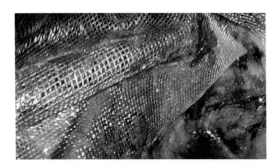

Fig. 16.4 Laparoscopic view of TiMESH® during pre-peritoneal placement of the mesh

Biological materials are also used in inguinal hernia repair. There are two main types of biologic prosthetics available currently. Those originating from human tissues are called allografts and those originating from animal tissue are called xenografts. The origin of the currently available xenografts are either porcine or bovine. The meshes differ from the species of animals they are made and on what part is harvested. The commonly harvested parts are dermis, small intestinal submucosa, and pericardium. The role of biologic materials in any hernia repair has mainly been limited to infected surgical fields. The advantage of biologic prosthesis could be reduced post-operative pain and the disadvantage of these meshes is the risk of recurrence. In cases where biologic meshes are used in a bridging manner, recurrence rates up to 9% in inguinal hernia repair and up to 80% in incisional hernia repair have been reported [1]. But the number of cases and studies where biologic prosthetics are used in inguinal hernia repair are much less compared to incisional hernia.

16.3 Recommendations for Biomaterials in Inguinal Herniorraphy

The European hernia society guidelines recommends a tension-free repair with synthetic non-absorbable flat meshes or composite meshes with a non-absorbable component for the treatment of inguinal hernia in adult patients. For open inguinal hernia repair, the use of lightweight, material-reduced, large-pore (>1 mm) meshes can be considered as there's a potential advantage of decreased long-term discomfort, but possibly at the cost of increased recurrence rates due to inadequate fixation and overlap [30].

A lightweight monofilament mesh with a pore size of at least 1.0–1.5 mm consisting of a minimum tensile strength in all directions of 16 N/cm appeared to be the most suitable for inguinal hernia repair. And the use of these large pore polypropylene meshes in laparoscopic hernia repair is harmless concerning azoospermia [31].

16.4 Biomaterials for Ventral Hernia Repair

Biomaterials used in ventral hernia repair are similar to those used in inguinal hernia repair. An ideal biomaterial or mesh should be strong enough to withstand high burst pressures generated within the abdominal cavity. An ideal mesh should be chemically inert so that it prevents an inflammatory or a foreign-body reaction. It should not form any adhesions on the visceral side and should not be carcinogenic. It should not initiate allergic reactions or hypersensitivity reactions. An ideal mesh should be easy to manufacture with a minimal cost and should have unique mechanical properties that allows modifications such as trimming and folding without compromising its shape and tensile strength. It should allow for sterilization, should be resistant to infection and should be easily maneuverable intra-operatively [1].

Polypropylene, polyester and expanded polytetrafluoroethylene (ePTFE) are the main materials used in ventral hernia repair. The initial polypropylene materials used in ventral hernia repair were heavyweight with small and dense pore design (>90 g/m²). These characteristics of the heavyweight meshes lead to an intense foreign body reaction which resulted in rigid scars with granuloma formation between pores and complications such as mesh extrusion, extensive adhesions and entero-cutaneous fistula formation [32]. Lightweight polypropylene meshes were introduced to overcome the issues faced with the heavyweight version but the studies showed similar results and higher failure rates due to mesh displacement or rupture during the early postoperative period [1, 33, 34].

Polyethylene terephthalate (PET) or polyester is another hernia mesh used commonly before and known to cause a considerable inflammatory reaction with gross tissue ingrowth into the macroporous interstices of the mesh which results in variable degrees of scar formation. To minimize the effects of inflammatory response, manufacturers started coating these PET meshes with various compounds [1]. Examples of coated PET meshes include C-Qur (Atrium) coated with Omega-3 fatty acid, Parietex composite (Covidien) coated with collagen-polyethylene glycol-glycerol, Proceed (Ethicon) coated with oxidized regenerated cellulose, Sepramesh IP composite (Bard) coated with hydrogel layer, Ti-Mesh (Biomet, Inc.) which has covalently bonded tetanized surface and PolyPro Mesh (STS) coated with polyether urethane urea.

PTFE is another biomaterial used for ventral hernia repair. Modifications were made to expand PTFE in 1960s to produce a uniform structure with enhanced mechanical strength (ePTFE). Gore-Tex (W. L. Gore) soft tissue patch was the first ePTFE mesh introduced for intra-peritoneal use. In 1993 this mesh was modified to have a more porous design to facilitate better tissue ingrowth and became commercially available as the MycroMesh (W. L. Gore). The two-sided DualMesh (W. L. Gore) was introduced in 1994 and it was subsequently modified with large interstices and an irregular "corduroy-like" surface on the parietal side to increase tissue ingrowth. The DualMesh (W. L. Gore) also became available with incorporated antimicrobial agents (silver clorhexidine film, type "Plus"). MotifMESH (Proxy Biomedical) is a new macroporous non-woven mesh of condensed PTFE (cPTFE) for intraperitoneal application. Although the mesh is macroporous, theoretically it has an anti-adhesion barrier because of the PTFE content. The MotifMESH is 90% thinner compared with older ePTFE meshes [35]. Omyra® mesh (Aesculap AG) is another example for a cPTFE mesh which is currently available. Figure 16.5

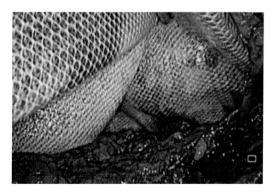

Fig. 16.5 Laparoscopic view of Omyra® mesh during intra-peritoneal placement of the mesh

shows an Omyra® mesh being deployed during a laparoscopic ventral hernia repair performed at our institution.

Resorbable meshes are also used in ventral hernia repair. These meshes are usually made of copolymerized forms of polylactic acid, polyglycolic acid, polyglactin or polycaprolactone. The degradation rate in these absorbable materials can pose a significant risk for recurrence. An example for a resorbable mesh is the TIGR Matrix surgical mesh (Novus Scientific). TIGR mesh is knitted with two polymers with different resorbable rates. One polymer has a fast degradation rate and the other has a considerably slower degradation rate, which secures the integrity of the mesh during the phase of initial inflammatory response. GORE BIO-A (W.L. Gore) is another resorbable mesh which became available later on. Compared to the TIGR matrix mesh, the GORE BIO-A mesh is microporous and has a faster resorption profile [1].

Biological meshes are also available for ventral hernia repair. These are acellular materials with an intact extracellular matrix which can be either allografts or xenografts. These materials can become vascularized and therefore poses a theoretical ability to clear infections. Acellular porcine dermal collagen and porcine small intestinal submucosa (Surgisis—Cook® Medical) has been used in laparoscopic ventral hernia repair with acceptable results. Bovine tunica vaginalis and bovine pericardium (Lyoplant®—B. Braun Aesculap) are also tested as biomaterials in animal studies for abdominal wall hernia repair [35]. A potential risk of using animal tissue in hernia repair could be immunologic rejection; however, this risk is minimal when allogenic acellular dermal matrix (AlloDerm—LifeCell Corporation) is used as a biomaterial.

16.5 Choice of Biomaterial and Recommendations for Ventral Herniorraphy

The optimal mesh for a ventral hernia repair should be chemically inactive and should be non-carcinogenic. It should not cause an inflamma-

tory reaction and the characteristics of the mesh should not change after tissue contact. An optimal mesh should not cause any allergic reaction or any hypersensitivity reaction and should be resistant to physical manipulation and should allow for sterilization. It should not cause any adhesion formation with bowel or abdominal organs and should allow adequate tissue ingrowth with minimal shrinkage to facilitate better incorporation to the host tissue. It should be resistant to infections and should not affect the abdominal wall compliance. An ideal mesh for ventral hernia repair should be easily maneuverable, reproducible and affordable as well [35].

Adhesion formation is a common phenomenon after laparoscopic ventral hernia repair and it can be due to scar formation after dissection and surgical trauma and also could be due to foreign body reaction to mesh materials and fixation devices. All techniques and devices used for ventral hernia repair can cause some degree of adhesion formation and at least for now it is not possible to completely prevent this from taking place. Dense adhesions can form between the abdominal organs and the mesh particularly if polypropylene and polyester is used as a mesh material and this can subsequently result in significant risk of bowel injury especially during revision surgeries. Revision surgeries in these patients are also known to pose a significant risk for entero-cutaneous fistula formation. An attempt has been made to reduce this risk by using ePTFE or textile meshes made of polyvinyl difluoride (PVDF), polypropylene or polyester with an additional coating or barrier function of another material, such as titanium, collagen, cellulose, hyaluronic acid or polydioxanon [36].

During laparoscopic ventral hernia repair the placement of an intra-peritoneal mesh is safe, provided that the mesh is specifically made for this purpose as mentioned earlier. Similar to the meshes used in inguinal hernia repair, most mesh materials used in ventral hernia repair also undergo some degree of shrinkage due to contraction of the deposited fibrous tissue after the intra-peritoneal positioning. No significant differences have been shown for adhesion formation and shrinkage for different mesh types specifically designed for intra-peritoneal placement [37].

International Endo-hernia Society guidelines recommend the use of only the materials approved for use in the abdominal cavity such as PTFE, PVDF and composite meshes for laparoscopic incisional and ventral hernia repair [36]. The guidelines also recommend that elective laparoscopic repair of incisional and ventral hernias should not be performed with the use of non-cross-linked biological mesh with a bridging technique because of the risk of high recurrence rates. Biological meshes are not impervious to infection and laparoscopic repair of incisional and ventral hernias in an infected or potentially contaminated surgical field can be performed with non-cross-linked biological meshes but the defect should be closed with sutures [36].

Key Points
- There is a wide range of biomaterials available for abdominal wall hernia repair. They may differ in their chemical characteristics, physical properties like fiber size, pore size, weight and pliability. They may also behave differently when in contact with host tissue due to the various modifications made to them. Different companies make various types of meshes using the same compound; however, the current available literature for inguinal hernia repair supports lightweight meshes as it gives fewer symptoms in the short term but for long-term outcomes the benefits seem to be less apparent as heavyweight meshes have shown satisfactory results when used by experienced hands. This observation proves that the surgical technique and experience can be more important than the type, size, weight, pore size and the make of the mesh in treating inguinal hernia [1].
- The literature shows that the minimally invasive approach with laparoscopic or robotic techniques have significantly improved the surgical morbidity associated with ventral hernia repair. There have been reports of major complications such as fistulas and mesh infec-

tions, but the incidence of these complications seems relatively low compared to open repair, regardless of the type of mesh used. Usage of polypropylene meshes inside the abdominal cavity needs to be evaluated again with the addition of new lightweight, large pore composite meshes. These meshes have shown to cause less inflammation and less postoperative pain due to less implanted mesh material which subsequently results in fewer adhesions. Currently the literature is unable to give general recommendations for choice of mesh based on randomized controlled trials and no difference seems to exist in relevant outcome parameters from clinical series between different mesh materials [35]. The final choice of the ideal biomaterial for abdominal wall hernia repair will therefore typically be based on surgeons' preference and cost, till the results of further randomized controlled clinical trials and their meta-analysis appear in the literature.

References

1. Jacob BP, Ramshaw B. The SAGES manual of hernia repair. New York: Springer; 2013.
2. Shillcutt SD, Clarke MG, Kingsnorth AN. Cost-effectiveness of groin hernia surgery in the Western Region of Ghana. Arch Surg. 2010;145:954–61.
3. Scott NW, McCormack K, Graham P, et al. Open mesh versus non-mesh for repair of femoral and inguinal hernia. Cochrane Database Syst Rev. 2002;(4):CD002197.
4. Nieuwenhuizen J, van Ramshort GH, Ten Brinke JG, et al. The use of mesh in acute hernia: frequency and outcome in 99 cases. Hernia. 2011;15(3):297–300.
5. Atila K, Guler S, Inal A, et al. Prosthetic repair of acutely incarcerated groin hernias: a prospective clinical observational cohort study. Langenbeck's Arch Surg. 2010;395:563–8.
6. Babcock WW. The range of usefulness of commercial stainless steel cloths in general and special forms of surgical practice. Ann West Med Surg. 1952;6:15–23.
7. Moloney GE, Grill WG, Barclay RC. Operations for hernia: technique of nylon darn. Lancet. 1948;2:45–8.
8. Handley WS. A method for the radical cure of inguinal hernia (darn and stay-lace method). Practitioner. 1918;100:466–71.
9. Lichtenstein IL, Shulman AG. Ambulatory outpatient hernia surgery. Including a new concept, introducing tension-free repair. Int Surg. 1986;71:1–4.

10. Muldoon RL, Marchant K, Johnson DD, et al. Lichtenstein vs. anterior preperitoneal prosthetic mesh placement in open inguinal hernia repair: a prospective randomized trial. Hernia. 2004;8(2):98–103.

11. Kurzer M, Belsham PA, Kark AE. The Lichtenstein repair. Surg Clin North Am. 1998;78:1025–46.

12. Wolstenholme JT. Use of commercial Dacron fabric in the repair of inguinal hernias and abdominal wall defects. Arch Surg. 1956;73:1004–8.

13. DeBord JR. The historical development of prosthetics in hernia surgery. Surg Clin North Am. 1998;78:973–1006.

14. Langenbach MR, Schmidt J, Zirngibl H. Comparison of biomaterials: three meshesand TAPP for inguinal hernia. Surg Endosc. 2006;20:1511–7.

15. Cobb WS, Peindl RM, Zerey M, et al. Mesh terminology 101. Hernia. 2009;13:1–6.

16. Weyhe D, Belyaev O, Muller C, et al. Improving outcomes in hernia repair by the use of light meshes—a comparison of different implant constructions based on a critical appraisal of the literature. World J Surg. 2007;31:234–44.

17. Bringman S, Wollert S, Osterberg J, et al. Three-year results of a randomized clinical trial of lightweight or standard polypropylene mesh in Lichtenstein repair of primary inguinal hernia. Br J Surg. 2006;93:1056–9.

18. Nikkolo C, Lepner U, Murruste M, et al. Randomized clinical trial comparing lightweight mesh with heavyweight mesh for inguinal hernioplasty. Hernia. 2010;14:253–8.

19. O'Dwyer PJ, Kingsnorth AN, Molloy RG, et al. Randomized clinical trial assessing impact of a lightweight or heavyweight mesh on chronic pain after inguinal hernia repair. Br J Surg. 2005;92:166–70.

20. Post S, Weiss B, Willer M, et al. Randomized clinical trial of lightweight composite mesh for Lichtenstein inguinal hernia repair. Br J Surg. 2004;91:44–8.

21. Coda A, Lamberti R, Martorana S. Classification of prosthetics used in hernia repair based on weight and biomaterial. Hernia. 2012;16(1):9–20.

22. Kingsley D, Vogt DM, Nelson T, et al. Laparoscopic intraperitoneal onlay inguinal herniorrhaphy. Am J Surg. 1998;176:548–53.

23. Amid PK. Classification of biomaterials and their related complications in abdominal wall hernia surgery. Hernia. 1997;1:15–21.

24. Champault G, Barrat C. Inguinal hernia repair with beta glucan coated mesh: results at two-year follow up. Hernia. 2005;9:125–30.

25. Champault G, Bernard C, Rizk N, et al. Inguinal hernia repair: the choice of prosthesis outweighs that of technique. Hernia. 2007;11:125–8.

26. Bringman S, Wollert S, Osterberg J, et al. One year results of randomized controlled multi-centre study comparing Prolene and Vypro II-mesh in Lichtenstein hernioplasty. Hernia. 2005;9:223–7.

27. Khan N, Bangash A, Sadiq M, et al. Polyglactine/polypropylene mesh vs. propylene mesh: is there a need for newer prosthesis in inguinal hernia? Saudi J Gastroenterol. 2010;16:8–13.

28. Bell RCW, Price JG. Laparoscopic inguinal hernia repair using an anatomically contoured three-dimensional mesh. Surg Endosc. 2003;17:1784–8.

29. Pajotin P. Laparoscopic groin hernia repair using a curved prosthesis without fixation. Le Journal de Celio-Chirurgie. 1998;28:64–8.

30. Simons MP, Aufenacker T, Bay-Nielsen M, et al. European Hernia Society guidelines on the treatment of inguinal hernia in adult patients. Hernia. 2009;13(4):343–403.

31. Bittner R, Montgomery MA, Arregui E, Bansal V, Bingener J, Bisgaard T, et al. Update of guidelines on laparoscopic (TAPP) and endoscopic (TEP) treatment of inguinal hernia (International Endohernia Society). Surg Endosc. 2015;29(2):289–321.

32. Schmidbauer S, Ladurner R, Hallfeldt KK, et al. Heavy-weight versus low weight polypropylene meshes for open sublay mesh repair of incisional hernia. Eur J Med Res. 2005;10(6):247–53.

33. Weyhe D, Schmitz I, Belyaev O, et al. Experimental comparison of mono file light and heavy polypropylene meshes: less weight does not mean less biological response. World J Surg. 2006;30(8):1586–91.

34. Gemma Pascual G, Rodrıguez M, Gomez-Giln V, et al. Early tissue incorporation and collagen deposition in lightweight polypropylene meshes: bioassay in an experimental model of ventral hernia. Surgery. 2008;144(3):427–35.

35. Eriksen JR, Gögenur I, Rosenberg J. Choice of mesh for laparoscopic ventral hernia repair. Hernia. 2007;11(6):481–92.

36. Bittner R, Bingener-Casey J, Dietz U, Fabian M, Ferzli G, Fortelny R, et al. Guidelines for laparoscopic treatment of ventral and incisional abdominal wall hernias (International Endohernia Society [IEHS])—Part III. Surg Endosc. 2014;28(2):380–404.

37. Silecchia G, Campanile FC, Sanchez L, Ceccarelli G, Antinori A, Ansaloni L, et al. Laparoscopic ventral/incisional hernia repair: updated guidelines from the EAES and EHS endorsed Consensus Development Conference. Surg Endosc. 2015;29(9):2463–84.

Laparoscopic Incisional and Ventral Hernia Mesh Repair

17

Davide Lomanto and Hrishikesh P. Salgaonkar

17.1 Introduction

Surgical practice has been revolutionized by the advent of minimal invasive surgery by imparting the ability to avoid major abdominal-wall incisions [1, 2]. Thus, laparoscopic surgery by utilizing smaller incisions is expected to reduce the burden of incisional hernias, but such morbidity of the era of conventional, open surgery is likely to remain a common problem for the foreseeable future. It is well-established that repair of sizeable incisional hernias with a mesh is associated with significantly reduced incidence of recurrence of hernia as compared to suture-repair without mesh [3]. Also, the mechanical superiority of mesh-placement in the pre-peritoneal or retro-muscular space (sublay or underlay) over onlay is conceptually apparent [4, 5]. Following Pascal's law, the description of laparoscopic ventral hernia repair (LVHR) was published over 20 years ago and this technique involves either an intra-peritoneal onlay mesh (IPOM) or pre-peritoneal mesh-placement (PPOM) as in the open sublay repair.

LVHR has gained sufficient popularity to be considered as one of the procedure of choice in selected cases and several systematic or randomized comparative clinical trials have showed its benefits. The reliability of repair, measured by the clinical outcome e.g. recurrence and complications as compared to the vast popular open mesh repair has shown similar or at times better clinical outcomes [6, 7]. Definitive comparison is difficult because of heterogeneity in case-mix, technique as well as length and accuracy of follow-up. But overall, LVHR appears to be at least as secure as open mesh repair; this impression is consistent with the similar prevalence of operations for recurrent incisional hernia before and after the introduction of LVHR, in a large population [8]. The well-established benefits of a minimally invasive approach, such as early recovery after surgery, reduced pulmonary complications, decreased risk of wound infection particularly in patients with higher body mass index (BMI) and better cosmesis favours the continuing increase in practice of LVHR.

17.2 Indications and Contra-indications for LVHR

Ventral and incisional hernias are operated mainly due to symptoms i.e. pain, discomfort, cosmesis or to prevent complications i.e. strangulation, respiratory dysfunction, skin problems. It

D. Lomanto (✉)
Minimally Invasive Surgical Centre, KTP Advanced Surgical Training Centre, Yong Loo Lin School of Medicine, National University Health System, National University of Singapore, Singapore
e-mail: davide_lomanto@nuhs.edu.sg

H. P. Salgaonkar
Department of Surgery, Minimally Invasive Surgical Centre, National University Health System and Yong Loo Lin School of Medicine, National University of Singapore, Singapore

© Springer Nature India Private Limited 2020
P. Chowbey, D. Lomanto (eds.), *Techniques of Abdominal Wall Hernia Repair*,
https://doi.org/10.1007/978-81-322-3944-4_17

is still unclear, whether asymptomatic ventral and incisional hernias should be treated surgically and whether the indication for surgery should be influenced by the size of the hernia or the age of the patient. According to the International Endolaparoscopic Hernia Society (IEHS) Guidelines here the Indications and Contraindications **(IEHS Guidelines) note** [9].

Indications:

- Primary ventral hernia with defect size varying from 3 to 15 cm
- Incisional hernia below 15 cm
- Patients with multiple defects ("Swiss cheese" type)

Contra-indications:

- Loss of domain
- Previous peritonitis
- Defect size greater than 15 cm
- Contra-indications for general anaesthesia e.g. severe cardiomyopathy, pulmonary disease

Relative contra-indications:

- Multiple previous surgery
- Multiple previous mesh repair with extensive adhesions
- Acute and sub-acute intestinal obstruction
- Ascitis and portal hypertension

Advanced age is no longer considered a contraindication for LVHR. In fact the Cochrane review [10] showed a clear and consistent result of reduced risk for surgical site infections with laparoscopic surgery in elderly patients.

It is debatable if defects <3 cm should be repaired with laparoscopy or by using mesh as many surgeons still repair these small defects without mesh. This, even after significant message from Burger et al. [11] after their long-term randomized clinical trial (RCT), showed that ventral hernia repair with only suture at 10-year follow-up had a recurrence rate of 63%. Similarly, in 2010 a meta-analysis of RCTs and an extensive review by Aslani et al. [12] favour mesh repair regarding recurrence. A guideline published by Italian

Consensus Conference recommended that hernias with a defect size <3 cm should not be approached laparoscopically [13]. This recommendation was based on expert opinion and a survey showing that less than 10% of surgeons used prosthetics in defects less than 3 cm; it was, therefore, deemed "an indirect indication of a minimum size limit for laparoscopy" [13]. But the recent published literature did not reveal any evidence in support of this recommendation. Therefore, additional evidence is needed before a minimum size for laparoscopic repair can be defined.

17.3 Pre-operative Evaluation

A detailed history and complete physical examination during the initial surgical consultation needs to be emphasized. This helps to identify patient risk factors such as diabetes, obesity and smoking, which cause peri-operative morbidity and mortality.

Routine use of radiological imaging (Computed tomography {CT} or Magnetic resonance imaging {MRI}) for diagnosis and planning is not required. CT scan can be used in selected cases, particularly in those with a recurrent hernia, complex hernias, multiple hernias, hernias in uncommon or challenging locations and when physical examination is unrevealing or limited due to Obesity.

Strict control of blood sugar levels in diabetics may help in reducing wound infections. Similarly, cessation of smoking needs to be emphasized. Some centres perform urine cotinine test evaluating compliance with smoking cessation.

In complex hernia with large contents, it is useful to assess respiratory functions in case of planning bridging or defect closure.

17.4 Surgical Technique

17.4.1 OT Layout and Patient Positioning: (Fig. 17.1)

The procedure is performed under general anesthesia. All pressure points are well padded and the patient is secured to the operating table with

Fig. 17.1 Operation theatre layout

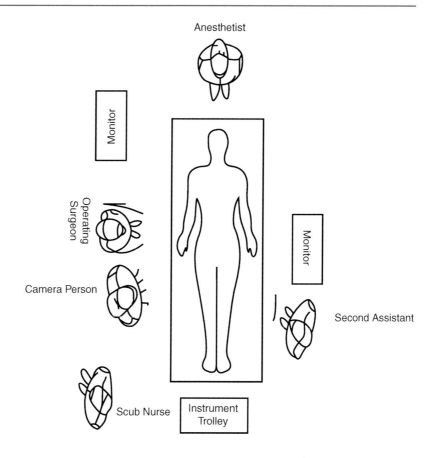

safety belts. The patient is placed in supine position with a slight elevation of the ipsilateral side in non-midline hernias. The operating surgeon and the first assistant (camera person) are positioned either on the left or right side facing the patient. The scrub nurse stands at the foot end of the operating table. The primary monitor is placed on the opposite side in line with the operative site. It is preferable to have at least one additional monitor on ipsilateral side especially in complex cases. Urinary bladder may be catheterized in lower abdominal hernia or if length of surgery is anticipated to be prolonged beyond 90 min.

17.4.2 Abdominal Access and Port Positioning: (Fig. 17.2)

Either Veress needle, open technique (Hasson) or optical viewing trocar can be utilized for abdominal cavity access. In case of previous abdominal surgery access can be done in Palmar's point (left subcostal midclavicular line at the lateral edge of the rectus abdominus muscle) using Veress or optical viewing trocar. In patients with multiple previous surgeries open technique is advisable because of intra-abdominal adhesions. Lately 3D cameras enhance the vision especially in complex cases where severe adhesions or multiple defects need to be repaired.

For subxiphoid defects the patient is given a modified lithotomic position with the surgeon standing in between the patient's legs. The camera port is placed at the umbilicus, and a 5-mm trocar on either side provides good triangulation around the hernia. For suprapubic defects with patient in Trendlenbergs position trocars can be placed on the opposite side if defect is lateral.

In most cases 3-trocars with a primary 10–12 mm-trocar and one or two 5 mm trocars are inserted depending on the intra-abdominal anatomical situation [14]. Most surgeons

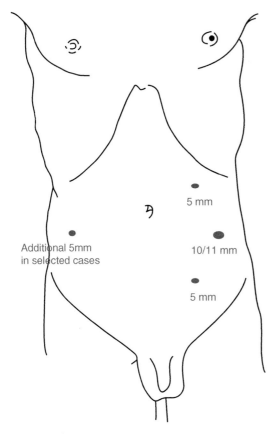

Fig. 17.2 Port placement

5 mm

Additional 5mm
in selected cases

10/11 mm

5 mm

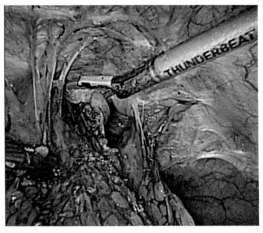

Fig. 17.3 Adhesiolysis

frequently choose the port positions depending upon the intra-abdominal anatomy, many insert instruments from the side of the patient in direct opposition to the viewing laparoscope for allowing a better viewing of all the adhesions [15]. Additional trocar on the opposite side may facilitate the mesh fixation even though they produce paradoxical movement.

17.4.3 Reduction of Hernia and Adhesiolysis

It is safe to use blunt and sharp dissection for adhesiolysis. Use of monopolar diathermy may lead to an injury due to lateral thermal spread and which is usually not visualized at the time of surgery and patient may present with a delayed leak. Alternative energy source like ultrasonic shears, bipolar or combined (Thunderbeat, Olympus, Japan) should be considered in diffi-

cult and complex repair to improve hemostasis and optimize operative time (Fig. 17.3).

Adhesiolysis is at high risk of bowel injury, from simple serosal tear to complete injury. Sharp dissection is recommended or bipolar or ultrasonic device in case of dense omental adhesions. It is important to achieve complete adhesiolysis of the abdominal contents to allow adequate overlap of mesh. A complete adhesiolysis may help in identification of other multiple defects (Swiss cheese). Hernias other than the palpable ones are not infrequently identified. In hernias over lower abdominal wall or suprapubic region this may require to enter the pre-peritoneal layer and to expose the Cooper's ligament for a better mesh fixation. Similarly, superiorly this may require division of the falciform ligament to facilitate mesh fixation. In extreme and difficult adhesiolysis a partial or complete preperitoneal dissection may facilitate the lysis and avoid bowel injury.

For subxiphoid hernias it is important to dissect the retroxiphoidal space. Space should be dissected from the dorsal aspect of the xiphoid process by blunt dissection and if necessary followed by detachment of the diaphragm's sternal portion and finally separation of the pericardium from the sternum. This step is mandatory for safe and effective mesh positioning with sufficient overlap.

In case of dense bowel adhesions if no progress is made, a combined open approach can be used with a skin incision made over the hernial defect to help in reducing the contents. If not it is wiser to convert to an open approach or a dissection above the peritoneum in the retromuscular plane.

17.4.4 Mesh Repair and Size

Mesh size matters as an inadequate overlap of the defect, is the key factor for recurrences. The general consensus is to achieve an overlap of at least 3–5 cm all around the defect with more overlap (6–7 cm) if patients are obese. The reason being mesh shrinkage, increased mesh-abdominal wall interface. By Pascal's principle larger the mesh, better the chances of mesh attaching to the abdominal wall due to intra-abdominal pressure. Irrespective of material used, all meshes are reduced in size with time, thereby exposing the defect. On the other hand in incisional hernia importance should be given to cover the entire previous scar in order to avoid a weak area, potential site for development of recurrence or a new hernia [16]. In our experience 5 cm or more overlap is the preferred size.

The hernia defect should be measured after lowering the pneumoperitoneum pressure (10–11 mmHg). In obese patients it is preferable to measure the defect intra-corporeally as the discrepancy between the intra-abdominal and external measurements may be significant. Once measured an adequate overlap of at least 5–7 cm all over the edge of the defect (3–5 cm in routine patient) with established margin in case of obese patients is necessary.

17.4.5 Choice of Mesh

Three main types of mesh are feasible to be used in IPOM technique: polypropylene, polyester or polytetrafluoroethylene (PTFE) based. The first two types of mesh are known to cause bowel adhesions and so are coated with various agents to provide an anti-adhesive barrier. PTFE is available in expanded (e PTFE) and condensed (OMYRA, B Braun, Germany) with the latter having large pore to improve tissue in growth and reduce seroma but further clinical data is needed to compare.

The role of biological meshes is their suitability for use in a contaminated and infected surgical field as these meshes produce less-pronounced foreign body reaction and get incorporated into the host tissue. But there is paucity of data in literature on the use of biological meshes for incisional hernia repair with some showing high recurrence rates. It would be premature to comment on its efficacy. The only acceptable indication so far is its use in a contaminated or infected environment.

17.4.6 Mesh Insertion and Fixation

The mesh should be rolled tightly and inserted through the 10/12 mm port. For larger-sized meshes a larger port may be used. Mesh should be opened just before its use and avoid contact with the skin to reduce contamination with *Staphylococcus aureus*.

Mesh fixation technique has been a debatable topic in LVHR, today either tackers or transfacial suture (TS) or combinations of both are used. In the last year we noticed a shift from permanent fixation or tackers to absorbable materials because of postoperative chronic pain and recurrence.

In the International Endohernia Society (IEHS) Guidelines, which evaluated the outcomes of 23 studies with more than 5000 patients, a cumulative recurrence rate of 3.95% for all 3 (sutures + tacks, sutures only, and tacks only) groups was reported during a median follow-up period of 35.5 months. The 3 groups did not differ significantly in terms of recurrence rates or follow-up periods [9]. Similarly, Guidelines of EAES (European Association for Endoscopic Surgery and other interventional techniques) and the EHS (European Hernia Society) reported that, at present, there are no adequate clinical studies about the use of absorbable devices, and they could not make any recommendation [17].

17.4.7 Bridging or Augmentation

Another topic of debate in LVHR is whether closure of defect should be attempted in all hernias or is mesh bridging acceptable. The major proponents of defect closure are of the view that it increases the mesh to abdominal wall interface and also restores the physiology of the abdominal muscles. The proposed advantages are reduced recurrence and reduced seroma formation. Such repair combines the closure of the musculo-aponeurotic defect with the intra-peritoneal onlay mesh placement in the form of an "augmentation repair" (or IPOM-Plus). Multiple techniques have been proposed for defect closure [18–23].

Orenstein et al. [24] in 2011 presented the shoe-lacing technique for physiological abdominal wall reconstruction. To enable the defect closure in large hernias some authors have suggested additional operative steps commonly known as Hybrid procedures [25–27]. In our experience multiple interrupted, non-absorbable transfascial sutures in combination with or without intracorporeal suturing are utilized to approximate the defect in IPOM plus technique [28].

By not closing the defect and bridging the mesh in IPOM we create an area which is functionally adynamic. This increases the risk for bulging, seroma formation and possible wound infection. Moreover, the defect closure increases the total surface area of mesh abdominal wall interface for future tissue in-growth and improves the solidity of fixation.

17.4.8 Port Closure

All 10–12 mm should be closed to reduce the risk of developing a port site hernia [29]. This may be accomplished in a variety of ways. Ideally, the fascia is directly visualized with the aid of retractors, the edges grasped and sutured with interrupted or continuous suture. A number of specialized instruments have been devised for fascial closure at the port site. The benefit of these devices is yet to be proven.

17.4.9 Novel Approach

The International Endohernia Society (IEHS) Guidelines [30] suggests that laparoscopic preperitoneal abdominal wall hernia repair via the transabdominal preperitoneal [TAPP] and totally extraperitoneal [TEP] repair techniques in small- and medium-sized primary and incisional abdominal wall hernias is feasible and has minimal morbidity.

The advantages are:

1. Cost-effective due to use of standard polypropylene or polyester mesh;
2. Hernia sac excised and removed;
3. Mesh is extra-peritoneal;
4. The defect is closed and the abdominal wall reconstructed anatomically.

However, the technique is more demanding, takes longer to perform than standard procedures and few clinical studies are available on its clinical outcomes.

17.4.10 Endoscopic Component Separation (ECS)

In large and complex ventral hernia component separation (CS) may be added to achieve closure of defect. Advancement of layers of abdominal wall by separating the lateral muscular layers is performed. In case of abdominal wall reconstruction augmentation with prosthesis is necessary (IPOM plus). By performing an ECS 10–15 cm advancement of defect margin is possible.

Technique of ECS involves a small incision below the coastal margin. The external oblique is split in the line of its fibers and a standard inguinal hernia balloon dissector is placed in between the external and internal oblique muscles, pointing towards the pubis. Standard trocars are then placed in the space created and dissection done extending from pubis to few centimeters above the coastal margin. After identifying the linea semilunaris the external oblique is incised from beneath staring 2–3 cm lateral to the linea semilunaris and muscle released from pubis to few centimeters above the coastal margin. The procedure is repeated on the other side. Although this relatively new technique is feasible, the long term data of its equivalence to OCS are lacking.

17.5 Post-operative Care

Routine antibiotic prophylaxis in ventral hernia repair is recommended [9]. Except in selected complex cases, use of antibiotics post-operatively is not recommended. Similarly, thromboembolic prophylaxis should be given in accordance with the presence of risk factors for the individual patient [9].

Most patients will go home the same day of surgery, while some stay few days more post-operatively mainly due to pain. Frequently, patients will require analgesics for few days. The surgeon may at times extend the hospital stay depending on the extent of the operative procedure.

At home, patients are encouraged to engage in all routine activities. Most patients are able to get back to their normal activities in a short period of time. These activities include showering, driving, walking up stairs, work and sexual intercourse.

Patient and relatives should be counseled to call the surgeon immediately if they have fever, chills, vomiting, are unable to urinate, or experience drainage from the incisions. Also, in case of prolonged soreness and no relief with the prescribed analgesics, they should notify their surgeon.

Patients need to be counseled about possibility of seroma formation and that this will disappear on its own with time. If not, then it may need aspiration. Use of abdominal binder needs to be stressed particularly in large hernias.

17.6 Complications and Clinical Outcomes

17.6.1 Mesh Infections

Perhaps the greatest advantage of LVHR is lower wound infection rate than open hernia repair. It is one of the most serious complication and equally difficult to treat. An infected mesh may lead to disastrous consequences e.g. entero-cutaneous fistula, abdominal wall and intra-abdominal wall abscess, sepsis. If ePTFE mesh gets infected it requires removal. With other meshes conservative trails can be attempted such as parenteral and local antibiotic treatment, with drainage of infected area, wound debridement, partial mesh removal and vacuum dressing application. At any point if infection is not getting controlled, it warrants complete mesh removal. The resultant morbidity of remnant defect, which most surgeons will close under tension, will inevitably lead to recurrence.

17.6.2 Seroma

In LVHR, the hernial sac is not resected and hence a seroma is a common occurrence. In most cases these seromas will resolve over a time as the mesh gets incorporated on the hernia sac. It is important to counsel patients pre-operatively that it is imperative to expect a temporary seroma after LVHR. We reserve aspiration only in symptomatic patients or if seroma is persistent after 6–8 weeks. But by repeated aspirations we may expose the patient to infection.

17.6.3 Enterotomy Intra-operative or Occult

Injury to bowel during adhesiolysis can be catastrophic. Controversy exists in managing an intra-operatively identified bowel injury. Management depends on the segment of intestine injured i.e. small or large bowel, amount of spillage and surgeon's skills. Options may range from aborting the surgery, closure of enterotomy followed by an open mesh repair (sublay or onlay), using an intra-peritoneal biologic mesh or delayed mesh repair after 3–4 days. As a principle if there is gross contamination, the use of synthetic mesh is not advisable.

An occult bowel injury is invariably identified late and ultimately may lead to wound infection with subsequent need for mesh removal. Although it appears that there is a greater risk of bowel injury during laparoscopic hernia repair, but clearly, more data is needed. The increased risk compared with the open approach seems relatively low and acceptable.

17.6.4 Pain

Theoretically laparoscopic surgery should be associated with minimal post-operative pain. In contrast, early post-operative abdominal pain is a regular finding in LVHR. The use of transfascial sutures and tacks can cause substantial early postoperative pain as well as chronic pain months to years after surgery. A Cochrane review [10], comprising 880 patients, measured pain after surgery. They reported that the intensity of pain between the open and laparoscopic repair groups was similar. As a rule, excessive pain after laparoscopic surgery is a reliable indicator of a serious intra-abdominal complication. But the specificity of pain as a marker of occult bowel injury cannot be applied to LVHR. Correctly interpreting excessive post-operative pain is important. There is no evidence in literature to guide us on this issue.

17.6.5 Recurrence

There is paucity of data in literature regarding the rates of recurrence following LVHR in comparison to open mesh repair. Most trails and studies have a short follow-up period with small number of patients. Laparoscopy allows us to inspect the entire incision and area around the defect. This allows us to cover it with adequate mesh overlap, thus reducing the probability of recurrence. But most surgeons do not close the defect and hence rely completely on the tensile strength of the mesh and its fixation. Further randomized control trails with larger patient size are required to validate these assumptions. LVHR has gained sufficient popularity to be considered as a standard procedure.

17.6.6 Hospital Stay

Hospital stay serves as an indirect indicator of multiple post-operative variables such as acute complications, post-operative pain, return of bowel movements and early mobilization. Hospital stay is shorter after laparoscopic inci-

sional and ventral hernia repair, as compared to open repair.

The Cochrane review [10] reported a significant advantage for LVHR in term of reduced hospital stay. Similar findings were reported by two meta-analysis by Forbes et al. [31] and Sajid et al. [32].

17.6.7 Return to Work

Return to activity and to work is an indirect measurement of the economic and social impact of any procedure or technique. In the Cochrane review [10], two RCTs reported on return to activity. Itani et al. [33] showed that time to work was shorter in laparoscopic group as compared to open repair group. But, Pring et al. [34] did not find any significant difference between the two groups. Olmi et al. [35] in his RCT reported that patients in laparoscopic group had a significantly shorter time of return to work. Hence, it would be safe to assume that return to work is shorter or equivalent in LIVHR as compared to open repair.

17.6.8 Quality of Life (QOL)

Patient satisfaction after any procedure is important and gives us an indication of post-operative quality of life and overall cosmetic outcome of any procedure. In the Cochrane review [10], no significant difference was reported in open and LVHR. Mussak et al. [36] in his study on QOL did not find any significant difference in between the two groups. Whereas Hope et al. [37] reported LVHR to be better in most parameters in his study on QOL as compared to open repair. It is reasonable to assume that minimal invasive techniques give better or equivalent patient satisfaction and QOL in comparison to open repair.

17.7 Summary

The laparoscopic approach is a safe and viable technique for the treatment of ventral and incisional hernias. It has an equivalent or lower recurrence rate than conventional open repair and better clinical outcomes compared to published literature. It should be strongly considered as a feasible primary option for repair of ventral and incisional hernias. As with any other advanced laparoscopic procedure, safe adoption of the technique requires appropriate training and patient selection.

Key Points
- Proper case selection is important while offering patient LVHR
- Role of LVHR for defect smaller than 3 cm is debatable
- Use of Imaging e.g. CT scan only in complex cases
- Antibiotic prophylaxis is suggested
- Safe trocar entry
- Adequate adhesiolysis using sharp dissection or safe energy sources
- Adequate mesh overlap (atleast 5 cm) and more in obese patients
- Mesh fixation can be done by sutures, tackers, glue or a combination of these techniques
- Closure of defect where possible (particularly if defect >5 cm) to restore functional physiology of abdominal wall
- Close all ports 10 mm or larger
- Use of abdominal binder in post-operative period may reduce severity of seroma

References

1. Sarela AI, Miner TJ, Karpeh MS, Coit DG, Jaques DP, Brennan MF. Clinical outcomes with laparoscopic stage M1, unresected gastric adenocarcinoma. Ann Surg. 2006;243:189–95.
2. Sarela AI, Murphy I, Coit DG, Conlon KC. Metastasis to the adrenal gland: the emerging role of laparoscopic surgery. Ann Surg Oncol. 2003;10:1191–6.
3. Luijendijk RW, Hop WC, van den Tol MP, de Lange DC, Braaksma MM, IJzermans JN, et al. A comparison of suture repair with mesh repair for incisional hernia. N Engl J Med. 2000;343:392–8.
4. Stoppa RE. The treatment of complicated groin and incisional hernias. World J Surg. 1989;13:545–54.
5. Wantz GE. Incisional hernioplasty with Mersilene. Surg Gynecol Obstet. 1991;172:129–37.
6. Cassar K, Munro A. Surgical treatment of incisional hernia. Br J Surg. 2002;89:534–45.
7. Cobb WS, Kercher KW, Heniford BT. Laparoscopic repair of incisional hernias. Laparoscopic surgery: beyond mere feasibility. In: Patel NA, Bergamaschi R, editors. Surgical clinics of North America. Philadelphia: Saunders; 2006. p. 91–103.
8. Flum DR, Horvath K, Koepsell T. Have outcomes of incisional hernia repair improved with time? A population-based analysis. Ann Surg. 2003;237:129–35.
9. Bittner R, Bingener-Casey J, Dietz U, Fabian M, Ferzli GS, Fortelny RH, Köckerling F, Kukleta J, Leblanc K, Lomanto D, Misra MC, Bansal VK, Morales-Conde S, Ramshaw B, Reinpold W, Rim S, Rohr M, Schrittwieser R, Simon T, Smietanski M, Stechemesser B, Timoney M, Chowbey P, International Endohernia Society (IEHS). Guidelines for laparoscopic treatment of ventral and incisional abdominal wall hernias (International Endohernia Society (IEHS)-part 1). Surg Endosc. 2014;28:2–29.
10. Sauerland S, Walgenbach M, Habermalz B, Seiler CM, Miserez M. Laparoscopic versus open surgical techniques for ventral or incisional hernia repair. Cochrane Database Syst Rev. 2011;(3):CD007781.
11. Burger JW, Luijendijk RW, Hop WC, Halm JA, Verdaasdonk EG, Jeekel J. Long-term follow-up of a randomized controlled trial of suture versus mesh repair of incisional hernia. Ann Surg. 2004;240(4):578–83. discussion 583–5.
12. Aslani N, Brown CJ. Does mesh offer an advantage over tissue in the open repair of umbilical hernias? A systematic review and meta-analysis. Hernia. 2010;14(5):455–62.
13. Cuccurullo D, Piccoli M, Agresta F, Magnone S, Corcione F, Stancanelli V, Melotti G. Laparoscopic ventral incisional hernia repair: evidence-based guidelines of the first Italian Consensus Conference. Hernia. 2013;17(5):557–66.
14. Heniford BT, Park A, Ramshaw BJ, Voeller G. Laparoscopic ventral and incisional hernia repair in 407 patient. J Am Coll Surg. 2000;190(6):645–50.
15. LeBlanc K. Herniorrhaphy with the use of transfascial sutures. In: LeBlanc K, editor. Laparoscopic hernia surgery. London: Arnold; 2003. p. 115–24.
16. Wassenaar EB, Schoenmaeckers EJ, Raymakers JT, Rakic S. Recurrences after laparoscopic repair of ventral and incisional hernia: lessons learned from 505 repairs. Surg Endosc. 2009;23(4):825–32.
17. Silecchia G, Campanile FC, Sanchez L, Ceccarelli G, Antinori A, Ansaloni L, Olmi S, Ferrari GC, Cuccurullo D, Baccari P, Agresta F, Vettoretto N, Piccoli M. Laparoscopic ventral/incisional hernia repair: updated guidelines from the EAES and EHS endorsed Consensus Development Conference. Surg Endosc. 2015;29:2463–84.

18. Palanivelu C, Jani KV, Senthilnathan P, Parthasarathi R, Madhankumar MV, Malladi VK. Laparoscopic sutured closure with mesh reinforcement of incisional hernias. Hernia. 2007;11:223–8.

19. Chelala, et al. The suturing concept for laparoscopic mesh fixation in ventral and incisional hernias: preliminary results. Hernia. 2003;7:191–6.

20. Chelala E, Thoma M, Tatete B, Lemye AC, Dessily M, Alle JL. The suturing concept for laparoscopic mesh fixation in ventral and incisional hernia repair: mid-term analysis of 400 cases. Surg Endosc. 2007;21(3):391–5.

21. Chelala E, Debardemaeker Y, Elias B, Charara F, Dessily M, Allé JL. Eighty-five redo surgeries after 733 laparoscopic treatments for ventral and incisional hernia: adhesion and recurrence analysis. Hernia. 2010;14(2):123–9. Epub 2010 Feb 14.

22. Agarwal BB, Agarwal S, Mahajan KC. Laparoscopic ventral hernia repair: innovative anatomical closure, mesh insertion without 10-mm transmyofascial port, and atraumatic mesh fixation: a preliminary experience of a new technique. Surg Endosc. 2009;23:900–5. https://doi.org/10.1007/s00464-008-0159-7.

23. Sharma D, Jindal V, Pathania OP, Thomas S. Novel technique for closure of defect in laparoscopic ventral hernia repair. J Minim Access Surg. 2010; 6(3):86–8.

24. Orenstein SB, Dumeer JL, Monteagudo J, Poi MJ, Novitsky YW. Outcomes of laparoscopic ventral hernia repair with routine defect closure using "shoelacing" technique. Surg Endosc. 2011;25:1452–7.

25. Barnes GS, Papasavas PK, O'Mara MS, Urbandt J, Hayetian FD, Gagn DJ, Newton ED, Caushaj PF. Modified extraperitoneal endoscopic separation of parts for abdominal compartment syndrome. Surg Endosc. 2004;18:1636–9.

26. Griniatsos J, Yiannakopoulou E, Tsechpenakis A, Tsigris C, Diamantis T. A hybrid technique for recurrent incisional hernia repair. Surg Laparosc Endosc Percutan Tech. 2009;19(5):e177–80.

27. Mathes SJ, Steinwald PM, Foster RD, Hoffman WY, Anthony JP. Complex abdominal wall reconstruction: a comparison of flap and mesh closure. Ann Surg. 2000;232(4):586–96.

28. Lomanto D, Iyer SG, Shabbir A, Cheah WK. Laparoscopic versus open ventral hernia mesh repair: a prospective study. Surg Endosc. 2006; 20:1030–5.

29. Johnson WH, Fecher AM, McMahon RL, Grant JP, Pryor AD. Versa Step trocar hernia rate in unclosed fascial defects in bariatric patients. Surg Endosc. 2006;20:1584–6.

30. Bittner R, Bingener-Casey J, Dietz U, Fabian M, Ferzli G, Fortelny R, et al. Guidelines for laparoscopic treatment of ventral and incisional abdominal wall hernias (International Endohernia Society [IEHS])-Part III. Surg Endosc. 2014;28:380–404. https://doi.org/10.1007/s00464-013-3172-4.

31. Forbes SS, Eskicioglu C, McLeod RS, Okrainec A. Meta-analysis of randomized controlled trials comparing open and laparoscopic ventral and incisional hernia repair with mesh. Br J Surg. 2009; 96:851–8.

32. Sajid MS, Bokhari SA, Mallick AS, Cheek E, Baig MK. Laparoscopic versus open repair of incisional/ventral hernia: a meta-analysis. Am J Surg. 2009;197:64–72.

33. Itani KM, Hur K, Kim LT, Anthony T, Berger DH, Reda D, Neumayer L, for the Veternas Affairs Ventral Incisional Hernia Investigators. Comparison of laparoscopic and open repair with mesh for the treatment of ventral incisional hernia: a randomized trial. Arch Surg. 2010;145:322–8.

34. Pring CM, Tran V, O'Rourke N, Martin IJ. Laparoscopic versus open ventral hernia repair: a randomized controlled trial. ANZ J Surg. 2008;78:903–6.

35. Olmi S, Scaini A, Cesana GC, Erba L, Croce E. Laparoscopic versus open incisional hernia repair: an open randomized controlled study. Surg Endosc. 2007;21:555–9.

36. Mussack T, Ladurner R, Vogel T, Lienemann A, Eder-Willwohl A, Hallfeldt KK. Health-related quality-of-life changes after laparoscopic and open incisional hernia repair: a matched pair analysis. Surg Endosc. 2006;20:410–3.

37. Hope WW, Lincourt AE, Newcomb WL, Schmelzer TM, Kercher KW, Heniford BT. Comparing quality-of-life outcomes in symptomatic patients undergoing laparoscopic or open ventral hernia repair. J Laparoendosc Adv Surg Tech A. 2008; 18:567–71.

Laparoscopic Pre-peritoneal Onlay Mesh (PPOM) Repair for Ventral and Incisional Hernia

18

George Pei Cheung Yang

Leblanc described the laparoscopic mesh repair of incisional hernia in 1993 [1]. It involves placing a PTFE the mesh with fixation by staples in the posterior abdominal wall in the peritoneal cavity covering the hernia orifice. This technique is known as intra-peritoneal onlay mesh repair (IPOM). The IPOM+ [2] technique involves the addition of closing the hernia defect with suture before placement of the mesh in the intra-peritoneal cavity. Laparoscopic repair for ventral hernia has undisputed advantages. Being able to place a large mesh through just several small tiny 5–10 mm wounds minimized tissue dissection and hence lowers the risk of wound infection. With low rate of wound infection, the risk of mesh infection also reduced. Secondly it clearly identifies the site and size of all hernia defects and avoids missing out multiple defects in some patients. However, but having the mesh placed in the peritoneal cavity creates one problem—mesh-induced visceral complications. This is a result of foreign body reaction to the synthetic materials and the tackers, or chemical degradation reaction to those re-absorbable components of the mesh like the coating barriers or absorbable tackers. This chronic foreign body tissue reaction, if persist long enough, will leads to bowel erosion and fistulation, and in some cases migration of the mesh into the internal lumen of the bowel causing distal obstruction. Some even reported spontaneous passage of the mesh through rectum [3]. This is more than just usual post-operative adhesion. The severity of this reaction is difficult to predict. Some may exhibit extensive reaction leading to adhesion, fistulation and obstruction. On the other hand, others might have mild reaction only. It is impossible to predict who will have problem and who will not. Needless to say there is no clinical parameter allowing us to predict the future progress of the patient after IPOM repair. The true incident of mesh-induced visceral complications is not known. The complexity of such event and subsequent management can be a surgical nightmare. It is this mesh-induced visceral complication drives the search for alternative laparoscopic approach for ventral and incisional hernia repair.

The newer laparoscopic techniques for ventral and incisional hernia explore the possibility of placing the mesh within different planes of our abdominal wall. In retro-muscular plane like those described in endoscopic mini/less open sublay (eMILOS), endoscopic totally pre-peritoneal ventral hernia repair (eTEP) and laparoscopic transversus abdominis release (TAR) [4–7]. In pre-peritoneal plane

G. P. C. Yang (✉)
Hong Kong Adventist Hospital,
Happy Valley, Hong Kong
e-mail: george.yang@hkah.org.hk

© Springer Nature India Private Limited 2020
P. Chowbey, D. Lomanto (eds.), *Techniques of Abdominal Wall Hernia Repair*,
https://doi.org/10.1007/978-81-322-3944-4_18

like Pre-peritoneal onlay mesh repair (PPOM) [8]. In this chapter, we will discuss about the technique pre-peritoneal onlay mesh (PPOM) repair for ventral and incisional hernia.

As we learned from open surgery, onlay and inlay methods have inferior results. To place the mesh extra-peritoneally within the abdominal wall, the two preferable options are either having the mesh place in the retro-muscular or preperitoneal planes. The retro-rectus space at the central abdomen is limited by its fascial compartment. The linea alba needs to be disconnected, incised and repaired to allow the mesh to place across the right and left retro-rectus space. Still the unified right and left retro-rectus compartment limits the size of the mesh to be placed. If a larger mesh is needed we have to extend laterally beyond the lateral border of the rectus fascial compartment. There is an important neurovascular bundle running posterior to the internal oblique muscle. So the preferable way for lateral extension is to incise the transversus abdominis component thus allowing us to enter the pre-peritoneal space; this becomes the laparoscopic TAR (Fig. 18.1). It is also important to stress that the size of the mesh used should be calculated according to the original hernia defect size with adequate overlapping margin, not according to the closed hernia orifice under tension.

On the other hand, the idea of PPOM is to place the mesh in the pre-peritoneal plane. Similar idea to laparoscopic transabdominal pre-peritoneal (TAPP) repair for groin hernia [9]. The term PPOM was first coined in 2016 [8]; this is a laparoscopic transabdominal pre-peritoneal placement of mesh for ventral and incisional hernia. The term PPOM readily allows the recognition that this is a laparoscopic ventral and incisional hernia repair technique. The term PPOM also allows easier search in database for research purpose. It is because the term laparoscopic transabdominal pre-peritoneal repair may be confused with groin hernia repair, and for ventral and incisional hernia some literatures actually include both pre-peritoneal and also retro-muscular mesh placement [10]. Nowadays, with so many different techniques, it is important to specify which layer we are talking right from the beginning for easier analysis in the future.

Our abdominal wall not only involves in holding the abdominal viscera but also assists in urination, defecation, respiration, and most importantly maintain stability of our body during static position or movement like running and climbing.

We have to understand that the function of our abdominal wall is influenced by many other factors as well, including effect from spinous muscle

Fig. 18.1 Dotted line indicates the lateral extension from retro-rectus space to pre-peritoneal space avoiding injury to the neurovascular bundle

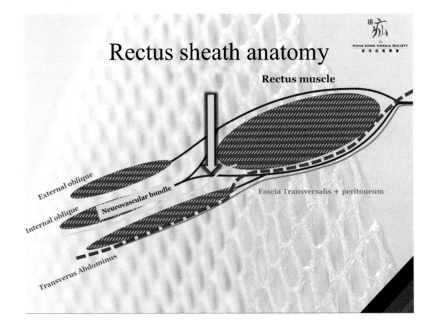

and upper and lower limb muscles. Thus measuring the abdominal wall function is extremely difficult and complex, and time factor has to be taken into account because the problem may not surface until other parts of the body deteriorate in the future as we age. Will unilateral component separation cause more burden to our body mechanism compared to bilateral component separation? The long-term effect of component separation on our abdominal wall functional mechanism is still waiting to be answered. Therefore component separation should really only be reserved for major hernia with abdominal wall distortion.

PPOM in this sense causes the least structural disruption of our abdominal wall architecture. The peritoneum itself plays a little role in the structural strength of our body. The mesh placement in PPOM-induced adhesion between the peritoneum and posterior fascia, whereas in retro-muscular, the mesh causes adhesion between the muscle and fascia compartment, where normally the muscle should be freely gliding within this space. Thus PPOM is probably the least disruptive technique and causes the least structural instability as compare to component separation.

PPOM may be the preferred alternative technique to IPOM for small- to medium-size ventral and incisional hernia, since it causes the least disruption to our abdominal wall and keep our abdominal wall architecture balanced and intact. In this chapter, we describe the PPOM technique.

18.1 PPOM (Pre-peritoneal Onlay Mesh Repair)

The surgical steps of PPOM include:
1. Diagnostic laparoscopy;
2. Skin marking for: the hernia defect/s, mesh size, and the incision line for peritoneum and your working ports sites
3. Laparoscopic adhesiolysis;
4. Creation of the peritoneal flap;
5. Placement of the mesh in the pre-peritoneal plane; and
6. Closure of the peritoneal flap and any other defect.

Surgical steps in details:
1. Diagnostic laparoscopy:
   Diagnostic laparoscopy is important. The first trocar site should be well away from the site of the hernia and previous surgical scar. Alternatively if the umbilical area is not involve, one can still use the subumbilical site for first port diagnostic laparoscopy, and later move away from this and use different working ports. Either way, whichever is the safest should be employed with one important point that the first trocar should never be inside the hernia defect vicinity. With diagnostic laparoscopy, the surgeon should assess the extent of adhesion, the number and sizes of the hernia defects and their location, therefore to plan the subsequent operation.
2. Surface skin marking:
   This step is vital. It allows you to plan your working trocar sites better in order to maximize the efficacy of your surgery. You should mark out the size and site of all hernia orifices, and decide on the size of the mesh to be used and its position to be placed under the hernias. Then you mark out the peritoneal pocket size required for the placement of the mesh, and thus the incision line of the peritoneal. Your working trocar sites should be 3–4 cm away from this peritoneal incision line (Fig. 18.2).

   In this step you should decide whether you are going to utilize single-directional dissection approach or bi-directional dissection

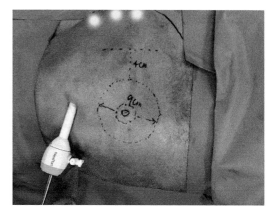

Fig. 18.2 Surface marking with yellow dots showing the planned placement site for working trocars

Fig. 18.3 Single-
directional dissection
approach

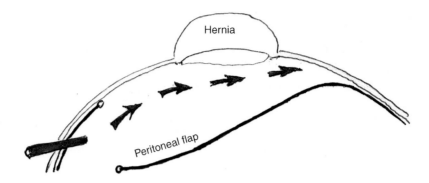

approach to create the peritoneal pocket.
Single-directional (uni-directional) dissection
approach means we create the peritoneal
pocket totally along one single direction of
dissection (Fig. 18.3). The incision on the
peritoneum should be 2–3 cm away from the
edge of the mesh you marked out on the abdomen. In complicated, multiple hernias, or
large-size hernia defect, one might consider
the bi-directional dissection approach. This
involves making the peritoneal incision along
the edge of the hernia, and dissects the peritoneum away from the hernia in both dissections (Fig. 18.4). Finally, after the placement
of the mesh, the peritoneum is suture-closed.
The bi-directional approach has the advantage
when you need to create a bigger size peritoneal pocket because the view near the working
trocar will be compromised due to of the lack
of distance and space.

3. Laparoscopic adhesiolysis:
   After skin marking and insertion of working
   ports under direct vision, we proceed to laparoscopic adhesiolysis. Adhesiolysis should be
   carefully done, with gentle blunt and sharp
   scissor dissection. Energy devise should be
   avoided to prevent collateral bowel wall injury
   by the heat created [11]. After complete adhesiolysis, the exact number and the size of the
   hernia defects with the mesh to be used should
   be rechecked and correlated with our initial
   planning.

   Adhesiolysis is one of the essences of laparoscopic ventral hernia surgery, and the surgeon should master this skill before starting

on this type of surgery. Bowel injury should
be avoided because it can contaminate the
synthetic mesh.

4. Creation of the peritoneal flap:
   The next step is the creation of the peritoneal
   flap or pocket to house the synthetic mesh.
   Having marked the position of the hernia
   defect and the mesh the surgeon should decide
   whether a uni-directional or bi-directional dissection approach is to be employed. This
   depends on the available working space, the
   size of the hernias and the peritoneal pocket
   required. For small simple hernia defect, uni-
   directional approach is suitable because the
   area of dissection is relatively small and
   straight forward. For complex hernia and large
   size defect, the bi-directional approach may
   be considered.

   In *uni-directional dissection approach*;

   The incision on the peritoneum should be
   around 2–3 cm away from the edge of the
   mesh to avoid inadequate space to house the
   mesh, the working ports should be another
   3–4 cm away from the intended peritoneal
   incision line. So in total the distance from the
   port to the edge of the mesh may be 5–7 cm.
   With access to the pre-peritoneal space, the
   peritoneum is carefully dissected off from the
   abdominal wall posterior fascia. The thinnest
   part of the peritoneal attachment is around
   central abdomen and at the lateral margin of
   the rectus abdominis muscle, the semilunar
   line. It is still feasible with careful and meticulous dissection to free off the peritoneum from
   this area. Most often blunt dissection can sep-

Fig. 18.4 Bi-directional dissection approach; opposite port (blue color) should be within the peritoneal flap to avoid obscure view by the loose peritoneal flap

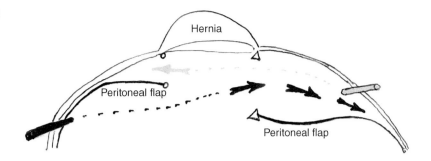

arate the thin peritoneum away from the posterior abdominal fascia. Traversing small vessels will be encountered in this plane; they are best controlled with energy dissecting devise like ultrasonic dissector to minimize blood which can obscure the operative view. The hernia sac can either be completely reduced or ligated and transected. The most important point here is to avoid injury to the overlying skin during the dissection at the site of the hernia. This is to avoid leakage of seroma and potential risk of exposing the mesh and mesh infection.

In *bi-directional dissection approach*:

This may be suitable for major hernia or swiss-cheese hernia defect in which freeing the peritoneal sac from the hernia is difficult and the laparoscopic working space is limited. The peritoneal incision will be around the edge of the hernia orifice and continue laterally to create the pre-peritoneal pocket on each side of the hernia. The hernia sac can either be carefully dissected away from hernia, or leave alone. The working port position should be well away from the edge of the mesh. Careful surface marking of the defect site and mesh size with its position should be done before the peritoneal dissection. After finished dissecting on one side, the ports insertion on the opposite side can be performed under direction vision and should be within the dissected peritoneal sac such that the dropped down peritoneal flap would not obstructed the laparoscope view when perform dissection from the opposite side (Fig. 18.4).

There are several techniques to separate the thin peritoneum from the posterior fascia. The peritoneum is at its thinnest around the seminular line at the umbilical level. Using veress needle, we can inject air or saline to develop the pre-peritoneal plane, therefore making dissection of pre-peritoneal pocket easier. The upper and lower abdomen is technically much less demanding. Below the arcuate line, both the retro-muscular and pre-peritoneal spaces are actually the same. This is the area we perform our TAPP for groin hernia repair, therefore most hernia surgeons should be familiar with it. In upper abdomen such as epigastric and sub-diaphragmatic areas, and also right at the para-umbilical area the presence of pre-peritoneal fat will also make dissection easier. In case there is a breach of the peritoneum, this should be closed with direct suturing in order to preserve the area of peritoneal flap, instead of using tacker overlapping the peritoneum. Preserving the peritoneum from the hernia sac will also help.

Dissecting the peritoneum (hernia sac) away from the hernia itself can be challenging sometime. It is because the plane between the hernia sac and the skin can be very thin. Since the mesh is underneath the hernia defect, any damage to the skin above will potentially expose the mesh. Also this creates a portal for seroma to track through. So it may be wise to leave the sac alone in case the sac has fibrotic adhesion. The surgeon should maintain correct orientation during dissection at all time, especially with the patient tilted sideway. Fortunately the important structures in the pre-peritoneal space are in the lower abdomen, the inferior epigastric vessels, the iliac vessels and nerves down in the pelvis, which the laparoscopic hernia surgeons should all be familiar with in their TEP or TAPP training.

5. Placement of the mesh in the pre-peritoneal space (Fig. 18.5):

This section comprises (a) orientation of the mesh in the space, (b) positioning the mesh in the planned position and (c) fixation of the mesh.

At this stage of the surgery, the surgeon should change to a new pair of sterile gloves before handling and introduce the mesh into the peritoneal cavity. Surgeons should develop the habit of double gloving; thereby making the change of the outer gloves less contaminating when compare to those using only single pair of gloves. The handling of the mesh should be kept minimal, avoiding unnecessary personnel touching the mesh. In PPOM, if the peritoneal flap is completely intact, a simple polypropylene or polyester mesh can be used. If the peritoneal flap is large and might have small defect, a coated mesh is recommended still. In this way small millimeter defects in the peritoneal flap need not to be closed completely. Also this allows maximal adhesion at the parietal side, and minimal adhesion to the peritoneum, in case we need to go back into this plane in the future.

Orientation of the mesh:

A transfixing stay suture should be applied to the parietal surface of the mesh if not already available ex-factory. This transfixing suture should be at least 3–4 cm inwards away from the edge of the mesh. In

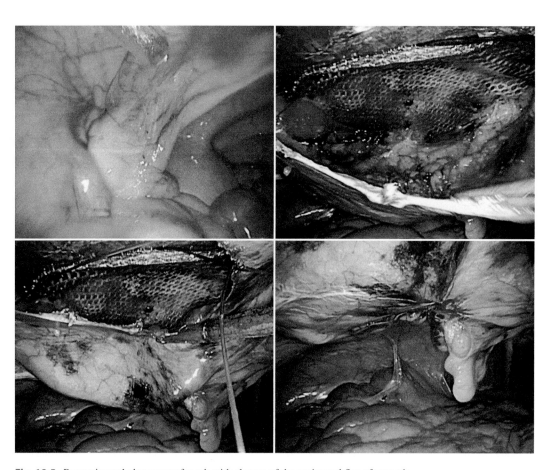

Fig. 18.5 Pre-peritoneal placement of mesh with closure of the peritoneal flap afterwards

this way, when we sling up the mesh, there will be at least 3–4 cm additional coverage at the edge of the hernia orifice. Two stay sutures at 12:00 and 06:00 o'clock position on the mesh at its parietal surface will help us to orientate and center the mesh over the hernia defect.

Positioning the mesh:

After inserting the mesh, the surgeon should orientate the mesh in its correct parietal and visceral side if a coated mesh is used. The stay suture should be grasped with transcutaneous grasper like Endoclose devise, through a tiny needle-size stab incision, about 2 cm away from the edge of the planned mesh landing zone. After sling up the mesh with the transcutaneous stay suture, the center of the mesh can be easily position over the hernia with the adjustment of these two slings up stay sutures. This is very important in large and complex hernia case because at this stage it is sometime impossible to accurately access the coverage of the mesh against the hernias, and also this prevents shifting of the mesh during fixation.

Fixation of the mesh:

Contrary to IPOM, we don't need to apply so many fixation tackers around the edge of the mesh. Some authors in the retromuscular technique avoid using fixation all together. It is because there is no chance for the mesh to fall down into the peritoneal cavity, and there is also no chance for the bowel to trap between the mesh and our abdominal wall provided the peritoneal incision is close properly. However, the mesh can still crumble up during friction upon abdominal wall movement, even if the peritoneal pocket is roughly the same size as the mesh. Three to four tackers are enough to prevent crumbling of the mesh and ensure flat deployment even during abdominal wall

movement in the early post-operative phase to allow tissue ingrowth. Since the purpose of the tacking is only to bridge the period until tissue ingrown to establish, a non-permanent material like absorbable tacker is preferred [12].

6. Closure of the peritoneal incision and defect: The peritoneal incision should be closed with running suture, especially with the bi-directional dissection approach. This is to avoid any bowel to adhere to the mesh and slip into the pre-peritoneal space. Alternatively, in uni-directional dissection technique the surgeon might close the peritoneal flap with absorbable tackers along its incision.

Recheck laparoscopy on the peritoneal flap should be performed at the end. Any major peritoneal flap defect should also be closed. And before concluding the surgery, it is wise to place the omentum underneath the operative site to separate the bowel from operative area.

Post-operative care:

Apart from usual advice on avoiding heavy lifting; it is always advisable for the patient to wear an abdominal binder for extra-abdominal wall support (Fig. 18.6). This will provide support for their abdominal wall during movement, and sandwich the mesh against the posterior fascia for theoretically better tissue ingrowth. The usual advice is to wear it during day time for 4–6 weeks post-operatively, and then wear it while they are doing sports.

18.2   Indication for PPOM /ePOM/ RePOM

Like the indication for laparoscopic iPOM, those with simple ventral or incisional hernia should be the best candidates for this approach.

Fig. 18.6 Post-
operative abdominal
binder for support

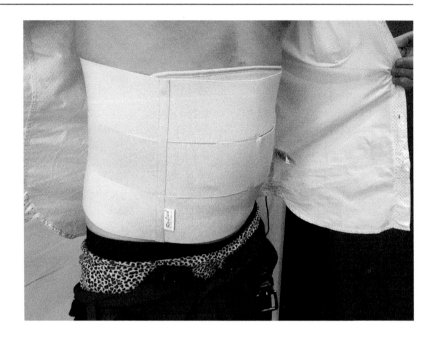

References

1. LeBlanc KA, Booth WV. Laparoscopic repair of incisional abdominal hernias using expanded polytetrafluoroethylene: preliminary findings. Surg Laparosc
Endosc. 1993;3(1):39–41.
2. Chelala E, Gaede F, Douillez V, Dessily M, Alle
JL. The suturing concept for laparoscopic mesh fixation in ventral and incisional hernias: preliminary
results. Hernia. 2003;7(4):191–6.
3. Horzic M, Vergles D, Cupurdija K, Kopljar M, Zidak
M, Lackovie Z. Spontaneous mesh evacuation per
rectum after incisional ventral hernia repair. Hernia.
2011;15:351–2.
4. Schwarz J, Reinpold W, Bittner R. Endoscopic mini/
less open sublay technique (EMILOS)—a new technique for ventral hernia repair. Langenbeck's Arch
Surg. 2017;402:173–80.
5. Novitsky YW, Elliott HL, Orenstein SB, Rosen
MJ. Transversus abdominis muscle release: a novel
approach to posterior component separation during
complex abdominal wall reconstruction. Am J Surg.
2012;204:709–16.
6. Miserez M, Penninckx F. Endoscopic totally preperitoneal ventral hernia repair. Surgical technique and
short-term results. Surg Endosc. 2002;16:1207–13.
7. Belyanshky I, Zahiri HR, Park A. Laparoscopic transversus abdominis release, a novel minimally invasive
approach to complex abdominal wall reconstruction.
Surg Innov. 2015;23(2):134–41.
8. Yang GPC, Tung KLM. Preperitoneal onlay mesh
repair for ventral abdominal wall and incisional
hernia: a novel technique. Asian J Endosc Surg.
2016;9(4):344–7. ISSN 1758-5902.
9. Antoniou SA, Pointner R, Granderath FA. Current
treatment concept for groin hernia. Langenbeck's
Arch Surg. 2014;399:553–8.
10. Prasad P, Tantia O, Patle NM, Khanna S, Sen
B. Laparoscopic ventral hernia repair: a comparative
study of transabdominal preperitoneal versus intra-
peritoneal onlay mesh repair. J Laparoendosc Adv
Surg Tech A. 2011;21(6):477–83.
11. Polychronidis A, Tsaroucha AK, Karayiannakis AJ,
Perente S, Efstathiou E, Simopoulos C. Delayed
perforation of the large bowel due to thermal injury
during laparoscopic cholecystectomy. J Int Med Res.
2005;33(3):360–3.
12. Colak E, Ozlem N, Kucuk GO, Aktimur R, Kesmer
S, Yildirim K. Propsective randomized trial of mesh
fixation with absorbable versus nonabsorbable tacker
in laparoscopic ventral incisional hernia repair. Int J
Clin Exp Med. 2015;8(11):21611–6.

Laparoscopic Repair of Peripheral Abdominal Wall Hernias

19

Anil Sharma

19.1 Introduction

Peripheral abdominal wall hernias are located in the peripheral zones of the abdominal wall and include subxiphisternal, subcostal, lumbar, and suprapubic hernias. These are difficult hernias to repair because of their close proximity to anatomically important structures like bone, nerves, major vessels, and bowel. Moreover, it is difficult to obtain a mesh overlap of more than 4–5 cm from the hernial defect, particularly from the distal margin in these hernias. Accordingly, the surgical repair of peripheral hernias would normally involve some additional maneuver to implant the mesh prosthesis in place.

19.2 Indications

Subxiphisternal, subcostal, lumbar, and suprapubic hernias.

A. Sharma (✉)
Max Institute of Minimal Access, Metabolic and Bariatric Surgery, Max Super Speciality Hospital (East Block), Saket, New Delhi, India

19.3 Contraindications

Absolute Contraindications
- Medically unfit for GA.
- Uncontrollable coagulopathy.
- Giant hernia with major loss of abdominal domain.
- Acute abdomen with abdominal distension and gross bowel dilatation.
- Major abdominal sepsis.
- Strangulated bowel as hernial content.
- Abdominal wall hernia in children (<12 years).

Previous surgery usually produces abdominal wall musculature denervation causing disruption of normal anatomy and large bulging defects that occupy most of the lumbar region [1, 2]. These patients may not be suitable for laparoscopic repair.

19.4 Operative Procedure

Bowel preparation is only required if a segment of large bowel is known to be content or is in close proximity to the hernial sac.

Lumbar Hernias
- The patient is placed in a semilateral position on the OT table.

Fig. 21.3 Key steps of component separation technique

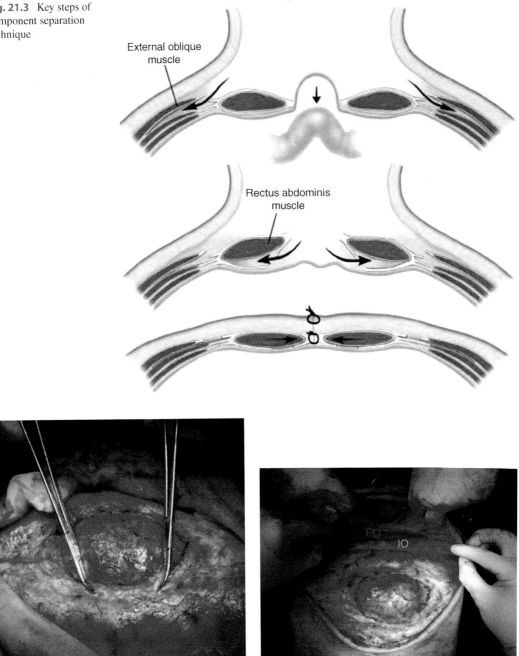

External oblique muscle

Rectus abdominis muscle

Fig. 21.4 Elevation of skin flaps

Fig. 21.5 Incision of EO aponeurosis

Following completion of mobilization, a check is made, bringing the 2 opposite ends together to ensure that the defect can be covered. We routinely place two 15Fr blake drains attached to closed suction in the subcutaneous plane to prevent any post-operative fluid collection in the subcutaneous plane following the extensive dissection (Fig. 21.8).

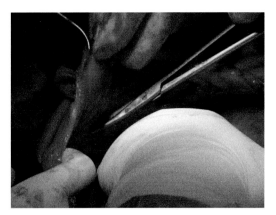

Fig. 21.6 Incision of posterior rectus sheath

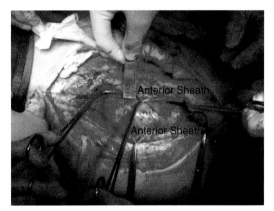

Fig. 21.7 Advancement to the midline

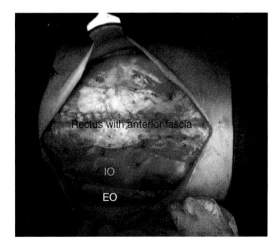

Fig. 21.8 Completion of CST and abdominal closure

At this point, if a defect remains in the mildine, consideration is made for the addition of a mesh in a non-contaminated environment. If a mesh is not required, the midline is closed with a monofilament suture with a long half-life or alternatively with a non-absorbably suture, e.g. Nylon. We use loop polydiaxone (PDS II, Ethicon J&J) for the closure. Additional tension band sutures can be added to reduce tension forces in the midline. The skin is closed with either surgical staples or a non-absorbable monofilament suture. Dressing is done and an abdominal binder is applied.

21.5.1.1 Operative Pearls

The technical success of the CST requires the following to allow abdominal wall closure:

1. Adequate mobilization of the musculofascial layer in the craniocaudal and lateral aspects.
2. Complete lateral fascial and posterior fascial division from the subcostal margin superiorly to the iliac crest inferiorly.
3. Mobilization of the musculofascial layers should be performed bilaterally rather than unilaterally to allow for centralization of the abdominal wall forces as opposed to skewing it to either side with the resultant undue tension.

It is critical that mobilization is completed as described above. A partial mobilization will result in closure under high tension which will result in a recurrence.

During closure of the fascia, communication with the anaesthetist is important, looking out for any increase in peak airway pressure greater than 5 mmH$_2$O. This increase in peak airway pressure can be associated with a restriction of respiratory efforts, prolonged ventilation and possible development of abdominal compartment syndrome. In such a situation, if despite fascial release an increase in peak airway pressure persists, consideration should be given to the deployment of a mesh to repair the ventral wall defect.

21.5.2 Modified Open Components Separation Technique

Since the original description by Ramirez et al., numerous descriptions of modifications to the technique have been described to address the shortcomings from the original technique.

Fig. 21.9 Modified
component separation
technique

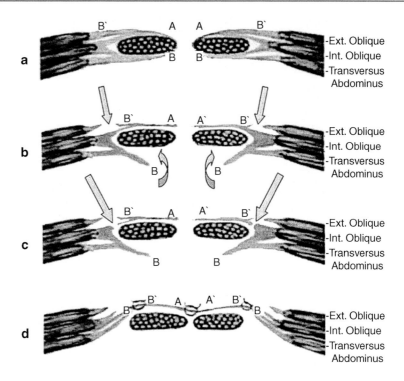

Fig. 21.9 Modified
component separation
technique

The modification technique described by Jernigan et al involved further releasing incisions: the IO aponeurosis of the anterior rectus sheath is divided down the arcuate line. Following this, the medial border of the posterior sheath is suture approximated to the lateral border of the anterior sheath.

The main purpose of the extra step in the modification is to provide further advancement to close the ventral wall defect. With this modification, additional 50% mobilization e.g. extra 15 cm in the mid-abdomen is possible. This makes it possible to close defects as large as 30 cm in the mid-abdomen without the need of a mesh (Fig. 21.9).

Additional Advancement Distance
- Epigastric: 8–10 cm
- Mid-abdomen: 10–15 cm
- Suprapubic: 6–8 cm

21.5.3 Endoscopic Components Separation Technique

Open CST is not without risks. The creation of large spaces and a potentially ischaemic skin flap can predispose the development of seromas/haematomas and surgical site infections. The endoscopic method of CST (ECST) was developed to mitigate the potential complications of the open approach.

ECST differs from the open CST in the following areas:

Summary of Additional Key Steps
1. Division of IO aponeurosis from the anterior sheath.
2. Suture apposition of the posterior sheath to the lateral aspect of the anterior sheath.

1. The skin and subcutaneous flaps area are raised for a distance of 1 cm laterally. This is to avoid disruption of the perforator vessels from the rectus muscles to the skin flaps.

2. Short 1.5–2 cm skin incisions are made approximately 5 cm medial to the anterior superior iliac spine (ASIS) along the anterior axillary line. It is vital that the surgeon stays lateral to the rectus abdominis muscle. An initial space between the external and internal oblique muscles is created bluntly.

3. Starting unilaterally, a balloon dissector is inserted into the avascular plane that was initially developed. Similar to laparoscopic total extraperitoneal hernia repair, the balloon is inflated under direct vision of 30° laparoscopic camera to develop the vertical plane.

4. Two additional 5 mm ports are inserted: one below the costal margin and another medial to the first port site. The external oblique aponeurosis is incised with a cautery device (laparoscopic hook or scissors) longitudinally from the costal margin to the level of the inguinal ligament. The process is repeated on the contralateral side.

21.5.3.1   Operative Pearls

In the obese patient, development of the plane between the external and internal oblique muscles can prove to be a challenge. The use of an optical trochar combined with a laparoscope allows much quicker and precise development of the avascular plane under direct vision.

In our experience, sequential unilateral dissection as opposed to synchronous bilateral dissection allows for a more controlled dissection. Nonetheless, this is at the discretion of the surgeon performing the procedure.

In a recent systematic review and meta-analysis, Switzer et al. compared outcomes of open vs. endoscopic. Sixty-three studies were analysed: 7 controlled studies and 56 case series. From the study, open CST was associated with higher overall post-operative fascial dehiscence (0.4% vs. 0%) rates and longer operative duration when compared with endoscopic CST. Most other types of wound complications (infection, seroma, haematoma, etc.) seemed to favour endoscopic CST although this did not reach statistical significance. Similarly, hernia recurrence rates appeared to favour endoscopic CST over open

CST (11.1% vs. 15.1%) although this did not reach statistical significance. The choice to perform either approach hinges on the individual surgeon's experience with either technique. Neither technique has been proven to be superior to the other.

21.5.4 Robotic Components Separation Technique

Recently, a few reports have emerged describing the usage of the Da Vinci® robotic system (Da Vinci Surgery) for a CST. This is performed using a 3 port trans-abdominal approach. The purported benefits relate to better camera optics, and stable visualization and instrumentation for the performance of this precision surgery. Further studies will need to be conducted to validate the benefits of the novel robotic CST approach compared to ECST, especially with an increased cost in using the robotic system.

21.6   Additional Considerations

21.6.1 Mesh Insertion

The principles of hernia repair are applicable to CST. The original description of CST involved a tension-free sutured repair. Hence, there exists the potential for appreciable recurrence as no mesh reinforcement is utilized. The addition of a mesh may reduce recurrence rates in complex ventral hernia repairs.

The main indications for mesh deployment include:

- a very large defect (>20 cm) that renders tension-free closure via CST alone improbable.
- relatively thinned-out fascial and peritoneal layers.

Contraindications to mesh insertion would include the presence of ongoing infection, a contaminated field, presence of malignancy.

An absorbable mesh was initially described as an adjunct to CST for complex ventral hernia closure. Since then other types of meshes including non-absorbable and biologic meshes have been described. However, these approaches result in hernia recurrence and re-operations. If possible, mesh placement in a non-contaminated environment is preferred.

Mesh can be positioned in an onlay, inlay or sublay fashion. Our preference is to place the mesh in the sublay position (in the preperitoneal plane just beneath the posterior rectus sheath medially and the transversus abdominis muscle laterally) and to cover the defect edges by more than 5-cm in all directions. In this case, a large piece of plain medium-weighted mesh can be used. However, in the case of intraperitoneal placement of mesh, a dual-layered mesh is used (Fig. 21.10).

The mesh is anchored laterally with non-absorbable transfascial sutures to the TA and IO, as shown in Figs. 21.11 and 21.12.

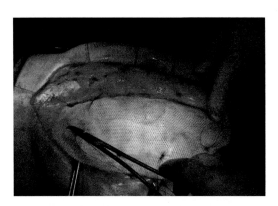

Fig. 21.10 Retromuscular composite mesh placement

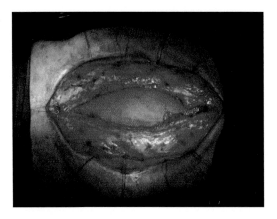

Fig. 21.11 Mesh secured with transfascial sutures

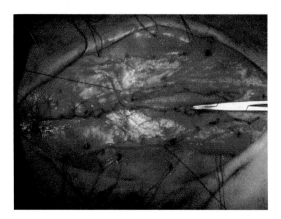

Fig. 21.12 Closure of anterior sheath over the mesh

21.6.2 Presence of a Stoma

The presence of an ileostomy, colostomy, or ileal conduit in singularity or in various combinations poses another challenge to CST.

Modifications to the technique would include:

- External oblique aponeurosis divided via two separate lateral incisions without dissection of the skin and subcutaneous layer from the rectus sheath. The stoma is subsequently advanced together with the rectus flap.
- Taking down the existing stoma with closure of the fascial defect, performing CST as described earlier followed by re-siting of the stoma.

A concern is that the shear/movement forces that can develop with the freed skin flap over the myofascial units could potentially affect the function of the stoma.

21.7 Post-operative Care

If the patient can be extubated, care can be continued in the general ward. However, if a period of controlled ventilation is needed, care is continued in the intensive care unit.

Good pain control in the post-operative period is important as there would have been a large area of dissection associated with some degree of muscle spasm. We routinely place patients on patient controlled analgesia (PCA) for pain control.

Initiation of post-operative feeding is at the discretion of the surgeon. Early post-operative feeding would be possible depending on the degree of bowel manipulation intra-operatively and the expected duration of ileus.

Early mobilization, chest physiotherapy and regular incentive spirometry are important components in the immediate post-operative period to minimize complications such as deep venous thrombosis and pneumonia.

Full length TED stockings are routinely worn for thromboprophylaxis. In addition, consideration is given to medical thromboprophylaxis with low molecular weight heparin depending on the patient's body habitus, anticipated mobility weighing this against the risk of post-operative bleeding. The post-operative abdominal binder is kept on at all times.

Closed suction drains are kept until drainage becomes minimal (<50 mL per day) and removed prior to discharge. If tension band sutures are used, these are left in place for a duration of 2–4 weeks.

On discharge patients are given advice on continued usage of an abdominal binder and to avoid strenuous and heavy-lifting activities for at least 3 months.

21.8 Complications and Results

21.8.1 Wound Infection

This represents the most common complication following CST and can be as high as 40%. Obese and diabetic patients are at higher risk of developing wound infections. Most infections are superficial and can be treated conservatively with antibiotics.

21.8.2 Seroma and Haematoma

Seven percent of patients develop clinically significant collections in the subcutaneous plane owing to the large area of dissection performed during a CST. Most usually resolve when treated conservatively. Larger or infected collections may require drainage which potentially puts a mesh at risk especially if used in the onlay position.

21.8.3 Skin Flap Necrosis

There is a 7% risk of developing skin flap necrosis during open CST largely due to the division of the perforating vessels originating within the rectus sheath that supply the anterior abdominal wall skin.

This can be mitigated by attention to the preservation of the perforators where possible during open CST. Endoscopic CST may reduce this risk as there is less anterior flap dissection and perforators can usually be preserved.

21.8.4 Hernia Recurrence

As with any hernia repair, this represents a significant source of concern and potential morbidity for the patient and the surgeon. Various retrospective reviews investigating open and endoscopic techniques reveal a wide spectrum of recurrence rates from 1 to 53% when followed over a 1–7-year period. A recurrence following CST poses a significant surgical challenge to repair and restore functional anatomy. Hernia recurrence can occur in the original defect area, or in the potentially weakened area laterally where the EO aponeurosis was incised. Placement of mesh reduces hernia recurrence, from 22 to 4% as shown by Ko et al. (Archives of Surgery, 2009).

21.9 Conclusion

CST is an effective technique for the treatment of complex ventral hernias or defects utilizing the patient's own autologous tissues. In cases where primary closure by itself is insufficient to bridge the defect, the addition of a mesh will be required to reconstruct the abdominal wall. The technique is associated with a low recurrence rate and represents an important surgical technique for restoration of complex defects of the abdominal wall.

Parastomal Hernia

22

Kai He and Qiyuan Yao

22.1 Introduction

Parastomal hernia (PSH) is a common and major clinical problem after abdominal ostomy, which may adversely affect quality of life, psychological well-being, and healthcare resources [1]. In the US, an estimated 450,000 people are living with a stoma and 120,000 new stomas are created each year [2], and similar data shows there are 102,000 people living with a stoma and around 20,000 new stomas are fashioned annually in the UK [3]. A meta-analysis estimated the incidence of PSH to be in the region of 1.8–28.0% for end ileostomy and 4.8–48.1% for colostomy [4], but some surgeons believe that PSH is an inevitable consequence of stoma formation [5].

A variety of open and laparoscopic approaches to repair parastomal hernia have been reported in the past 50 years [6], but with a similar recurrence rates up to 50%. Laparoscopic parastomal hernia repair is safe and appears to be associated with better short-term outcomes compared to open approaches [7, 8], and the "Sugarbaker" technique appears to be superior to the "Keyhole" technique when a laparoscopic approach is used.

Prophylactic mesh reinforcement during primary stoma formation appears to reduce the parastomal herniation rate according to many papers [9, 10] and might be the less costly and more effective strategy compared to no mesh to prevent PSH in patients undergoing abdominoperineal resection with permanent colostomy for rectal cancer [11].

Prophylactic mesh reinforcement during primary stoma formation and PSH repairing approaches have similar repairing methods, but lead to different outcomes of recurrence. We found the difference between them is the condition of the abdominal quadrant where the stoma locates in, and the PSHs always consist of a hernia defect in abdominal wall, a subcutaneous hernia sac, and a zigzagging stoma bowel in common once they form.

Based on above all, we designed the "Lap-re-Do" technique in a scheme to restore the primary parastomal anatomical structure, which consists of two main parts including popular laparoscopic PSH repairing approaches and rebuilding the parastomal area with closing hernia defect, removing hernia sac, resecting overlong stoma bowel, and reostomy in situ respectively through open approaches. We started to perform our "Lap-re-Do" technique to repair PSHs, especially for paracolostomy hernias (PCSHs) in May 2009. Since then, our hernia center has accumulated our series for more than 100 patients with primary or recurrent PCSHs,

K. He · Q. Yao (✉)
Department of General Surgery, Hernia Center,
Huashan Hospital, Shanghai Medical College,
Fudan University, Shanghai, China
e-mail: stevenyao@huashan.org.cn

© Springer Nature India Private Limited 2020
P. Chowbey, D. Lomanto (eds.), *Techniques of Abdominal Wall Hernia Repair*,
https://doi.org/10.1007/978-81-322-3944-4_22

and we would like to share our experience with the surgeons who may concern with the treatments of PSHs.

22.2   Main Content

- Indications
  Surgical indications of paraileostomal hernia and paracolostomal hernia are ill-fitting appliances causing leakage, pain, discomfort, and cosmetic complaints. Treatment is mandatory when incarceration or strangulation of hernia content occurs.
- Contraindications
  - Evidences of carcinoma recurrence are certificated on PSH patients preoperatively or being detected during the surgical procedures.
  - Patients accompany with any infective symptoms including pneumonia, urinary infection, FUO, parastomal skin bacterial infection, those who run a high risk on potential postoperative infection.

- Patients are unable to tolerate a general anesthesia or procedures because of cardiopulmonary dysfunctions, hepatic dysfunctions, or bleeding and coagulation dysfunctions.
- Preoperative preparation
  A bowel preparation and intravenous prophylactic antibiotics such as cefuroxime are routinely given preoperatively.

  The patient is placed in a supine position under general anesthesia with endotracheal intubation. Two Foley catheters are normally placed, one in the bladder and another in the stoma bowel, to assist with correct localization when dissecting adhesions.

  The operative field is prepared and draped including the colostomy in a standard fashion: The stoma is covered with sterile gauze, and the stoma-located abdominal quadrant is recovered with transparent adhesive drape.
- O.T layout
  The surgeon and the cameraman stand contralateral to the stoma site, while another assistant stands at the stoma site. O.T layout refers to Fig. 22.1.

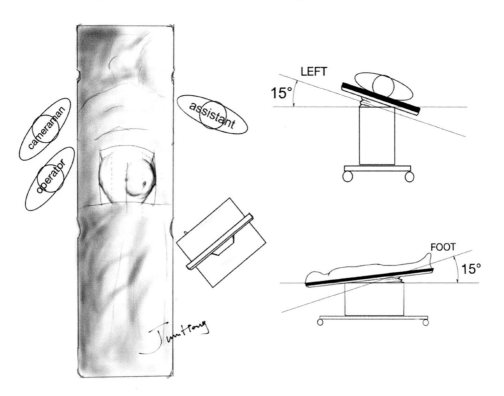

Fig. 22.1 O.T.layout

- Surgical Technique of Laparoscopic approaches to repair PSHs
  - Common Steps
    - The Hasson cannula or a 12-mm optical trocar is inserted at anterior axillary line and 3 cm below the costal margin in the right upper quadrant to create the pneumoperitoneum to a pressure of 12 mmHg with a 30° laparoscope utilized, and another two 5-mm trocars are placed under direct vision in the same quadrant as Fig. 22.2. All the trocars are placed away from the hernia defect to facilitate surgical manipulation.
    - Surgeons sometimes will meet very difficult situation to deal with during laparoscopic adhesiolysis. Sharp scissors are recommended to separate adhesion mixed with small intestine, stoma

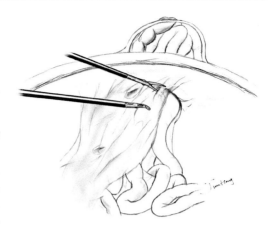

Fig. 22.3 Laparoscopic adhesiolysis

bowel, omentum and scar tissues (Fig. 22.3). Then the hernia contents can be reduced by a combination of external pressure and internal traction. After adhesiolysis and reducing the hernia contents, the hernia defect should be measured to determine the size of the mesh that would allow 3–5 cm of overlap circumferentially (Fig. 22.4).

  - Keyhole Technique
    - Keyhole technique was reported by BME. Hasson [12]. An e-PTFE patch is fashioned with a central keyhole of 2 cm and two radial incisions of 5 mm, thus creating a funnel-like shape for fixation to the bowel. Then the mesh is inserted, unrolled, and tacked to the abdominal wall with titanium tacks placed at 1-cm interval around the circumference of the patch and in the central part around the central hole. The cylindrical part of the mesh forms a collar covering the stoma bowel and is stitched to the bowel wall with two seromuscular U-stitches using nonabsorbable sutures (Fig. 22.5).
  - Sugarbaker Technique
    - This technique mimics that of the open repair being described by Sugarbaker in 1985 [13], under which the stoma bowel is lateralized along the abdominal wall by sutures and an anti-adhesion prosthesis is then placed to cover the bowel and the hernia defect (Fig. 22.6). We applied

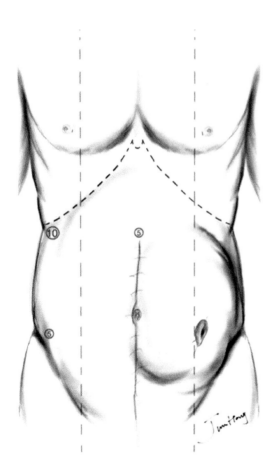

Fig. 22.2 Trocars for laparoscopic PCSH repair and on the contrary for PISH repair

Fig. 22.4 Laparoscopic measure the hernia defect

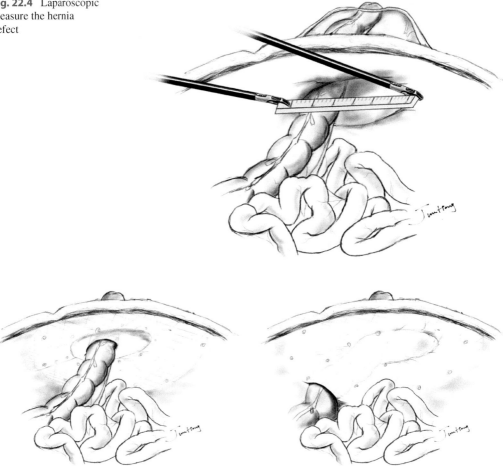

Fig. 22.5 Laparoscopic Keyhole technique

Fig. 22.6 Laparoscopic Sugarbaker technique

Sugarbaker technique not only for paracolostomal hernia (PCSH), but also for paraileostomal hernia (PISH) caused by ileal conduit (Fig. 22.7).

– Sandwich Technique
  o D. Berger reported "Sandwich" technique with two pieces of Dynamesh-IPOM (FEG-Textiltechnik, Aachen, Germany), a type of large pore-size anti-adhesion mesh, which was combined with "Keyhole" technique and "Sugarbaker" technique in 2007 [14].
– Lap-re-Do Technique
  o **Step 1. *Laparoscopic approach.*** After adhesiolysis, reducing the hernia contents and measuring the hernia defect,

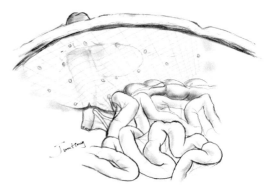

Fig. 22.7 Laparoscopic Sugarbaker technique for PISH after ileal conduit

we continue to dissociate the stoma bowel cautiously until closing to the anterior abdominal dermal or subcutaneous layer as possible. The relationships and the length ratio between the colostomal bowel and its mesentery should be also observed, which will indicate to apply Lap-re-Do Keyhole with a limitation of stomal bowel length or Lap-re-Do Sugarbaker technique with abundant stomal bowel length to repair hernia defect with an anti-adhesion prosthesis afterwards.

o **Step 2. *Open approach*.** Then, we transfer to make a round incision alongside the original stoma to pull through the stoma bowel (Fig. 22.8), which is sealed by a sterilized glove and deligated at once to prevent contamination (Fig. 22.9).

  After re-sterilizing the stoma operative field, if the Keyhole technique would be performed, we shall utilize the Dynamesh-IPST mesh (FEG-Textiltechnik, Aachen, Germany) with a pre-shaped and elastic 3-D funnel device in the center of it which the stomal bowel can be pulled through. We sew up the stomal bowel to the pre-shaped and elastic 3-D funnel device by 3–0 anti-bacteria Vicryl (Ethicon, New Jersey, USA). Then we put the mesh into the abdominal cavity with its polypropylene side to abdominal wall and the PVDF side to viscera, and sew up to close hernia ring with Surgilon (Covidien, Mansfield, USA), a type of nonabsorbable stitches, to an appropriate size to let stomal bowel pass through without entrapment (Fig. 22.10). But if Sugarbaker technique is applied to repair PCSH, during this operative step

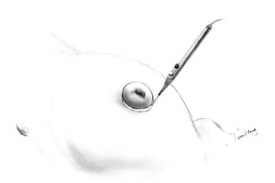

Fig. 22.8 Lap-re-Do Technique: Round incision alongside the stoma

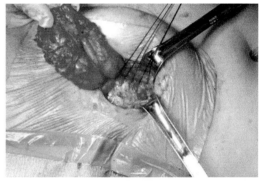

Fig. 22.10 Lap-re-Do Technique: Sew up the hernia ring

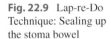

Fig. 22.9 Lap-re-Do Technique: Sealing up the stoma bowel

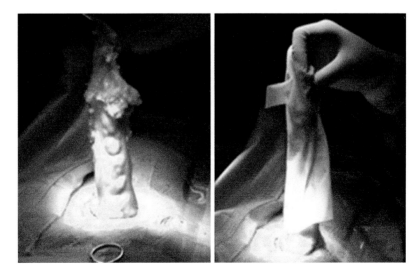

we only need to deal with the hernia defect just like we have introduced above and the anti-adhesion prosthesis would be put into the abdominal cavity through the 10-mm trocar.

o **Step 3.** *Laparoscopic approach.* After unfolding the transparent or semi- transparent mesh flatly and adjust its position around the stoma bowel in abdominal cavity, we fix the Dynamesh-IPST mesh as a Keyhole technique, or an anti-adhesion prosthesis as Sugarbaker technique to the abdominal wall with ProTack (Covidien, Mansfield, MA, USA) or Absorbable screws (Ethicon, New Jersey, USA) (Figs. 22.11 and 22.12). Drainage is recommended with

potential risk of unrecognized enterotomy when a serious adhesiolysis is performed during the operation.

o **Step 4.** *Open approach.* Finally, we remove the hernia sac, reduce the subcutaneous space and suture the stomal bowel to abdominal wall with 3–0 antibacteria Vicryl stitches (Ethicon, New Jersey, USA) interruptedly, sometimes even with local vacuum sealing drainage to prevent potential parastomal seroma or infection, resect and cut off the redundant stoma bowel, rebuild a stoma in situ (Fig. 22.13), We also suggest our patients to be wrapped up with a belt around the lower abdominal wall for at least 3 months postoperatively.

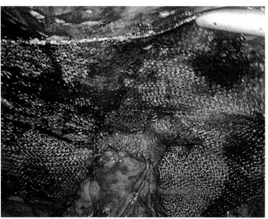
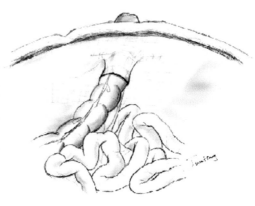

Fig. 22.11 Lap-re-Do: Keyhole technique

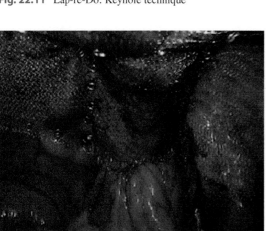
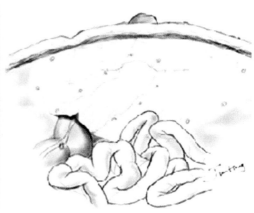

Fig. 22.12 Lap-re-Do: Sugarbaker technique

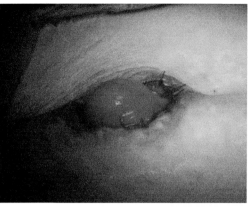
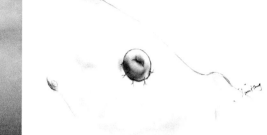

Fig. 22.13 Lap-re-Do: Re-colostomy in situ

- Postoperative care
  - The patient can drink water 6 h after the operation, have full liquid diet on the first postoperative day, and eat semi-liquid diet after postoperative exhaust.
  - The rebuilt stoma in situ should be observed very carefully to evaluate its blood supply after operation.
  - The amount and nature of the fluid drainage should be recorded and observed every day postoperatively.
  - Postoperative analgesia treatments are applied in all the patients to relieve the pain caused by patching mesh.
  - Postoperative early ambulation is recommended to all the patients to prevent deep vein thrombosis and pneumonia.
- Postoperative complications
  - Intraoperative Complications
    - *Intestinal injuries and bleeding* are significant events that may occur during the dissection of the intestine or adhesiolysis during any bowel surgery. Incidence of Intraoperative intestinal injuries is approximately 1–3% [12]. The management of a recognized enterotomy is somewhat controversial; a part of surgeons will terminate the hernia repair procedure and only repair the injury either laparoscopically or by a conversion to the open operation [13]. More recently, we agree with the reports indicating that the repair of the recog-

nized intestinal injury and completion of the intended hernia repair may be safe because of application of the anti adhesion prosthesis without e-PTFE [14]. Meanwhile we also recommend applying the Harmonic Scalpel to lyse the omentum adhesions to prevent bleeding.
  - Postoperative Complications
    - *Unrecognized enterotomy* is a serious complication that occurs in less than 1% patients [15]. This is often caused by a traction injury from the grasping instruments or a burn from the use of an energy source to lyse the adhesions during the procedures.
    - *Stoma-related complications* including ischemia, collapse, and stenosis of the stoma bowel have been observed in our series of Lap-re-Do technique. We dealt with all the stoma-related complications without re-operation, but the surgeon who may apply the Lap-re-Do technique should pay attention to the procedure of re-ostomy and care must be taken to avoid injury of stoma bowel and its mesentery.
    - *Ileus* includes adhesive intestinal obstruction and stoma obstruction. It is one of the most reported postoperative complications in nearly every literature about PSH with an incidence of approximately 6.3% [4]. Most of ileus can be

healed up with conservative treatment without re-operation.

○ *Infection* is another kind of common postoperative complication including mesh infection, wound infection, pneumonia, and urinary infection. Mesh infection in the laparoscopic approach was reported in 3.7% lower than in open hernia repair [16].

○ *Seroma* There has been a series of patients that were evaluated by ultrasonic study found the incidence of seroma is 100% because the hernia sac is not removed and its peritoneal membrane surface will secrete the fluid which can be contained by the prosthetic mesh [17]. If the seroma occurs, a puncture under ultrasonic location is recommended. We designed the Lap-re-Do technique to remove the hernia sac even with local subcutaneous vacuum sealing drainage to prevent potential parastomal seroma.

22.3 Summary

It is well known that most ostomates face sensitive physical, social, and psychological problems, and severe stoma-related issues often impair their quality of life. The parastomal hernia, known to be

a common complication, often causes stoma care problems, such as leakage and skin irritation, and can lead to rare but severe complications including obstruction, bowel incarceration, and perforation.

Obesity, chronic lung disease, type II DM, advancing age, malnutrition, renal failure, malignancy, steroid treatment, jaundice, radiotherapy, chemotherapy, and oral anticoagulant use are considered to be patient-related factors that increase the risk of developing an incisional hernia [18]. In addition to these factors, the site of stoma placement, the peritoneal route used for colostomy creation (extraperitoneal or transperitoneal) and the size of the fascial opening are reported to be risk factors for parastomal hernia development [19].

A variety of open and laparoscopic approaches to repair parastomal hernia with mesh have been reported in the past 50 years. Open approaches include onlay, sublay, and IPOM technique, and laparoscopic approaches include common repairs like Keyhole or Sugarbaker technique and case report as Sandwich, Double Patch, and Scroll technique. The recurrence of different approaches with a range of 0–62.5% and complications can be referred from many literatures and meta-analysis of PSHs [20–34] (Table 22.1). We have performed Laparoscopic Sugarbaker technique on 11 PISH patients after ileal conduit since April 2005, and no recurrence occurred afterwards.

Table 22.1 Follow-up of PSH repairs (No > 10)

Study	Year	No of repairs	Technique	Recurrence (%)	Infection (%)	Follow-up (months) (mean)
Luning	2009	16	Open onlay	19	6.2	6–110 (33)
Valdivia	2008	25	Open onlay	8	8	8–24 (12)
de Ruiter	2005	46	Open onlay	15.9	6.6	12–156 (60)
Steele	2003	58	Open onlay	26.0	3.4	0.2–139 (50.6)
Geisler	2003	16	Open onlay	62.5	12.5	2–161 (39)
Egun	2002	10	Open sublay	0	20	22–69 (54)
Sprundel	2005	15	Open IPOM	13.3	0	5–52 (29)
Stelzner	2004	20	Open IPOM	15	5	3–84 (42)
Mizrahi	2011	29	Keyhole	46.4	3.4	12–53 (30)
Hansson	2009	54	Keyhole	37	1.8	12–72 (36)
Pastor	2009	12	Keyhole/sugarbaker	33.3	16.6	(13.9)
Muysoms	2008	24	Keyhole/sugarbaker	41.7	0	4–54 (21.2)
Berger	2007	41	Sugarbaker	19.5	4.5	3–72 (24)
		47	Sandwich	2.1	2.1	(20)
Craft	2007	21	Keyhole/sugarbaker	4.7	4.8	3–36 (14)
Mancini	2005	25	Sugarbaker	4.0	4.0	2–38 (19)
LeBlanc	2005	12	Keyhole/sugarbaker	8.3	0	3–39 (20)

We have performed Lap-re-Do technique on 102 PCSH patients from May 2009 to June 2015, including 93 primary PCSHs and 9 recurrent PCSHs. The mean operating time was 113 min and the mean length of postoperative hospital stay was 8 days. 16 patients were observed as recurrence (rate $\approx$ 15.7%) during a mean follow-up period of 39 months (range from 6 to 79). According to the follow-up, the PCSH patients with BMI over 26 run an obviously higher risk of recurrence of 31.8% postoperatively than whose BMI under 26 with a recurrence of only 1.8%. Different postoperative complications were observed in detailed on 21 patients in hospital and 18 patients after hospital discharge, including stoma-related complications on 15 patients, ileus and stoma obstruction on 19 patients in all, and 5 for others. Re-operation had to be performed on 2 patients because unrecognized enterotomy and mesh infection, and no patients died of procedure-related complications (Table 22.2).

Key Points
- Parastomal hernia is a difficult problem for surgeons to deal with because it is a special type of dynamic incisional hernia with stoma bowel as its hernia content, and there is lack of evidence on the ideal technique for stoma formation or surgical procedure for symptomatic parastomal hernias. Herein, large prospective controlled multicenter trials are required to compare different surgical techniques of laparoscopic parastomal hernia repair in reducing the postoperative complications and recurrence.
- Future research needs to address the pathogenesis of parastomal hernia formation, as until we have fully understood the mechanism of its formation, direct prevention, and treatment will always be unsatisfactory.
- Laparoscopic Sugarbaker technique has a good result on dealing with PISH patients after ileal conduit and appears to be superior to the "Keyhole" technique on PCSHs.
- "Lap-re-Do" technique is easy for surgeons to learn and handle according to our introductions and graphical representation. The summarized key-points of "Lap-re-Do" technique

Table 22.2 Follow-up of Lap-re-Do

	Series ($n = 102$)
Follow-up (mon)	39 (6~79)
Operating time (min)	113 (60~185)
Postoperative hospital stay (day)	6.5 (3, 66)
Hospitalized complications	
Re-ostomy complications	9
Peristomal abscess	1
Parastomal seroma	3
Stoma ischemia	3
Others	2
Ileus/stoma obstruction	10
Others	4
Unrecognized enterotomy	1
Patients with no complications (rate)	81 (79.41%)
Discharged complications	
Ileus	9
Stoma-related complications	6
Peristomal abscess	3
Colostomy stenosis	1
Stoma ischemia	1
Parastomal fistula	1
Others	3
Patients with no complications (rate)	84 (82.35%)
Recurrence(rate)	16 (15.69%)
Absorbable prosthesis(1)	1 (100%)
Nonabsorbable prosthesis (101 cases)	15 (14.85%)
Comparing by BMI	
BMI ≥ 26 (44 cases)	14 (31.82%)
BMI < 26 (57 cases)	1 (1.75%)
Different Lap-re-Do Types[a]	
Type A(32 cases)	8 (25%)
Type B(52 cases)	4 (11.5%)
Type C(17 cases)	1 (5.9%)

[a]**Type A:** "Lap-re-Do" Keyhole technique with slow-absorbable stitches "PDS-II" to close the hernia ring; **Type B:** "Lap-re-Do" Keyhole technique with nonabsorbable stitches "Surgilon" to close the hernia ring; **Type C:** "'Lap-re-Do" Sugarbaker technique with nonabsorbable stitches "Surgilon" to close the hernia ring

includes sewing up hernia defect with nonabsorbable stitches, repairing with no e-PTFE prosthesis, operating in detailed with aseptic concept, and shortening the length of time when the stoma of colon once being open.
- Lap-re-Do technique can be considered as another clinical choice for primary and recurrent PCSH therapy, especially on the patients with BMI under 26, but the open approach of Lap-re-Do technique to rebuild stomal area in situ shall be improved step by step to reduce the incidence of stoma-related complications.

References

1. Pringle W, Swan E. Continuing care after discharge from hospital for stoma patients. Br J Nurs. 2001;10:1275–88.
2. Turnbull GB. Ostomy statistics: the $64,000 question. Ostomy Wound Manage. 2003;49:22–3.
3. Brown H, Randle J. Living with a stoma: a review of the literature. J Clin Nurs. 2005;14:74–81.
4. Hansson BME, de Hingh IH, Bleichrodt RP. Laparoscopic parastomal hernia repair: pitfalls and complications. Hernia Repair Sequelae. 2010;3:451–5.
5. Moreno-Matias J, Serra-Aracil X, et al. The prevalence of parastomal hernia after formation of an end colostomy. A new clinic-radiological classification. Color Dis. 2009;11:173–7.
6. Hotouras A, Murphy J, Thaha M, Chan C. The persistent challenge of parastomal herniation: a review of the literature and future developments. Color Dis. 2013;15:202–14.
7. Halabi WJ, Jafari MD, Carmichael JC, et al. Laparoscopic versus open repair of parastomal hernias: an ACS-NSQIP analysis of short-term outcomes. Surg Endosc. 2013;27:4067–72.
8. Helgstrand F, et al. Risk of morbidity, mortality, and recurrence after parastomal hernia repair: a nationwide study. Dis Colon Rectum. 2013;56:1265–72.
9. Wijeyekoon SP, Gurusamy K, El-Gendy K, Chan CL. Prevention of parastomal herniation with biologic/composite prosthetic mesh: a systematic review and meta-analysis of randomized controlled trials. J Am Coll Surg. 2010;211:637–45.
10. Shabbir J, Chaudhary BN, Dawson R. A systematic review on the use of prophylactic mesh during primary stoma formation to prevent parastomal hernia formation. Color Dis. 2011;14:931–6.
11. Lee L, Saleem A, Landry T, et al. Cost effectiveness of mesh prophylaxis to prevent parastomal hernia in patients undergoing permanent colostomy for rectal cancer. J Am Coll Surg. 2014;218:82–91.
12. Hansson BME, van Nieuwenhoven EJ, Bleichrodt RP. Promising new technique in the repair of parastomal hernia. Surg Endosc. 2003;17:1789–91.
13. Sugarbaker PH. Peritoneal approach to prosthetic mesh repair of paraostomy hernias. Ann Surg. 1985;201:344–6.
14. Berger D, Bientzle M. Laparoscopic repair of parastomal hernias: a single surgeon's experience in 66 patients. Dis Colon Rectum. 2007;50:1668–73.
15. LeBlanc KA, Whitaker JM, Bellanger DE, et al. Laparoscopic incisional and ventral hernioplasty: lessons learned from 200 patients. Hernia. 2003;7:378–82.
16. Heniford TB, Park A, Ramshaw BJ, et al. Laparoscopic ventral and incisional hernia repair in 407 patients. J Am Coll Surg. 2000;190:645–50.
17. Berger D, Bientzle M, Muller A. Postoperative complications after laparoscopic incisional hernia repair. Surg Endosc. 2002;16:1720–3.
18. LeBlanc KA, Elieson MJ, Corder JM 3rd. Enterotomy and mortality rates of laparoscopic incisional and ventral hernia repair: a review of the literature. JSLS. 2007;11:408–14.
19. Pierce RA, Spitler JA, Frisella MM, et al. Pooled data analysis of laparoscopic vs. open ventral hernia repair: 14 years of patient data accrual. Surg Endosc. 2007;21:378–86.
20. Susmallian S, Gewurtz G, Ezri T, et al. Seroma after laparoscopic repair of hernia with ePTFE patch: is it really a complication? Hernia. 2001;5:139–41.
21. Pilgrim CH, McIntyre R, Bailey M. Prospective audit of parastomal hernia: prevalence and associated comorbidities. Dis Colon Rectum. 2010;53:71–6.
22. Funahashi K, Suzuki K, Nagashima Y, et al. Risk factors for parastomal hernia in Japanese patients with permanent colostomy. Surg Today. 2014;44:1465–9.
23. Luning TH, Spillenaar-Bilgen EJ. Parastomal hernia: complications of extra-peritoneal onlay mesh placement. Hernia. 2009;13:487–90.
24. Valdivia G, Guerrero TS, Laurrabaquio HV. Parastomal hernia-repair using mesh and an open technique. World J Surg. 2008;32:465–70.
25. Ruiter PD, Bijnen AB. Ring-reinforced prosthesis for paracolostomy hernia. Dig Surg. 2005;22:152–6.
26. Steele SR, Lee P, Martin MJ, et al. Is parastomal hernia repair with polypropylene mesh safe? Am J Surg. 2003;185:436–40.
27. Geisler DJ, Reilly JC, Vaughan SG, et al. Safety and outcome of use of nonabsorbable mesh for repair of fascial defects in the presence of open bowel. Dis Colon Rectum. 2003;46:1118–23.
28. Egun A, Hill J, MacLennan I, et al. Preperitoneal approach to parastomal hernia with coexistent large incisional hernia. Color Dis. 2002;4:132–4.
29. Sprundel ST, Hoop AG. Modified technique for parastomal hernia repair in patients with intractable stoma-care problems. Color Dis. 2005;7:445–9.
30. Stelzner S, Hellmich G, Ludwig K. Repair of paracolostomy hernias with a prosthetic mesh in the intraperitoneal onlay position: modified Sugarbaker technique. Dis Colon Rectum. 2004;47:185–91.
31. Mizrahi H, Bhattacharya P, Parker MC. Laparoscopic slit mesh repair of parastomal hernia using a designated mesh: long-term results. Surg Endosc. 2012;26:267–70.
32. Hansson BM, Bleichrodt RP, de Hingh IH. Laparoscopic parastomal hernia repair using a keyhole technique results in a high recurrence rate. Surg Endosc. 2009;23:1456–9.
33. Pastor DM, Pauli EM, Koltun WA, et al. Parastomal hernia repair: a single center experience. JSLS. 2009;13:170–5.
34. Muysoms EE, Hauters PJ, Van Nieuwenhove Y, et al. Laparoscopic repair of parastomal hernias: a multicentre retrospective review and shift in technique. Acta Chir Belg. 2008;108:400–4.

Muscle–Aponeurotic Plication Associated with Dermolipectomy in the Treatment of Ventral Hernias and Diastasis Recti: A Functional and Aesthetic Approach

23

Marco Aurelio Faria-Correa

23.1 Introduction

In the treatment of ventral hernias and diastasis recti, a functional and an aesthetic approach should be considered. The abdominal wall may be affected by pregnancies, weight variation, and previous abdominal surgical procedures [1–5]. The weakening of the muscle–aponeurotic layer is attributed to a congenital condition related to the ratio of collagen type I and III in the composition of the aponeurosis. It has been shown that aponeuroses with a high concentration of collagen type III are weaker than those with a higher number of type I fiber [6]. Also, there is a change in the relation of the rate of collagen types to the aging process, with an increasing number of collagen types III compared with type I [7]. The quality of the extracellular matrix of the skin, aponeurosis, and muscle has similarities in the same individual [8], which is why there is a straight relationship between the muscle–aponeurotic deformity and the excess skin of the abdomen. Patients presenting with a large amount of excess skin have more complex muscle–aponeurotic deformities [6].

Based on a representative number of more than 2560 patients, some with up to 20 years' follow-up presenting with successful results (Figs. 23.1, 23.2, 23.3, and 23.4) and a series of 182 secondary surgeries for repairing unsuccessful cases (Figs. 23.5 and 23.6), we present a study of our personal clinical experience. We also present a bibliographic review of the efficacy and durability of muscle–aponeurotic plication using various methods of plication with different suture materials, including absorbable and non-absorbable [9, 10]. The long-term evaluation was done with the use of clinical examination, in addition to abdominal wall CT and linear ultrasound [10–12]. Trans-operative findings in secondary cases were also analyzed, discussing the type of suture material and stitching technique used, in addition to the reason for failure.

23.2 Materials and Methods

During the last 30 years, we have been treating the small, medium and large cosmetic and functional abdominal wall deformities such as abdominal lipodystrophies associated with diastasis recti, and with umbilical, ventral, and hernias.

Our experience is approximately 2560 cases divided up as follows:

M. A. Faria-Correa (✉)
Dr Marco Faria Correa Plastic Surgery Pte Ltd,
Singapore, Singapore
e-mail: admin@drmarco.com, drmarco@drmarco.com

© Springer Nature India Private Limited 2020
P. Chowbey, D. Lomanto (eds.), *Techniques of Abdominal Wall Hernia Repair*,
https://doi.org/10.1007/978-81-322-3944-4_23

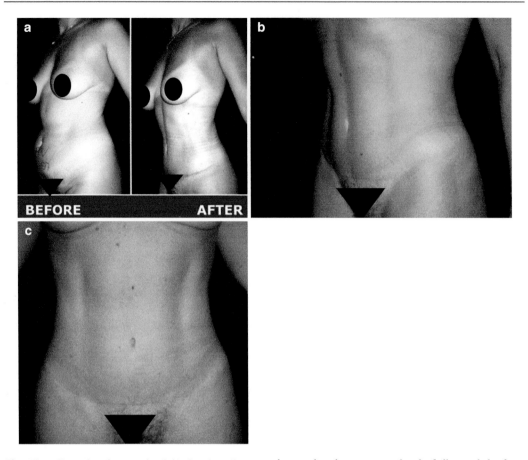

Fig. 23.1 Example of cosmetic abdominoplasty(lower abdomen + rectus plication). (a) Before and after 3 months—scar still visible. (b, c) After 3 years, we can observe that the scars are already fading and the functional and cosmetic results achieved are still present

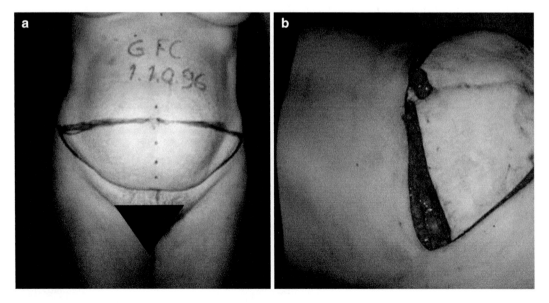

Fig. 23.2 (a) Lower abdominal dermolipectomy drawing. (b) Showing the full flap of skin removed. (c) Before and after 3 years, scar results

Fig. 18.2 (continued)

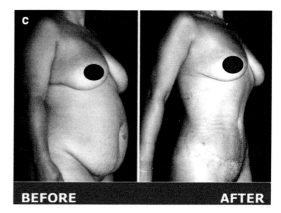

Fig. 23.3 Abdominoplasty
with plication performed
together with bilateral breast
lifting. (**a**, **c**) Pre-operatively.
(**b**, **d**) Post-operatively 10
months

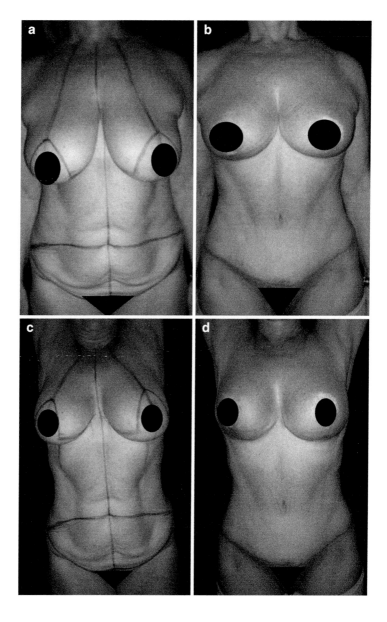

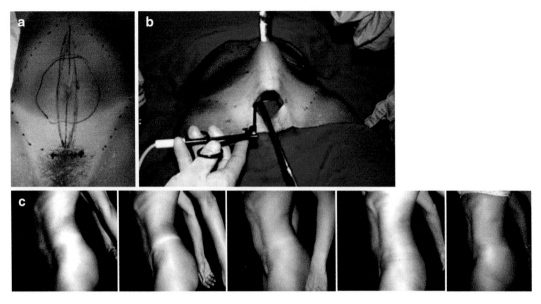

Fig. 23.4 Endoscopic abdominoplasty. (**a**) Operative drawing showing the minimally invasive muscle–aponeurosis rectus plication endoscopic abdominoplasty. (**b**) Intra-operatively—showing the minimally invasive surgery with a small hole. (**c**) Before, and the 6 months ,8 years, 15 years and 20 years follow-up showing the efficacy and longevity of the method

Fig. 23.5 Secondary abdominoplasty. (**a**) Pre-operatively. (**b**) Post-operatively 2 years. (**c**) Intra-operative findings: no hernia with epiploon content found. However, fats are growing incarcerated inside the previous rectus plication showing that fats were left behind at the midline area

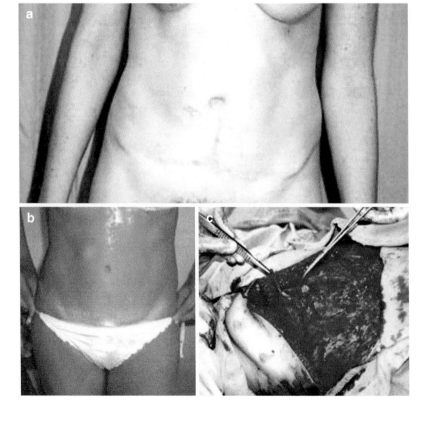

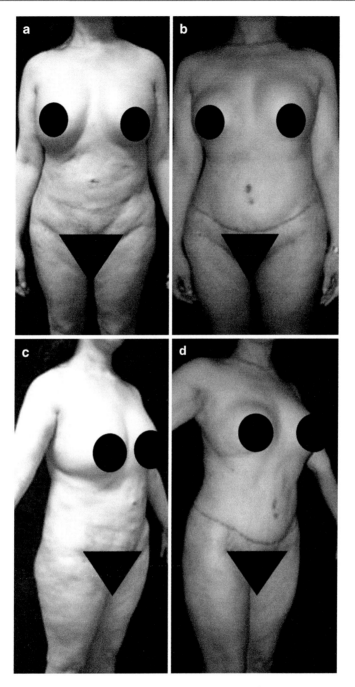

Fig. 23.6 Secondary abdominoplasty. Patient complained of poor cosmetic and functional results: flabbiness, bulging stomach, and pain in the umbilical area. We can observe in the post-operative period a significant improvement in the flabbiness and cosmetic results in the trunk and thigh area. Frontal view: (**a**) Pre-operatively, (**b**) Post-operatively 2 years; semi-profile view: (**c**) Pre-operatively, (**d**) Post-operatively 2 years; lateral view: (**e**) Pre-operatively, (**f**) Post-operatively 2 years. Intra-operative (**g**) Fat found inside the previous rectus plication and previous running suture partially open, (**h**) After trimming and removing the fats and previous sutures, preparing the diastasis recti for plication. (**i**) First layer of interrupted stitching with 2-0 mono-nylon. (**j**) Second layer of muscle–aponeurosis plication properly distributing the tension—interrupted 2-0 mono-nylon sutures. (**k**) Removing the excess skin from the previous scar down to the pubis and inguinal area causing a thigh lift

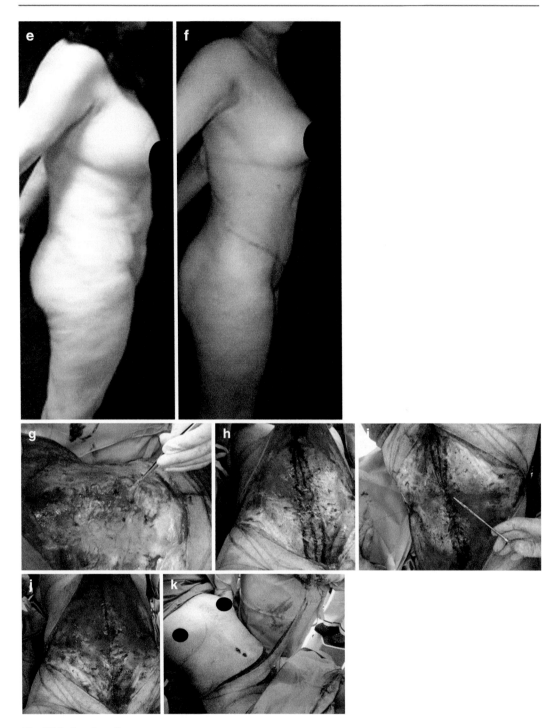

Fig. 18.6 (continued)

- 282 cases of small deformities (mini-abdominoplasty, endoscopic abdominoplasty, and robotic abdominoplasty (Fig. 23.4)
- Approximately 2100 cases of medium and large cases of primary dermolipectomy with diastasis recti or hernias (abdominoplasty and dermolipectomy with rectus plication with or without hernias) (Figs. 23.7, 23.8, and 23.9)
- Approximately 182 cases of secondary abdominoplasty (Figs. 23.5 and 23.6) for repairing various complaints such as a bulging stomach due to

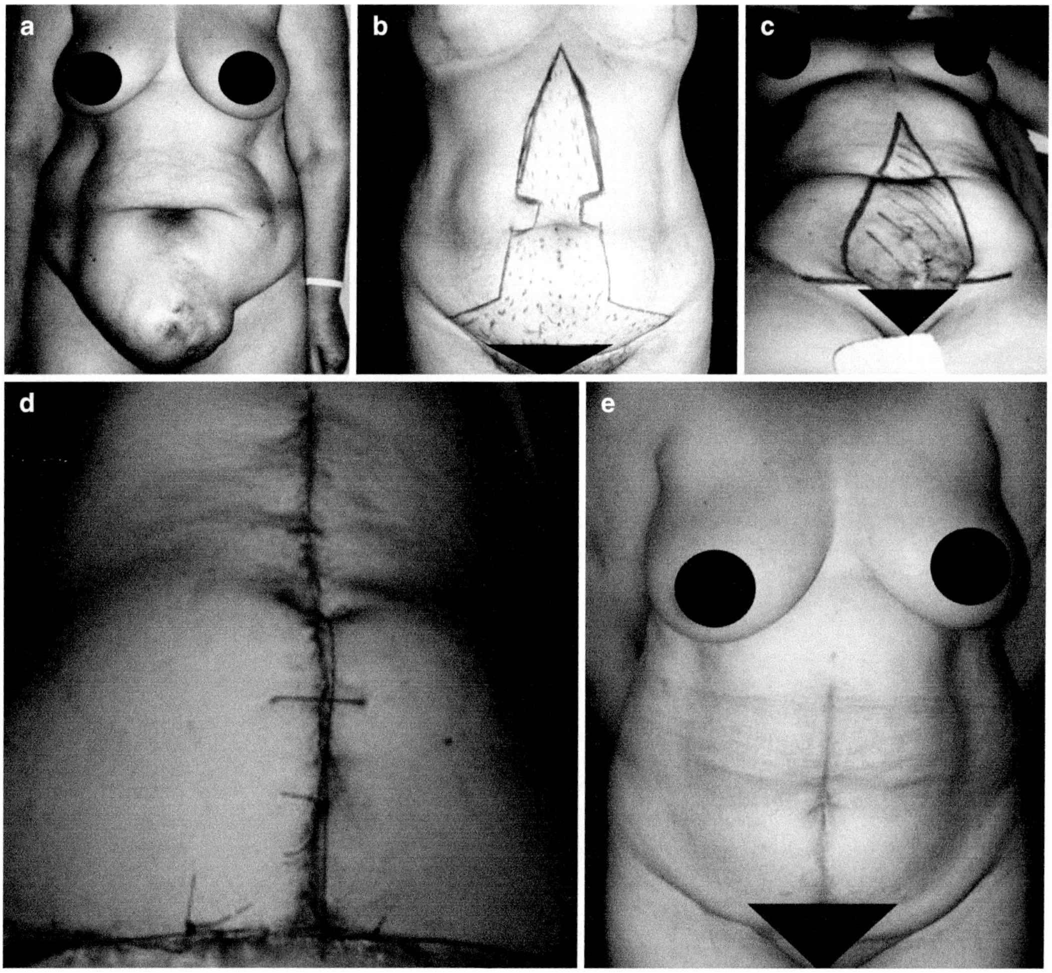

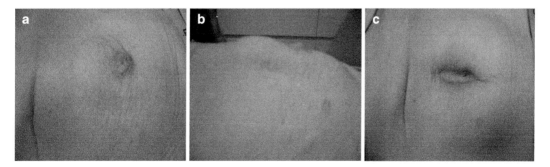

Fig. 23.7 Incisional hernia repair and vertical dermoli-pectomy. (**a**) Incisional hernia. (**b**) Vertical abdominal dermolipectomy. Drawing shows the area of skin to be removed. Note that the small flaps are used to reconstruct the new umbilical scar. (**c**) Beginning of the operation. (**d**) Immediate result. (**e**) Patient 2 years post-operatively with a successful result

Fig. 23.8 Clinical examination for diastasis recti, and ventral and umbilical hernia. (**a–e**) Pre-operatively. (**f**) Post-operatively 1 year. (**g**) Pre-operatively. (**h**) Post-operatively 1 year. (**i**) Pre-operatively. (**j**) Post-operatively 1 year. (**k**) Pre-operative drawing and planning. (**l**) Post-operatively 1 year. (**m**) Intra-operatively. (**n**) Marking the gap of the diastasis recti. (**o**) After two layers of muscle–aponeurosis plication performed using 0-0 mono-nylon

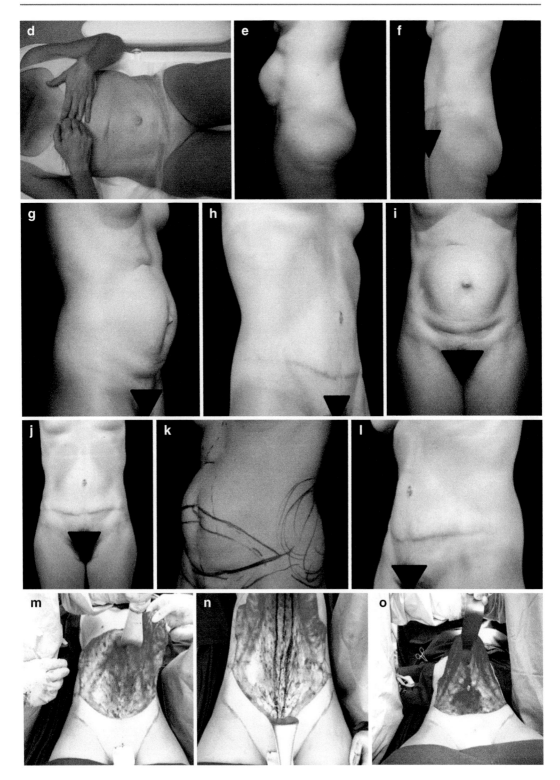

Fig. 18.8 (continued)

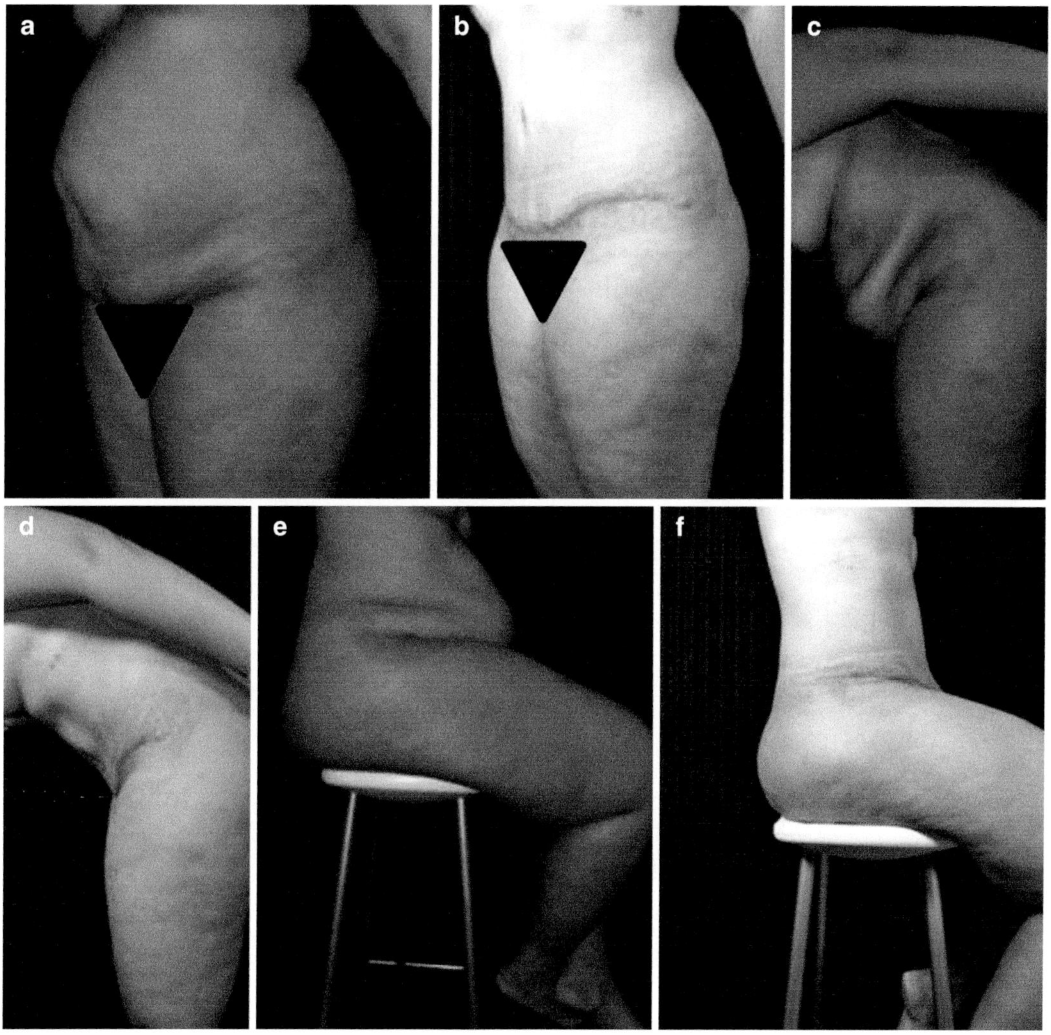

Fig. 23.9 Lower abdomen dermolipectomy and ventral hernia and diastasis recti repair. (**a**) Pre-operatively. (**b**) Post-operatively 1 year. (**c**) Pre-operatively. (**d**) Post-operatively 1 year. (**e**) Pre-operatively. (**f**) Post-operatively 1 year. (**g**) Pre-operative drawing. (**h**) Intra-operatively showing the eventration. (**i**) Two layers of xipho-pubic muscle–aponeurosis plication performed using interrupted 0-0 mono-nylon stitches. (**j**) Stitching down the skin flap to reduce the formation of a seroma. (**k**) Limited undermining and tunneling to preserve perforator vessels so as to reduce the risk of seroma and skin necrosis

poor or failed plication, repair of umbilical, incisional, or recurrent hernias, poor cosmetic results, a new tummy tuck after new pregnancy.

Since the beginning of my practice, I have always used non-absorbable (00-mono-nylon) sutures to perform the rectus plication, and the method of stitching has been interrupted inverted-X fashion buried stitches with a distance of 0.5–0.8 cm from each other, with one single layer of stitches in the plication. We used to take quite large sections (3–4 mm) of the muscle itself.

I observed that this method was effective and quite fast to perform, but patients use to complain of post-operative pain.

Trying to make the procedure faster, I also tried the running suturing method, taking 2–3 mm sections of the inner borders of the abdominal

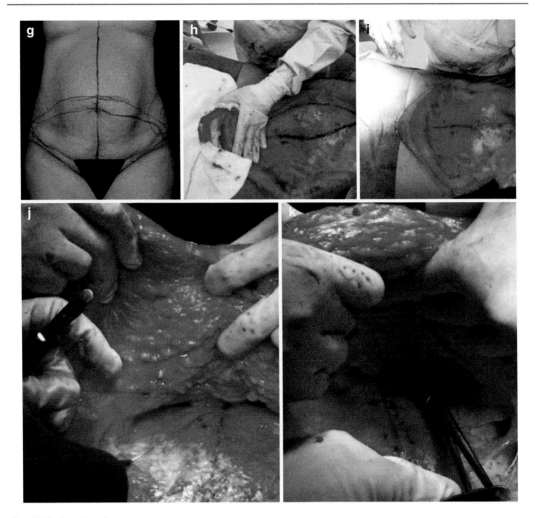

Fig. 18.9 (continued)

muscles and their aponeuroses, one running suture above and one below the umbilical stack. However, I abandoned this method after a few cases because I noted that my patients complained of more pain with this method than with the interrupted stitching method, mainly when they tried to walk straight. I realized that the sutures running over and over strangulate the muscle, causing pain when the patients straighten their body, and also because of the risk of rupturing the suture, causing the wound to open.

- What did I learn from my own mistakes?
- What did I learn from the findings in secondary cases that were performed by me or by others?

- What were the most common mistakes that caused the procedure to fail?
- What were the patients complaints?
- How to avoid the mistakes?
- How to make the procedure better and more successful?

The answers are:
- To be humble and learn from one's own mistakes
- To be humble and learn from others
- To be smart and learn from others' mistakes
- To be smart and learn from one's own successful cases
- To be smart and learn from others' successful cases and those from the literature.

23.3 Trans-Operative Findings in Secondary Cases

In most cases, failure of the rectus plication was due to the stitching method and the suture material and/or the presence of fat inside the plication (Figs. 23.5 and 23.6).

We noted that in many cases, the surgeon applied a running suture and in some cases I found that the suture ruptured and the diastases recurred (Figs. 23.5 and 23.6). In other cases, no sutures was found or only minimal signs of absorbable sutures were found and the diastasis recurred.

In many cases, there were large quantities of fat tissue inside the plication that caused the recurrence of the diastasis and the patient was in pain (Figs. 23.5c and 23.6g). There was one case in which the patient came to me complaining of pain and a mass at the midline of her lower abdomen at the peri-umbilical area after abdominoplasty performed elsewhere a few years earlier. She underwent CT, which reported "recti diastasis with fat and suspected hernia involving transversal colon + epiploon," but our trans-operative findings only showed the presence of fat inside the rectus plication. The patient mentioned that she had put on 3 kg after undergoing the abdominoplasty. I realized that the fat left inside the plication had grown as she put on weight and that this was the cause of the pain. The diastasis recti recurrence and the mass found on the CT had given the wrong impression of a hernia involving the epiploon.

Another cause of the recurrence of incisional and umbilical hernias that I found in secondary cases was the poor distribution of tension, with the repair limited to the hernia area without distributing the tension along the rectus. When we perform a xiphoid–pubic plication as a second layer of stitches, we increase the chance of success. In Figs. 23.5 and 23.6, we see the trans-operative findings of a secondary abdominoplasty for a recurrent umbilical hernia, repairing both the recurrent umbilical hernia and the rectus plication in a second layer of interrupted 0-0 nylon sutures from the xiphoid process to the pubic bone, providing a good distribution of the tension all along the rectus, supporting the umbilical her-

nia correction, and preventing recurrence before and after 2 years.

In Fig. 23.6, we see a case of the repair of a recurrent incisional hernia associated with dermolipectomy by performing a second layer of 0-0 mono-nylon interrupted plication from the xiphoid process to the pubic bone, with a smooth distribution of the tension in the suture line. We follow up this patient for 3 years without recurrence.

I believe that reducing the weight of the dermal–adipose flap on the abdominal wall, and the wide layer of collagen formed by the inner scar between the abdominal wall and the dermal–adipose flap, also contributes to the formation of a stronger and more reliable repair for hernias and rectus diastasis.

23.4 Bibliography Review

We found many articles in the literature in which different authors present studies using CT and linear ultrasound to evaluate the efficacy and longevity of muscle–aponeurotic rectus plication performed using different methods of plication such as: one layer of running sutures × one layer of interrupted sutures × two layers of sutures interrupted and running, using different suture materials, i.e., polydioxanone (PDS) versus mono-nylon, after 3 months, 1 year, and 3 years.

Studies of rectus plication with the use of different suture materials such as mono-nylon and PDS in different sizes and using different techniques of suturing such as running sutures and interrupted sutures in one or two layers were compared [4, 9, 13].

Some authors do not recommend absorbable suture such as PDS because it loses 50% of its strength in approximately 1 month, by which time the scar is not yet mature, which is why it is not the best choice for one layer of muscle–aponeurotic plication.

There are reports of successful experiences with the use of PDS 0-0 [9]; perhaps because of the thickness of the suture, it takes longer to be dissolved.

Mono-nylon 0-0 seems to be the best choice. Interrupted sutures are safer than continuous suturing.

One layer of plication with mono-nylon 0-0 was effective in some studies.

The longevity of the plication was evaluated after a few months, after 1 year, and after 3–5 years. The failure occurred more frequently during the first year. There were not many cases of failure after 3–5 years [6, 10, 11, 13].

23.5 Complications

The reasons for recurrences of hernia diastasis vary from surgical methods and materials to patients' post-operative care and instructions.

Complications caused by surgical methods are due to the variety of surgical plication techniques and also the choice of surgical sutures used.

Post-operative care is one of the most crucial sources of complications. Formation of a seroma

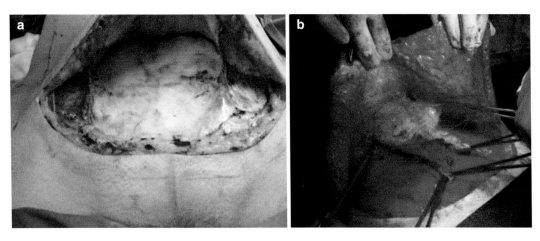

Fig. 23.10 Seroma complication. (**a**) Large seroma. (**b**) Removing the seroma cavity

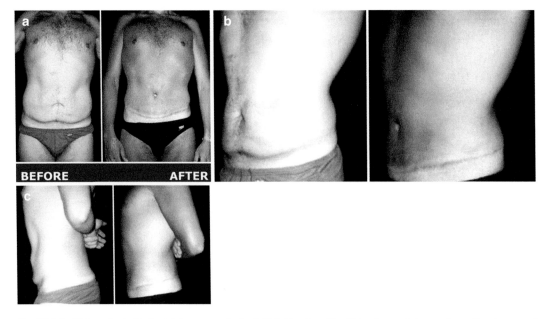

Fig. 23.11 Male patient after bariatric surgery. (**a, b, c**) Weight reduced by 45 kg, lower abdomen dermolipectomy, and rectus plication performed

used to affect more than 30% of patients (Fig. 23.10). After we adopted the method of stitching down [4] the dermal–subcutaneous flap to the abdominal wall (Fig. 23.9i, j), we reduced this complication to close to a maximum of 4–5% of our patients. The choice of suction drainage used and keeping the drainage for a minimum of 2–3 days, or a daily output of less than 30 mL daily, have also helped to reduce the percentage [4].

Use of an abdominal binder/surgical pressure garment versus not using it, early post-recovery movement, and returning back to exercise or carrying heavy things after 2–3 months also play a crucial part in the post-operative complications.

Skin necrosis is one of the most dangerous complications in dermolipectomy surgery because of the limited amount of skin left behind and the degree of tension that we administer for cosmetic purposes [14, 15].

We avoid operating on smokers and diabetics (Fig. 23.11).

Hematoma and deep vein thrombosis are also causative factors; mainly with regard to the time to start using anti-coagulants for high-risk patients, the use of a foot pump during the intra- and post-operative periods, and the encouragement of early leg movement.

23.6 Conclusions

After all that I have learned from my own experience of both primary and secondary cases and from the literature, I recommend:

Proper undermining of the dermal–adipose flap from the muscle–aponeurotic abdominal wall from the pubis to the xiphoid process, leaving no fat tissue in the midline, avoiding fat inside the plication. The plication is then free of fat tissue [1, 2, 4].

Using 0-0 mono-nylon sutures and performing interrupted stitches, inverted X, buried fashion, with a distance of 0.3–0.5 mm between them, in one or two layers, from the xiphoid process to the pubic bone, properly distributing the tension. Do not overcorrect. It is just enough to join the inner borders of the left and right rectus abdominis muscle.

Stitch the aponeurosis by simply taking minimal sections of the muscle itself, and mainly in the first layer of plication. If necessary, apply a second layer of stitching, then only taking the aponeurosis to reinforce and properly distribute the tension.

The xiphoid–pubic–rectus plications reconstruct the connection and balance between the anterior and posterior abdominal muscles.

Abdominal dermolipectomy with concomitant rectus plication and hernia repair eliminates the weight of the dermal–adipose flap over the suture line and also creates a wide area of subcutaneous scarring with a thicker layer of collagen that reinforces the scars and seems to be helpful.

References

1. Faria-Correa MA. Abdominoplasty: the South America style. In: Ramirez OM, Daniel RK, editors. Endoscopic plastic surgery. New York: Springer; 1995.
2. Faria-Correa MA. Abdominoplastia videoendoscopica (subcutaneoscopica). In: Atualizacao em Cirurgia Plastica Estetica e Reconstrutiva. Sao Paulo: Robe Editorial; 1994.
3. Faria-Correa MA. Videoendoscopic abdominoplasty (subcutaneouscopy). Rev Soc Bras Cir Plast Est Reconstr. 1992;7:32–4.
4. Faria-Correa MA. Videoendoscopic subcutaneous abdominoplasty. In: Endoscopic plastic surgery, vol. IV(16). 2nd ed. St. Louis, MO: Quality Medical; 2008. p. 559–86.
5. Faria-Correa MA. Videoendoscopy in plastic surgery: brief communication. Rev Soc Bras Cir Plast Est Reconstr. 1992;7:80–2.
6. Nahas FX, Ferreira LM. Concepts on correction of the musculoaponeurotic layer in abdominoplasty. Clin Plastic Surg. 2010;37:527–38. https://doi.org/10.1016/j.cps.2010.03.001.
7. Friedman DW, Boyd CD, Noton P, et al. Increases in type III collagen gene expression and protein synthesis in patients with inguinal hernias. Ann Surg. 1993;218(6):754–60.
8. Biondo-Simoes MLP, Whesthpal VL, de Paula JB, et al. Collagen synthesis after the implantation of polypropylene mesh in the abdominal all of young and old rats. Acta Cir Bras. 2005;20(4):300–4.
9. Birdsell DC, Gavelin GE, Kemsley GM, et al. Staying power—absorbable vs nonabsorbable. Plast Reconstr Surg. 1981;68(5):742–5.
10. Nahas FX, Ferreira LM, Augusto SM, Ghelfond C. Long-term follow-up of correction of rectus diasta-

sis. Plast Reconstr Surg. 2005;115(6):1736–41. https://doi.org/10.1097/01.PRS.0000161675.55337.F1.

11. Mastarasso A. Long term follow up of correction of rectus diastasis. Plast Reconstr Surg. 2005;115(6):1742–3.

12. Nahas FX, Ferreira LM, Ely PB, Ghelfond C. Rectus diastasis corrected with absorbable suture: a long-term evaluation. Aesthetic Plast Surg. 2011;35:43–8. https://doi.org/10.1007/s00266-010-9554-2.

13. Nahas FX, Augusto SM, Ghelfond C. Suture materials for rectus diastasis: nylon versus polydioxanone in the correction of rectus diastasis. Plastic Recons Surg. 2001;107(3):700–6. The division of plastic surgery and radiology, hospital Jaragua. Sao Paulo, Brazil.

14. Avelar JM. Uma nova tecnica de abdominoplastia-sistema vascular fechado de retalho subdermico dobrado sobre si mesmo combinado com lipoaspiracao. Rev Bras Cir. 1999;88/89(1/6):3–20.

15. Avelar JM. Umbilicoplastia-uma tecnica sem cicatriz externa. In: An do XIII Cong Bra de Cir Plast Porto Alegre; 1976. p. 81–2.

Faria-Correa_Minimally Invasive Subcutaneouscopic and Robotic Rectus Plication

24

Marco Aurelio Faria-Correa

24.1 Introduction

The cosmetic appearance of the abdomen is one of the most popular concerns in the modern society. We are seeing an increasing number of female and male patients presenting with small and medium-size abdominal cosmetic deformities coming to our clinics asking for minimally invasive and scarless procedures that can effectively improve the aesthetic appearance of the abdomen. In many cases the problem is not over-redundant skin, over-weight or abdominal lipodystrophy, but rectus diastasis (Figs. 24.1, 24.2, 24.3, and 24.4). They complain that despite working hard at losing weight, having a strict and rigorous workout regime, they cannot get rid of that bulging stomach and/or the peri-umbilical deformity. The weakening of the muscle aponeurotic abdominal wall due to congenital conditions, weight variation, aging, or pregnancy is a frequent cause of rectus diastasis and/or umbilical hernia that can alter the cosmetic aspect of the abdomen [1, 2]. The rectus abdominal muscle plays an important role not only in the cosmetic appearance of the abdomen but also in the stabil-

ity of the spine. Depending of the degree of the rectus diastasis it can lead to a vicious posture, spine problems, back pain, slipped disc etc. Rectus plication can effectively restore function providing a balance between the anterior and posterior muscle of the abdominal wall and improve the cosmetic appearance of the abdomen [1, 3]. The long-term evaluation by ultrasonography and CT-scan of the plication of the anterior rectus sheath [4, 5] as well as our long-term clinic follow-up (Fig. 24.3) has shown the efficiency of the recti plication when properly performed.

24.2 Objective

The goals of my work are: understanding what was wrong in the mini-abdominoplasty technique, the way I learned, the way I was performing it back to 1986, and how to improve it.

What I learned that time (and still nowadays we can see in the internet as a definition of mini-abdominoplasty) was the following: Small skin resection in the lower abdomen (mini-dermolipectomy), dissection limited to the lower abdomen, and also the rectus plication limited to the infra-umbilical area.

As a young plastic surgeon, I just follow what I learned, and I became disappointed with my results (Fig. 24.1). Then I started my novel in understanding the mistakes and in improving the mini-abdominoplasty technique.

M. A. Faria-Correa (✉)
Dr Marco Faria Correa Plastic Surgery Pte Ltd,
Singapore, Singapore
e-mail: drmarco@drmarco.com;
admin@drmarco.com

© Springer Nature India Private Limited 2020
P. Chowbey, D. Lomanto (eds.), *Techniques of Abdominal Wall Hernia Repair*,
https://doi.org/10.1007/978-81-322-3944-4_24

Fig. 24.1 Mini abdominoplasty with mini dermolipectomy done in 1986 caused an anatomical derfomity by lowering the umbilicus position

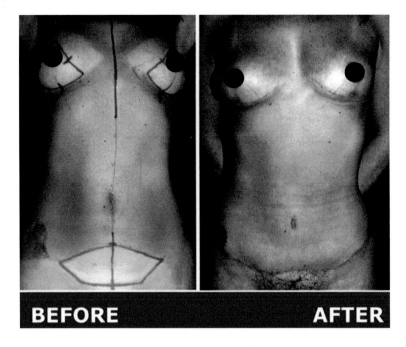

Fig. 24.2 Set of instrument develop by the author

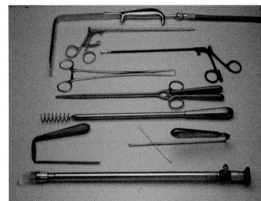

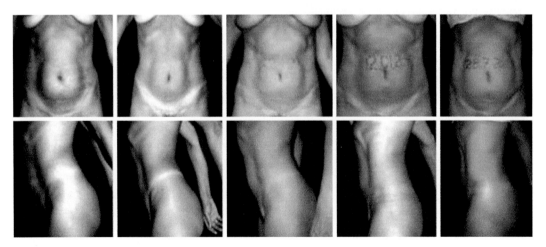

Fig. 24.3 Endoscopic abdominoplasty 20 years follow-up showing the maintenance of the result of the rectus plication even after patient aging 20 years and put on 8 kg

Fig. 24.4 Long-term follow-up of endoscopic abdominoplasty after 35 days showing a very fast recovery with minimal swelling. After 5 years showing maintenance of the result of the rectus plications and fat plication

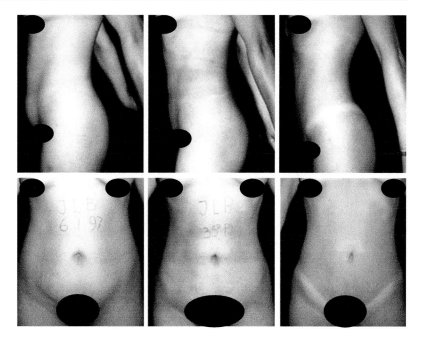

First understanding the mistakes:

- in many cases removing part of the lower abdominal skin is unnecessary and can cause more an anatomical deformity than a cosmetic improvement by the lowering of the umbilicus position.
- rectus plication limited to the lower abdomen can cause an unpleasant bulging in the upper abdomen.
- liposuction alone will not correct the rectus diastasis, that is functional and cosmetic deformity, that causes of the bulging abdomen and also is the cause of back pain due to spine instability.

24.3 Methods

In 1989 I started performing mini-abdominoplasty by just using the previous C-section scar, without removing any skin (when there is no over-redundant skin), performing a xyphoides—pubic rectus plication, and lipectomy (Fig. 24.5) that I called minimal scar abdominoplasty.

The beautiful results achieved by effectively treating the cosmetics and functional deformities through minimal incisions, without adding new scars but just using the previous scars and even improving it, gave me the enthusiasm for going to the next level, treating patients without previous C-section scars through even smaller incisions using endoscopic methods [6–9].

In 1991 at the University Hospital PUC Porto Alegre I started a research project to adapt endoscopic methods to the subcutaneous territory for treating patients presenting with rectus diastasis and no redundant skin, working through incisions as small as 4–5 cm hidden in the pubic hair-bearing area and inside the umbilical area [6–10] (Fig. 24.6). The problem to circumvent was using pressured gas in the subcutaneous to develop the optical cavity, the working space, due to the risk of gas embolism when cutting perforators veins during the flap dissection and also the gas dispersion causing the subcutaneous emphysema. For circumventing those risks I developed a set of instruments to gasless undermining the abdominal flap, tenting the flap, and stitching the muscle [6, 7, 9] (Fig. 24.2).

Attentive to the development of new instruments, machines, and methods in surgery that can facilitate and improve our task and result and with more than 20 years follow-up shows the effectiveness of the technique and the

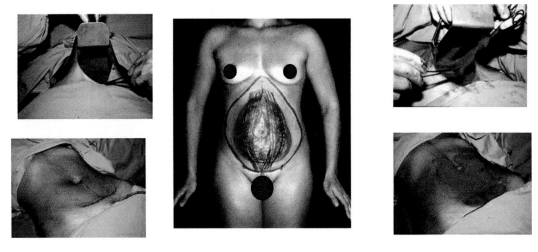

Fig. 24.5 Minimal scar abdominoplasty: Xifo-pubic rectus plication, lipectomy, and no skin removal

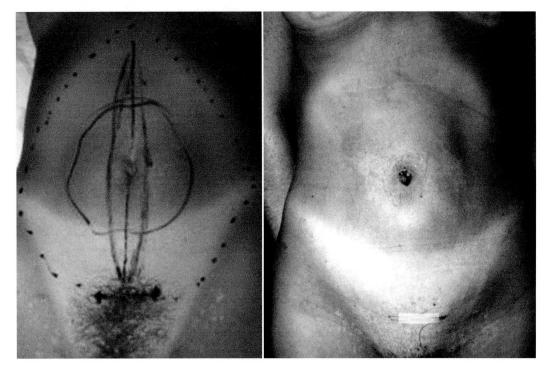

Fig. 24.6 Endoscopic abdominoplasty scars hidden inside the navel/umbilical and inside the pubic hair bearing area

beauty of restoring the original anatomy leaving minimal and inconspicuous scars (Fig. 24.6), in 2013 I started studying and training Robotic Surgery with the enthusiasm of going for the next level, using daVinci Robotic Surgery System to perform rectus plication in mini-abdominoplasty [1].

Robotic Surgery is becoming the gold standard of the minimally invasive surgery in many surgical fields. In urology, robotic prostatectomy is such a solid application, presenting so many advantages over the open methods as well as over the endoscopic methods [11, 12] that, if a patient has the chance to choose which methods to undergo, the best choice would be to go for robotics-assisted. In cardiothoracic surgery the surgical robots are also proving to be the key in transforming technically challenging open procedures like mitral valve repair and heart revascularization into technically feasible, minimally invasive procedures. In any institution where robotics "da Vinci surgical system" is available, the tendency for laparoscopic surgery (in gynecology, colon-rectum surgery, and general surgery) is being replaced by robotics-assisted surgery due to the many advantages that robotics-assisted surgery presents over laparoscopic method [1].

The robot high definition 3-dimentional view and the amplification of images gives us a much better depth sensation of the surgical field than the 2-D endoscopic view; it is even better than our naked eyes. Laparoscopic instruments have a limited range of motion; the robot endowrist range of movements is comparable to the human wrist. The surgeon's hand tremor is transmitted through the rigid laparoscopic instrument, this limitation makes delicate procedures more difficult [12, 13]. The superb precision and stability of the robot arms, surgical field and instruments, all controlled by the surgeon seated at the console in a comfortable ergonomic position, without the need of coordinating camera and instrument movement with a surgical assistant makes the surgery much easier, more precise and less stressful [1].

In many surgical fields robot is becoming a promising technology.

In reconstructive plastic surgery it has already being used for the harvesting of latissimus dorsi in breast reconstruction, super microsurgery, hand surgery [10, 14, 15], and hair transplant.

So far I didn't find in the literature any report of other applications of robotics in aesthetic plastic surgery [1].

As a cosmetic plastic surgeon I feel it is very interesting that there is fast growing trend for the use of robot for performing trans-axillary robotic thyroidectomy, robot retro-auricular submandibular gland resection [16, 17], procedures that are improved or tweaked to minimize visible scars or even relocate scars to other body areas that could be hidden. Yet little is done in the area of aesthetic plastic surgery, where scarring is of an important concern for patients [1].

My first case of muscle aponeurotic robotic core plication was done in April 2015 and since then 15 cases are done with no complication and very satisfactory results.

Surgical Robots—The equipment that we are using is the daVinci Surgical System SI. It consists of three components. The console where the surgeon sits to operate the robotic arms; the patient site robotic cart with 3 or 4 arms; the high-definition 3D vision system.

Is the surgeon operates. The robot system does not have autonomy to do anything by its own; every single movement is operated and controlled by the surgeon. Sited at the console are the joysticks. The surgeon drives the robot arms and endowrist instrument operating very precise miniaturized tools. With the feet, the surgeon controls the camera, zoom-in zoom-out, monopolar, bipolar cut, and cauterization, as well as switching use of the second and the third robot-working arms, without the need of coordinating the movements with an assistant [1]. There are a few different robot models presenting with different features, we are using the daVinci S and the daVinci SI. The daVinci XI still not available in my practice but is more versatile.

24.4 Surgical Technique and Results

Anesthesia—General anaesthesia is my preference. After docking in the robotic arms, the patient should stay still, in a state where she could move as a reaction to pain or other stimuli. There is a so called "remote centre" in the trocar that must stay in place to avoid tearing the skin. All the movement of the robot arms are around a fixed rotating point.

Infiltration—500 mL of saline solution and 1 mL of epinephrine (1:500,000) is infiltrated at the area to be undermined in between the fat tissue and the muscular aponeurosis to facilitate dissection and reduce bleeding as well as in the incisions sites.

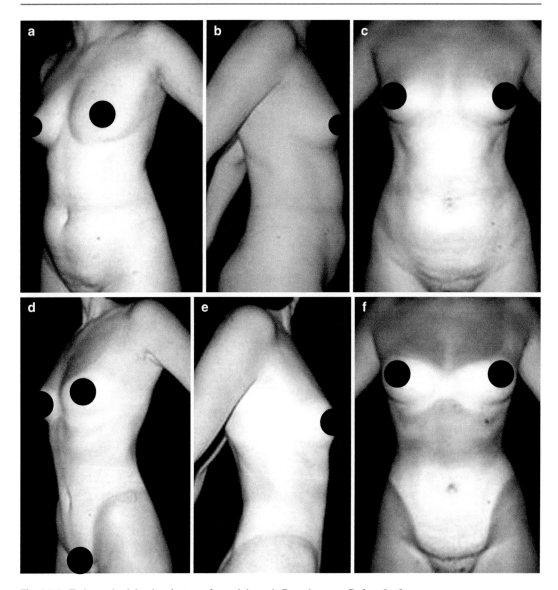

Fig. 24.7 Endoscopic abdominoplasty performed through C-section scar: Before & after

Incisions—If patient presents with previous scars from caesarean sections or other abdominal surgery (Fig. 24.7), the surgeon assesses the need to repair the scars as well as the possibility of using them for access [6, 9].

In Endoscopic Abdominoplasty Technique if there is no previous C-section scar, a 5 cm incision is made at the pubic hair bearing area and another one inside the umbilical scar (Fig. 24.8b).

In Robotic Abdominoplasty I use 2 incisions of 0.7 cm at the bikini line 20 cm far from each other to avoid instrumental collision, one incision for the camera arm at the midline of the patient's abdomen, inside the pubic hair bearing area at the pubic bone level, 3 cm above the vaginal furcula, measuring to 2 cm, and one Y-shaped incision is made within the umbilical scar (Fig. 24.9). The umbilical port is used for the introduction of retractors for tenting the abdominal flap, for supplying sutures and gauze into the operative field, and for the surgical assistant helping with laparoscopic instruments if necessary. Additional

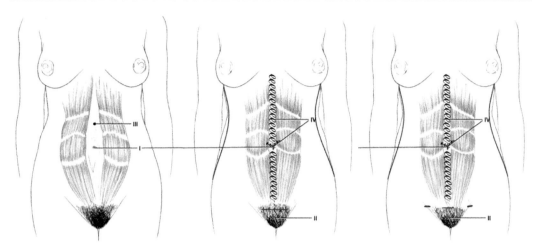

Fig. 24.8 (**a**) Rectus diastasis, (**b**) Rectus plication and incision in endoscopy abdominoplasty technique, (**c**) Rectus plication with the aid of robot. I—Y-shaped umbi-licus incision, II—Pubic incision, III—Rectus diastasis, IV—Rectus diastasis repair

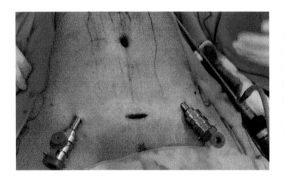

Fig. 24.9 The incisions: at the bikini line 3 incisions one at the mid line 2.5 cm for the robot endoscope and 2 at the bikini line 1 cm length distant 12 to 16 cm from each other for the robot arms and 1 at the navel for passing the sutures, gaze, suction, and helper instruments. Additional 0.5 cm incisions can be made at the iliac crest level each on bilateral sides, in cases of lipo-abdominoplasty when the lower back needs to be treated. These incisions can also be used extra port for the surgical assistant

0.5 cm incisions can be made at the iliac crest level each on bilateral sides, in cases of lipo-abdominoplasty (Fig. 24.9).

The skin of the umbilical scar is detached from its stalk. If there is an umbilical or para-umbilical hernia to be repair we do it before proceeding for the rectus plication The umbilical stalk is then transfixed using a 3–0 mono-nylon suture. The reinsertion of the umbilicus skin flaps is done after finishing the rectus plication, at its original site, deep inside the plication [9]. If there is redundant skin at the navel a Y-shaped incision is made generating 3 o triangular flaps [6, 9], the closure of it will leave inconspicuous converging scars, following Avelar original idea [18]. By resecting part of these triangular flaps we treat the redundant skin (Fig. 24.10) [1, 6, 9].

24.4.1 Dissection and Elevation of the Abdominal Flap

The undermining starts from the umbilicus progressing downwards through the midline towards the pubis and from the pubic incision upwards, or vice-versa, to meet each other. The procedure begins with the use of traditional methods with conventional instruments as far as our eyes, fingers, and instruments allow us to work safely and comfortably. With the aid of a 4 or 7 mm 30° endoscope, retractors and the "subcutaneous tomoscope" [9] or electrocautery we progress dissecting a tunnel from the pubic bone to the xiphoid process (Fig. 24.11), up to the outer borders of the rectus abdominal muscles to create the optical cavity. The undermining can be done endoscopically or with the aid of the robot

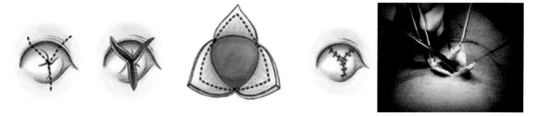

Fig. 24.10 The surgical sequence of umbilicoplasty technique is as follows: [19] Intraumbilical Y-shaped incision, [18] Three triangular flaps and a wide entrance port, [6] Partial resection of these flaps to treat flabbiness, [7] Closure leaving inconspicuous converging scars

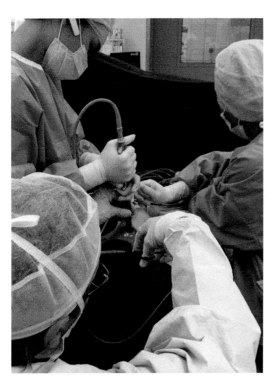

Fig. 24.11 Surgeon undermining the dermoadiposous abdominal flap from the muscle aponeurotic fascia, preparing for robotic rectus aponeurotic plication

system. If further undermining is necessary for a proper redistribution of the abdominal flap, we do a blunt dissection, creating tunnels, preserving vessels and nerves. Tunneling preserves the sensitive innervation of the abdominal wall and provides faster recovery with earlier reduction of the oedema [9], (Fig. 24.4). If there is any area that requires liposuction, the liposuction will be performed after the rectus plication. We aspirate only the deep surface of the derma-adipose flap.

In the undermined areas we use the cannula with the holes facing up. In the non-undermined areas we use the cannula with the holes facing down in the traditional way, liposuction of the deep fat tissue area, creating tunnels preserving vessels creating a closed vascular system like described by Avelar [19].

At this stage we are still doing the undermining in our conventional "subcutaneouscopic" method [6–10] (Fig. 24.11). I am working in developing dissectors and retractors (Fig. 24.12) to facilitate the keyhole gasless robotic subcutaneous techniques.

24.4.2 Recti Plication

We identify the rectus diastasis (Fig. 24.13a) and with a small cotton bud tinted with methylene blue, we demarcate the inner border of the rectus abdominal muscle aponeurosis to be plicated (Fig. 24.13b) Plication of the anterior rectus sheath is performed in two layers, the first layer using 2–0 or 3–0 nylon buried stiches 1.0 cm distant from each other (Fig. 24.13c), and the second layer of two continuous sutures using v-loc 00 nylon (Fig. 24.13d): one starting from the xiphoid process running till just above the umbilical stalk; another continuous running suture starting from just below the umbilical stalk to the pubic bone.

Supra-umbilical or peri-umbilical flabbiness is frequent finding (Fig. 24.14a). This deformity occurs during pregnancy when the abdominal muscles stretch and the subcutaneous fatty tissue attached to them is pulled away, creating a gap with

Fig. 24.12 The surgeon positioning the robot arms and camera

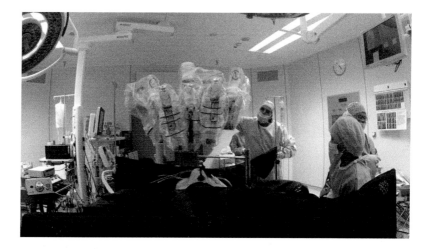

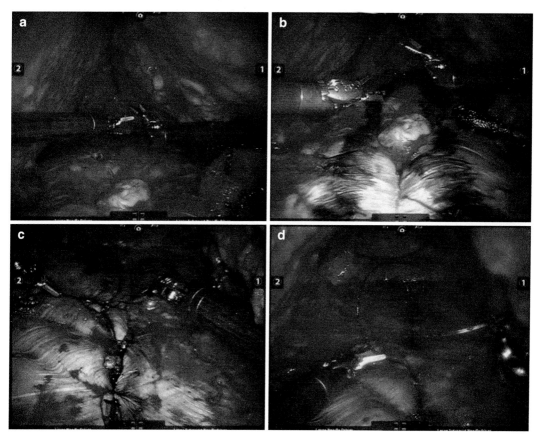

Fig. 24.13 Robot rectus aponeurotic plication. Surgeon's HD 3D view in the console. (**a**) Identify the rectus diastasis, (**b**) Drawing the inner border of the rectus abdominalis using a small cotton bud, (**c**) Plication starts using 2–0 nylon interruptive stiches 1 cm distant from each other, (**d**) A second layer of plication by using a 2–0 V-loc nylon running suture

skin flabbiness in the region. This subcutaneous fat gap is repaired by suturing the two edges of the fat tissue together with 4–0 monocryl interrupted sutures (Fig. 24.14b, c). A small hole is left between the edges to permit these small triangular umbilical skin flaps to pass through it for the reinsertion into the umbilical stalk, which was previously secured by the spare suture mentioned earlier [9].

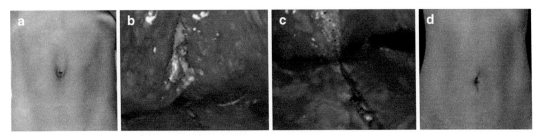

Fig. 24.14 Pre-op showing the rectus and peri-umbilical fat diastasis. (**a**) Intra operation, a view of repaired rectus diastasis and the mark of the edges of the subcutaneous fat gap to be repair, (**b**) Intra-op view of the rectus diastasis repaired and subcutaneous fat gap repaired, (**c**) Immediate post-operation result

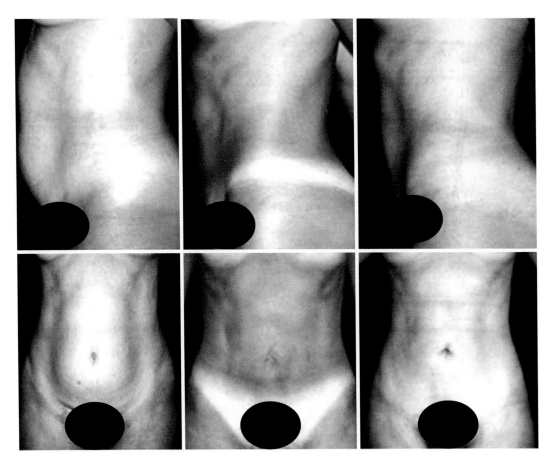

Fig. 24.15 The before photo showing patient had abdominal deformities after delivery twins and 4 kg over weight. 1 -year follow-up after patient cut down 8 kg. After 5 years post-op, patient put back 2 kg. We observe the long-term maintenance of the result

24.5   Results

I have done approximately 20 cases of Minimal Incision Abdominoplasty from 1989 till 1992. Approximately 300 cases of Endoscopic Abdominoplasty from 1992 till 2015 and 15 cases of Robotic Abdominoplasty From 2015 till now. Many patients I have the long-term follow-up up to 5 years (Figs. 24.4 and 24.15) and 20 years (Fig. 24.3).

The rectus plication shown effective and long lasting in most of the cases when the plication method was done using 2 layers of stitching, first layer interruptive stitches with nylon 00 and second layers running stitches. It failed in a few patients that didn't respect the proper downtime and started exercises before 6 months.

I converted it in a full abdominoplasty in about 20 cases. Some after a short period of time because they had some degree of flabbiness that they did not accept and in others after long-term because they kept putting on weight and due to the aging process that caused redundant skin.

Over all the results are very satisfactory when it is done in the right patients with no redundant skin and with realistic expectation, and that don't want scars.

24.6 Complications

We anticipate that complications would be similar to those encountered in endoscopic abdominoplasty. Seroma was the most common one. We manage to reduce the incidence of seroma by reducing as much as possible the undermining area, creating a closed vascular system [19], stitching the dermo-adiposous flap to the muscle fascia, and suction drainage would have to be maintained minimal for 2 or 3 days or until the drainage over 24 h is less than 30 cc [6, 9] (Figs. 24.16, 24.17, and 24.18).

24.7 Discussion

Minimally invasive surgery presents many advantages compared to open methods, like fast recovery, less pain, lower risk of infection, and minimal scars that are our goals in cosmetic surgery. But there are a number of limitations even though minimally invasive surgery appears attractive. The few most obvious limitations include loss of haptic feedback (force and tactile), natural hand-eye coordination, and dexterity. The daVinci System proves to be superior in compensating these aspects of limitations. Conventional endoscopy presents with a 2D image view whereas the daVinci system presents with a high definition precise 3D image that compensates the loss of haptic feedback [1].

Fig. 24.16 Left side endoscopic abdominoplasty, the patient and surgical team position with the video monitor and incisions. Right side showing doctor sited at the console and operating the robotic arms

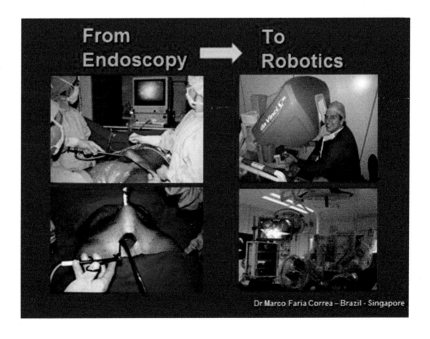

Fig. 24.17 Robot arms and camera docked in and positioned ready to start the rectus plication

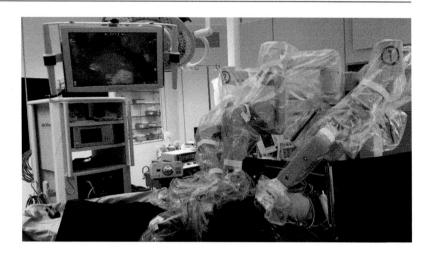

Fig. 24.18 Surgeon seated at the robot console distant about 4–5 m from the patient, operating the robot arms and camera with joysticks and pedals

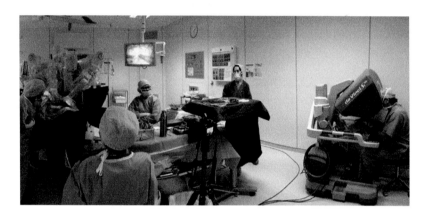

24.8   Conclusion

Robotics in aesthetic plastic surgery is still at its infancy stage but it is very promising considering its many advantages of minimally invasive surgery associated with high technology that helps us work through minimal scars with incisions at remotes sites, leaving inconspicuous scars that are the hallmark of plastic surgery. Over the past 30 years we are seeing an increasing number of female and male patients coming for the treatment of small and medium- size abdominal deformities. Many of them are presenting with rectus diastasis, no redundant folds of skin, good skin elasticity, with or without abdominal lipodystrophy. They demand for scarless procedures that can effectively correct it. Liposuction alone will not be effective enough in many cases. The long-

term evaluation of midline aponeurotic rectus plication, when properly performed, has proved its efficiency. Plastic surgeons are always looking for tools and instruments that can help us to better perform our procedures with more precision, efficacy, less trauma, faster recovery for our patients, and leaving minimal scars. Since 1991 I started using endoscopic methods for the treatment of the described deformities. The efficacy of the method in patients with more than 20 years follow-up gives me the enthusiasm of going for the next level. The gold standard of the minimal invasive video surgery, the use of Robot "daVinci Surgery System" for the plication of the rectus diastasis. In many areas of application like urology, gynecology, general surgery, neurosurgery, and heart surgery Robot surgery has proved to have many advantages over conventional endoscopic methods due to the Robot high definition 3-dimentional surgical view and amplification of images that makes it much more accurate than the 2-D view provided by the conventional endoscopic methods, the superb precision and a much larger range of motion of the robot endowrist instruments that are comparable to the human wrist, the stability of the surgical field, camera and instruments, all controlled by the surgeon seated at the console in a comfortable position [1].

References

1. Faria_Correa MA. Robotic procedure for plication of the muscle aponeurotic abdominal wall. In: New concepts on abdominolplasty and further applications, vol. 11. Berlin: Springer; 2016. p. 161–77.
2. Nahas FX, Ferreira LM. Concepts on correction of the musculoaponeurotic layer in abdominoplasty. Clin Plast Surg. 2010;37:527–38. https://doi.org/10.1016/j.cps.2010.03.001.
3. Nahas FX, Augusto SM, Ghelfond C. Suture materials for rectus diastasis: nylon versus polydioxanone in the correction of rectus diastasis. Plast Reconstr Surg. 2001;107(3):700–6. The division of plastic surgery and radiology, Hospital Jaragua. Sao Paulo, BR.
4. Nahas FX, Ferreira LM, Augusto SM, Ghelfond C. Correction of diastasis: long-term follow up of correction of rectus diastasis. Plast Reconstr Surg. 2005;115(6):1736–41. https://doi.org/10.1097/01.PRS.0000161675.55337.F1.
5. Nahas FX, Ferreira LM, Ely PB, Ghelfond C. Rectus diastasis corrected with absorbable suture: a long-term evaluation. Aesthetic Plast Surg. 2011;35:43–8. https://doi.org/10.1007/s00266-010-9554-2.
6. Faria-Correa MA. Abdominoplasty: the South America style. In: Ramirez OM, Daniel RK, editors. Endoscopic plastic surgery. New York: Springer; 1995.
7. Faria-Correa MA. Abdominoplastia videoendoscopica (subcutaneoscopica). In: Atualizacao em Cirurgia Plastica Estetica e Reconstrutiva. Sao Paulo: Robe Editorial; 1994.
8. Faria-Correa MA. Videoendoscopic abdominoplasty (subcutaneouscopy). Rev Soc Bras Cir Plast Est Reconstr. 1992;7:32–4.
9. Faria-Correa MA. Videoendoscopic subcutaneous abdominoplasty. In: Endoscopic plastic surgery, vol. IV(16). 2nd ed. St. Louis, MO: Quality Medical; 2008. p. 559–86.
10. Faria-Correa MA. Videoendoscopy in plastic surgery: brief communication. Rev Soc Bras Cir Plast Est Reconstr. 1992;7:80–2.
11. Lanfranco AR, Castellanos AE, Desai JP, Meyers WC. Robotic surgery: a current perspective. Ann Surg. 2004;239(1):14–21. https://doi.org/10.1097/01.sla.0000103020.19595.7d.
12. Lee HS, Kim D, Lee SY, Byeon HK, Kim WS, Hong HJ, Koh YW, Choi EC. Robot—assisted versus endoscopic submandibular gland resection via retroauricular approach: a prospective nonrandomized study. Br J Oral Maxillofac Surg. 2014;52(2):179–84. https://doi.org/10.1016/j.bjoms.2013.11.002.
13. Morris B.. Robotic surgery: applications, limitations, and impact on surgical education. All about robotic surgery. 2005. http://www.allaboutroboticsurgery.com/avrasurgicalrobotics.html.
14. Selber JC. The role of robotics in plastic surgery. St. Louis, MO: Quality Medical; 2009. http://www.plasticsurgerypulsenews.com/12/article_dtl.php?QnCategoryID=112&QnArticleID=236.
15. Selber JC, Baumann DP, Holsinger FC. Robotic latissimus dorsi flap for breast reconstruction. Plast Reconstr Surg. 2012;129(6):1305–12. https://doi.org/10.1097/PRS.0b013e31824ecc0b.
16. Lee J, Chung WY. Robotic thyroidectomy and radical neck dissection using a gasless transaxillary approach. Robot Gen Surg. 2014;24:269–70. https://doi.org/10.1007/978-1-4614-8739-5_24.
17. Mattei TA, Rodriguez AH, Sambhara D, Mendel E. Current state-of-the-art and future perspectives of robotic technology in neurosurgery. Neurosurg Rev. 2014;37(3):357–66. https://doi.org/10.1007/s10143-014-0540-z.
18. Avelar JM. Umbilicoplastia-uma tecnica sem cicatriz externa. In: An do XIII Cong Bra de Cir Plast Porto Alegre; 1976. p. 81–2.
19. Avelar JM. Uma nova tecnica de abdominoplastia-sistema vascular fechado de retalho subdermico dobrado sobre si mesmo combinado com lipoaspiracao. Rev Bras Cir, 1999; 88/89(1/6):3–20.

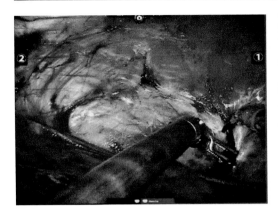

Fig. 25.4 Creating peritoneal flap

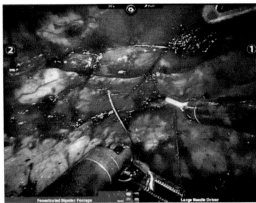

Fig. 25.5 Continuous suturing for defect closure

25.6.2 Defect Closure

There are several techniques available for closure of the defect, but the most common in practice is the transfascial closure or "shoelace technique." Before starting defect closure, decrease insufflations to 6–8 mmHg for reduction of tension on sutures.

Considering fascial closure with or without transfascial closure technique is debatable. In author's opinion, either can be used to close the defect (Fig. 25.5). Another way is to considering it as a temporary mean to facilitate the intracorporeal suturing. It depends on patient's criteria and surgeons choice as well. Some favors transfascial closure even in robotic repair despite flexibility of instruments and argue that it is better to bring tension of abdominal wall back to equilibrium so mesh can be placed in a nice way. Data suggest that defect closure in robotic hernia repair is far superior than its counterpart laparoscopic approach due to increased ergonomics and wrist flexibility. Defect closure is done with continuous non-absorbable monofilament suture in an interrupted way. Robot gives advantage of defect closure in a continuous fashion for small hernia using two sutures, starting from each end and meeting at center point.

25.6.3 Mesh Placement

There are two tissue planes which are more physiological and favors mesh placement: pre-peritoneal (i.e., transabdominal pre-peritoneal, or TAPP, repair) or intraperitoneal underlay (i.e., intraperitoneal onlay mesh, or IPOM, repair). Mesh is introduced through assistant port with a non-touch technique and is deployed at the defect site.

It is then oriented over the closed defect to cover almost 5 cm on each side of the defect (Fig. 25.6) keeping in view later contraction of mesh, and also preventing it to expose hernia defect which can be vulnerable for recurrence.

25.6.4 Mesh Fixation

This can be achieved by different methods like transabdominal or intracorporeal suturing, tacking, glues, or bone anchors as done in laparoscopic surgery. But, robotic surgery is superior to laparoscopic surgery for mesh anchorage because flexibility of instruments makes it possible to do intracorporeal suturing (Fig. 25.6). After placement of mesh, peritoneal flap is brought around to close the peritoneal defect as well. This can be achieved either using absorbable sutures in a continuous fashion or by using tacking technique. If the mesh is positioned in the pre-peritoneal or retromuscular plane, fixation may be avoided but we need long-term study to verify the efficacy of this approach. Care must be taken while tacking on lateral side because injury to nerves can cause devastating results. All port sites larger than 8 mm are closed with absorbable sutures for prevention of port site hernia.

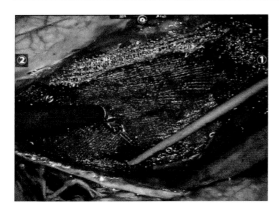

Fig. 25.6 Mesh placement and fixation

25.7 Conclusions

Robotic-assisted ventral hernia repair is comparable with laparoscopic and open repairs in terms of postoperative outcomes like pain and early recovery as per patient expectations; and regarding surgeon's satisfaction, "cure" is excellent. Pre-peritoneal mesh placement pushes robotic surgery towards summit of leading method because it not only allows to complete the task easily but also prevents mesh to be in direct contact with abdominal viscera. In a nutshell, robotic-assisted ventral repair should be considered instead of laparoscopic or open mesh repair for large or complex ventral hernia.

Acknowledgments None.

Conflicts of Interest: The authors have no conflicts of interest to declare.

References

1. Burger JW, Luijendijk RW, Hop WC, et al. Long-term follow-up of a randomized controlled trial of suture versus mesh repair of incisional hernia. Ann Surg. 2004;240:578–83; discussion 583–5.
2. Forte A, Zullino A, Manfredelli S, et al. Rives technique is the gold standard for incisional hernioplasty. An institutional experience. Ann Ital Chir. 2011;82:313–7.
3. Shahdhar M, Sharma A. Laparoscopic ventral hernia repair: extraperitoneal repair. Ann Laparosc Endosc Surg. 2018;3:79.
4. Bittner JG 4th, Alrefai S, Vy M, et al. Comparative analysis of open and robotic transversus abdominis release for ventral hernia repair. Surg Endosc. 2018;32:727–34.
5. Armijo P, Pratap A, Wang Y, et al. Robotic ventral hernia repair is not superior to laparoscopic: a national database review. Surg Endosc. 2018;32:1834–9.
6. Gonzalez A, Escobar E, Romero R, et al. Robotic-assisted ventral hernia repair: a multicenter evaluation of clinical outcomes. Surg Endosc. 2017;31:1342–9.
7. Orenstein SB, Dumeer JL, Monteagudo J, et al. Outcomes of laparoscopic ventral hernia repair with routine defect closure using "shoelacing" technique. Surg Endosc. 2011;25:1452–7.
8. Gonzalez AM, Romero RJ, Seetharamaiah R, et al. Laparoscopic ventral hernia repair with primary closure versus no primary closure of the defect: potential benefits of the robotic technology. Int J Med Robot. 2015;11:120–5.
9. Donkor C, Gonzalez A, Gallas MR, et al. Current perspectives in robotic hernia repair. Robot Surg. 2017;4:57–67.
10. Nguyen DH, Nguyen MT, Askenasy EP, et al. Primary fascial closure with laparoscopic ventral hernia repair: systematic review. World J Surg. 2014;38:3097–104.
11. Walker PA, May AC, Mo J, et al. Multicenter review of robotic versus laparoscopic ventral hernia repair: is there a role for robotics? Surg Endosc. 2018;32:1901–5.

Future Consideration

Davide Lomanto

Hernia has experienced a dramatic change in the last two decades. After *the golden age* with Bassini, Billroth, Mac Vay and all other pioneers in suture repair, the last two decades have acquired new knowledge in the physio-pathology and metabolism of the hernias; new discovery in biomaterial from synthetic, semi-absorbable to biological, a new concept in surgical repair called "tension-free repair" till the endo-laparoscopic and single or reduced port surgery. In the last few years the use of robotic-assisted surgery for ventral hernias and abdominal wall reconstruction seems to make it easy and is challenging all other alternatives.

All these greatest achievements on hernias have made hernia repair one of the most attractive surgical procedures today, lifting it from the role of "Cinderella" to a new and more specific role in the surgical world.

Interest has been growing among researchers, academia, industries and, more surgeons are attracted by the treatment of this disease that was once simply defined as "the most common operation" and too easy to treat.

The new knowledge on the disease and its anatomy and physiology, the development and challenges of new biomaterial with new concept of porosity, wound healing process, body response to prosthesis and its fabric; the growing numbers of procedures worldwide, the raising number of hernia centres in top academic institutions are the few symbols of the new role of hernia disease in surgery. The 1,500,000 abdominal wall repairs in the US, 2,000,000 in Europe, more than 10–15,000,000 repairs in China, India and in other countries have a great impact on both socio-economics and healthcare policies pushing all the players to find the best surgical treatment that reduces the risk for recurrence and improve the clinical outcome.

The hernia societies from all continents have published guidelines and recommendations, but lately they come together to publish the international guidelines, in which all the experts have taken into account the diversity of the various countries and continents, the accessibility to resources by the patients, the variety of healthcare systems to try to make uniform recommendations that fit to all. It is indeed a big effort of cooperation and certainly will bring benefits to patients from all over the world clarifying several contrasting issues from indications, classification, diagnosis and treatments.

It is probably the first time in which worldwide experts are not looking at the superiority of one treatment over the other but they are starting

D. Lomanto (✉)
Minimally Invasive Surgical Centre, KTP Advanced Surgical Training Centre, Yong Loo Lin School of Medicine, National University Health System, National University of Singapore, Singapore
e-mail: davide_lomanto@nuhs.edu.sg

© Springer Nature India Private Limited 2020
P. Chowbey, D. Lomanto (eds.), *Techniques of Abdominal Wall Hernia Repair*,
https://doi.org/10.1007/978-81-322-3944-4_26

to propose a "tailored approach" or "individualization of the treatment option" and in which is not the "ego of the surgeon" to be at the centre but, finally, the patient, and adopt the best repair for each patient.

Teaching, proficiency and hernia centre have become important today, because hernia is becoming a specialized disease due to the several aspects and techniques and also due to the more important role in the healthcare system. Population is aging worldwide, the incidence and number of hernia cases is on the rise together with the large number of repairs making hernia repair an import key player in all healthcare systems and attracting attention on the outcome by the insurances and governments. Day surgery, recurrence, chronic pain, convalescence and complications are becoming key indicators of performance in many hospitals worldwide. Local, national and continental registry are established to monitor data, quality of care and driven-value outcome.

Last but not least, should be a better understanding of the concept of physiopathology of the hernia disease. Today, we have achieved great results in terms of recurrence and post-operative sequelae, but still, for example, for ventral hernia or recurrent hernias we are far from reaching an optimal cure. We have a debatable area, for example, mesh positioning or mesh technology; from the position of the mesh intraperitoneally to rertomuscular or preperitonela, from the characteristic of synthetic mesh, the so-called lightweight to large pore, to the woven characteristic in terms of simple knitted or 3D fabric. Semisynthetic or partially absorbable are still under discussion, and the indication and when-to-use of biological mesh are still open issues. We should probably focus more on the nature and etiology of the disease to find the best cure. We have several types of surgical repair and hundreds of meshes to choose, but more information on the metabolic and biochemical changes in patients with hernias are needed. The role of collagen, matrix metalloproteinases, protease metabolism, nutritional deficiencies, wound healing process and the error in remodelling need to be investigated to find the ultimate best repair for all kinds of hernia. Probably the simple use of mesh is not enough to guarantee a definite cure to all hernia diseases.

A merging of knowledge on mesh technology and a better understanding of the hernia biology will be the future to find the cure for the best hernia repair.

Printed by Printforce, the Netherlands